W9-CBV-869

# Eat and Heal

By the Editors of FC&A Medical Publishing®

# Publisher's Note

The editors of FC&A have taken careful measures to ensure the accuracy and usefulness of the information in this book. While every attempt has been made to assure accuracy, errors may occur. We advise readers to carefully review and understand the ideas and tips presented and to seek the advice of a qualified professional before attempting to use them. The publisher and editors disclaim all liability (including any injuries, damages or losses) resulting from the use of the information in this book.

The health information in this book is for information only and is not intended to be a medical guide for self-treatment. It does not constitute medical advice and should not be construed as such or used in place of your doctor's medical advice.

"Jesus said to her, 'I am the resurrection and the life; he who believes in Me will live even if he dies, and everyone who lives and believes in Me will never die. Do you believe this?'"

— *John 11:25-26*

*Eat and Heal* and all material contained therein copyright ©2001 by Frank W. Cawood and Associates, Inc. All rights reserved. Printed in the United States of America.

This book or any portion thereof may not be reproduced or distributed in any form or by any means without written permission of the publisher. For information, or to order copies, contact:

FC&A
103 Clover Green
Peachtree City, GA 30269

Produced by the staff of FC&A

**Sixteenth printing August 2003**

ISBN 1-890957-52-6

# Table of contents

. . . . . . . . . . . . . . . . . . . . . . . . . . . .

# Nutrition building blocks for better health

· · · · · · · · · · · · · · · · · · · · · · · · · · · · · · · · ·

## 5 ingredients for a healthy diet

How do you choose the foods you eat? If you are like most people, taste, price, ease of preparation, and nutrition play a major role.

But chances are, eating nutritious foods is the one thing you care about most. You know making the right food choices can help prevent many health problems, including obesity, heart disease, diabetes, and cancer. But you hear so much confusing information, how do you know if you are choosing the right foods?

A good place to start is with these five characteristics of a healthy diet from nutrition experts Frances Sizer, M.S., and Eleanor Whitney, Ph.D., authors of the book, *Nutrition Concepts and Controversies.*

◆ **Adequacy.** Be sure your diet provides enough vitamins, minerals, and other nutrients to replace those you use up each day.

◆ **Balance.** Don't fill up on foods that are rich in some nutrients and ignore others that are equally important. Extra iron, for example, won't make up for too little calcium.

◆ **Calorie control.** Take in no more calories than you use. Those you don't burn get stored as fat, which can lead to obesity and other health problems.

◆ **Moderation.** Limit certain foods — like those containing fat, cholesterol, and sugar. Sizer and Whitney say, "Some people take this to mean that they must never indulge in a

delicious beefsteak or a hot-fudge sundae, but they are mis-
informed — moderation, not total abstinence, is the key."

◆ **Variety.** Eat a lot of different foods. You'll not only get all the
nutrients you need, you'll enjoy mealtimes more. Further-
more, many foods contain small amounts of toxins and con-
taminants your body doesn't notice unless you eat them a lot.
Wait a few days before repeating a food to reduce the chances
of any danger.

In this book, you'll find the information you need to plan
meals that meet these five requirements. You'll learn about the
basic nutrients — vitamins, minerals, proteins, carbohydrates,
fats, and water, as well as phytonutrients and fiber.

You'll also find more than 50 chapters on individual healing
foods, which will help add variety to your meals. The other chapters help you understand how specific conditions can be prevented
or treated with certain foods.

## 'Eyeball' a nutritious plate

You may have learned to ignore wild claims about fad diets,
but sometimes it's hard to understand advice from reliable sources.
The U.S. Department of Agriculture (USDA) food pyramid, for
example, can be confusing, especially if you forget it's three-
dimensional — with height, width, and depth. The base of the
pyramid represents a lot more rice, bread, cereal, and pasta than
you might realize if you view it as a triangle having only height
and width.

And keeping up with RDAs and DRIs, food groups, and serving sizes is enough to make you throw up your hands — or reach
for a bag of potato chips.

**Picture your plate.** To show you at a glance how a healthy
arrangement of food actually looks on your plate, nutritionists at

the American Institute for Cancer Research (AICR) created an eating plan called *The New American Plate.*

Vegetables, fruits, whole grains, and beans cover two-thirds or more of this plate. That's because a diet based mostly on plant foods lowers your risk of many diseases. Be sure you include hearty helpings of different vegetables and fruits. Don't fill all that space with pasta and whole grain bread.

Meat, fish, poultry, or low-fat dairy foods cover no more than one-third of *The New American Plate.* Stick to a recommended serving of no more than 3 ounces of meat by mixing it with vegetables, grains, and beans in a stir-fry, stew, or casserole.

**Size up a simple serving.** What you think you eat and what you really eat may be quite different. A USDA survey compared what people said they ate — with what they really ate. Most underestimated the amounts of some foods and overestimated others.

This confusion probably occurs because people don't understand how much food a serving really is. To make it clearer, the AICR suggests you measure out standard servings of foods and put them into your usual bowl or plate. One cup is the standard serving of most cereals, for example. You may be surprised at how it looks in your bowl. What you considered one serving may be closer to two.

Pay attention to portion sizes when you eat out, too. Many restaurants have switched from the traditional 10-inch to 12-inch plate, but you don't have to load it up. Here's another healthy idea — turn down the larger amounts in those fast-food deals like "value meals" and "super-sizing." Everybody likes saving a buck, but bad health is not a bargain.

**Stay slim with a lifetime eating plan.** *The New American Plate* was not designed to be a weight loss diet. "But it does show people how to enjoy all foods in sensible portions," says Melanie Polk, AICR Director for Nutrition Education. "Thus, it promotes a healthy weight as one aspect of an overall healthy lifestyle."

If you forget fad diets and stick to this plan, Polk believes, you won't have to worry about obesity. "All the fad diets with their high-protein, low-sugar, low-carbohydrate directives," she says, "have confused people about some basic principles."

Ignore any diet that encourages you to cut back on the fruits and vegetables that help prevent chronic disease. You don't want to put your long-term health at risk for short-term weight loss.

In addition to selecting healthy foods, pay attention to the calories you take in. "Once you suit your portions to your needs," says Polk, "you will find it easier to maintain a healthy weight for life."

---

### Serving sizes simplified

One way to make it easier to remember what a serving looks like is to compare it with something familiar. These examples should help.

| A single serving of: | is about the size of: |
| --- | --- |
| vegetables, raw | your fist |
| vegetables, cooked | the palm of your hand |
| pasta | one scoop of ice cream |
| meat | a deck of cards |
| grilled fish | a checkbook |
| butter, margarine, peanut butter, or cream cheese | your thumb (joint to tip) |
| snacks (pretzels, chips) | a handful |
| chopped fruit | a tennis ball |
| apple | a baseball |
| potato | a computer mouse |
| steamed rice | a cupcake wrapper |

Small changes can make a big difference. "Choosing the regular burger instead of the quarter-pound burger," Polk points out, "saves 160 calories."

If you'd like a free copy of *The New American Plate* brochure, call 800-843-8114, extension 22. More information is available on the AICR Web site at <www.aicr.org>.

## Menu for a long and healthy life

"Following the right diet can literally add years to your life," say Ronald Klatz, M.D., and Robert Goldman, M.D., in their book, *Stopping the Clock.* If you are looking for the best eating plan to take you all the way to your 100th birthday, be sure it meets their three requirements:

◆ It's nontoxic.

◆ It provides enough nutrients and fuel to satisfy your daily needs.

◆ It's made up of foods that are easy to digest and eliminate.

There's one thing you need to remember — food is not the whole story. If you want to sing a hearty "Happy Birthday" to yourself when you reach 100, get a lot of exercise and plenty of sleep, reduce your stress, don't smoke, limit alcohol, drive safely, and buckle your seatbelt.

> ### Real foods beat out pills
>
> Vitamin pills and mineral supplements are not your answer to a long and healthy life. "We know that consuming a healthy, varied diet offers more effective protection against disease than any pill could hope to," says AICR nutritionist Melanie Polk.
>
> Pills may seem more convenient, but nutritious eating can be simple, too. "People have to understand," says Polk, "that a healthy meal isn't necessarily an elaborate meal. A quick veggie stir-fry, or a simple salad, can get you in and out of the kitchen in minutes."

# Carbohydrates

Did you have the vitality to take a brisk walk this morning? If so, you can thank carbohydrates, your body's main source of energy. And if you were mentally sharp and in good spirits throughout the day, give them credit for helping your brain and nervous system operate at peak performance.

Carbohydrates are starches, sugars, and fibers that come mainly from plants. They seem so commonplace it's easy to overlook their importance. Yet, without them, not only would you lack energy and have a sluggish brain, your digestive system wouldn't work very smoothly, either.

## Choose whole and healthy carbohydrates

Nutritionists suggest you get at least 55 percent of your total calories from carbohydrates. There are two kinds — complex and simple — and a healthy diet contains a lot more of the first kind than the second.

**Complex carbohydrates.** Your body needs these important starches and fibers. You get them from grains, breads, pastas, and vegetables, like white or sweet potatoes, corn, and dried beans.

It's important to remember that commercial processing removes a lot of nutrients and fiber. For better nutrition, choose whole grains and avoid foods made with white flour. When you're cooking vegetables, don't overdo it. Lightly sautéing or steaming is best. And to increase your fiber intake, eat the skins, too.

**Simple carbohydrates.** These carbohydrates — which are sugars — give you quick energy. Milk, fruits, and juices contain simple carbohydrates. They bring nutrients, like water, vitamins, minerals, and sometimes fiber, to your table.

Refined sugar, found in soda, candy, desserts, and your sugar bowl, is also a simple carbohydrate. But it doesn't have any nutrients — just a lot of empty calories. And when you eat sugar in rich desserts, you usually get a great deal of fat, as well.

You might be surprised how much refined sugar shows up in processed foods. It's in everything from boxed cereals to jars of spaghetti sauce. When you're grocery shopping, read labels and avoid foods that list sugar among the first ingredients. Watch for words ending in *ose,* which means "sugar," or *saccharide,* meaning "sugar unit."

# Fats

• • • • • • • • •

Your body needs fats to stay healthy. They provide the raw materials for making hormones and bile. Other fats carry the fat-soluble vitamins — A, D, E, and K — in your bloodstream throughout your body.

Although fats add to the enjoyment of eating by making food tender, tasty, and pleasant-smelling, eating too much fat contributes to obesity, heart disease, high blood pressure, cancer, diabetes, and other diseases. And while fats contribute to feelings of fullness after a meal, they also stimulate your appetite.

That's why you should pay attention to the experts' recommendation to get no more than 30 percent of your calories from fat.

## Choose fats wisely

Almost all foods contain at least traces of fat. Nutritionists refer to fat as an energy-dense food. That's because 1 gram packs in nine calories, while 1 gram of carbohydrate or protein contains only four.

All fats are equal when it comes to calories, but there are big differences in how the three types — saturated, polyunsaturated, and monounsaturated — affect your health.

**Saturated fats.** These fats raise your cholesterol level. Most saturated fats come from animal sources, like meat, egg yolk, butter, and cheese. They are also present in coconut, coconut oil, and palm oil.

You can reduce the amount of saturated fat you eat by choosing low-fat or fat-free dairy products and sticking to lean cuts of meat. Trimming the fat off a pork chop, for example, can lower the saturated fat from 13 grams to 4 grams.

To protect your heart, limit saturated fats to less than 10 percent of your total calories.

**Polyunsaturated fats.** These fats lower bad LDL cholesterol, but they also lower good HDL cholesterol. A little bit of polyunsaturated fats, like safflower oil and sunflower oil, in your diet is all right, but don't overdo it.

Hydrogenated vegetable shortenings and margarines, processed from polyunsaturated fats, act like saturated fats in your bloodstream. The harder a fat is at room temperature, the more harmful it is to your arteries.

**Monounsaturated fats.** Olive oil is one of the best sources of the healthiest kind of fat — monounsaturated. Numerous tests prove it lowers LDL cholesterol and raises HDL cholesterol. It also helps prevent arthritis, high blood pressure, diabetes, and some cancers. Olive oil beats other oils at helping you feel full longer after a meal, and it even boosts your memory.

Canola oil, avocados, and peanuts are also high in monounsaturated fats. Use them to replace some of the unhealthy saturated fats in your diet. Slices of avocado are a good substitute for cheese on a veggie sandwich. Instead of cream cheese, spread a little natural peanut butter — made from 100 percent peanuts with no hydrogenated oils — on your bagel.

# Balance the fatty acids

The omega-3 fatty acids found in Alaskan salmon, albacore tuna, mackerel, and sardines help keep your blood from becoming too sticky and forming clots, which can cause heart attack and stroke. Omega-3 also keeps your heart healthy by lowering your bad cholesterol and triglyceride levels. These coldwater fish can also help protect you from diabetes, depression, cancer, and other diseases.

The American Heart Association recommends eating two servings of fish — particularly these fatty fish — every week. Wheat germ, walnuts, flaxseeds, and dark green leafy vegetables also provide some omega-3 but not nearly as much as fish.

Omega-6, another essential fatty acid, is much more abundant than omega-3 in the typical diet. Most people get 10 to 25 times more omega-6 — from vegetable oils, meats, milk, and eggs — than they do omega-3.

Some health experts believe the balance between these two is more important than how much you get of either one. This may be particularly important if you have problems with chronic pain or depression. Lowering the ratio of omega-6 to omega-3 to somewhere between 4-to-1 and 10-to-1 could help you feel a lot better.

Nutritionist Carl Germano, co-author of the book *Nature's Pain Killers* with orthopedic surgeon William Cabot, says, "It

---

### A word of caution

Don't let low-fat and fat-free desserts, pastries, and snacks fool you, advises Martin Katahn, Ph.D., author of *The T-Factor 2000 Diet*.

"Because these foods simulate the taste and texture of fat," says Katahn, "they can turn on your appetite just like the real thing." Unfortunately, the tempting creamy taste comes partially from certain fatty acids that, by law, don't have to be counted as fat.

Katahn also says many of these foods have more sugar and calories, but less nutrition, than the foods they were created to replace.

seems that you have nothing to lose and everything to gain by altering your diet to include more omega-3 fatty acids and fewer omega-6."

If you have arthritis, fibromyalgia, or other chronic pain, Germano suggests you lower the ratio to between 2-to-1 and 4-to-1. You'll feel better and need fewer anti-inflammatory drugs.

# Fiber

· · · · · · · · ·

Back in the 1940s, Dr. Denis Burkitt began to notice the importance of diet to good health. Working as a surgeon in East Africa, he rarely saw conditions, like constipation, hemorrhoids, and appendicitis, that were widespread in the Western world. He came to believe the amount of fiber, or roughage, people eat could explain why.

Fiber is the part of fruits, vegetables, and grains your body can't digest. There are two kinds, both important in keeping you healthy. Soluble fiber dissolves easily in water and becomes a soft gel in your intestines. Insoluble fiber remains unchanged as it speeds up your food's trip through your digestive system.

In his book, *Eat Right — To Stay Healthy and Enjoy Life More,* published over 20 years ago, Burkitt pointed out that people in developing nations tended to eat about 60 grams of fiber a day. In Western countries, the average amount was about 20 grams.

Today fiber intake is even lower. According to the National Institutes of Health, Americans eat only 5 to 20 grams of fiber a day. If you are among those eating the lowest amounts, you fall far short of the recommended 20 to 35 grams. Many nutritionists believe you'd be healthier with the higher amounts Burkitt recommended.

# 10 conditions you can fight with fiber

Bumping up the fiber in your diet can help you avoid these conditions — or deal with them in a healthier way.

**Diabetes.** Fiber helps improve the way your body handles insulin and glucose. That means you can lower your risk of diabetes by eating whole grains rather than refined carbohydrates. Dark rye bread, whole-wheat crackers, multi-grain bagels, and bran muffins are good choices.

**Heart attacks and strokes.** The soluble fiber in foods like oatmeal, okra, and oranges helps eliminate much of the cholesterol that can clog your arteries and cause a stroke or heart attack.

**Constipation and hemorrhoids.** "If fiber intake were adequate, laxatives would seldom be required," said Burkitt. Apples, sweet potatoes, barley, and pinto beans provide this roughage. Burkitt thought "softage" would be a better name for fiber, because it keeps the stool moist, soft, and easy to eliminate.

**Appendicitis.** "Keeping bowel content soft," said Burkitt, "seems to provide the best safeguard against the development of appendicitis." Treats like apricots and peaches are a tasty way to do this.

**Diverticulosis.** As your body processes fibrous foods, like peas, spinach, and corn, it tones up your intestinal muscles. This helps prevent pouches, called diverticula, which can cause abdominal pain if they become inflamed.

**Weight gain.** The best way to lose weight is to eat low-fat, low-calorie vegetables and grains. "The more bulky fiber-rich foods you eat," said Burkitt, "the less fat you will be consuming, and vice versa." And since the fiber swells, you'll feel satisfied faster. If you have room for dessert, choose fruits like plums or strawberries.

**Impotence.** You probably never imagined that navy beans, brussels spouts, and zucchini squash could improve your love life. But these fiber-filled vegetables help maintain strong blood flow to the penis by lowering your cholesterol and keeping your blood vessels unclogged. The beans, in addition, contain L-arginine, a protein that also helps improve potency.

**Cancer.** Burkitt believed a high-fiber diet defends against colon and rectal cancers in two ways. His cultural studies showed the more animal fat in a diet, the higher the incidence of bowel cancer. Eventually, he realized that the more bulky, fiber-rich foods people eat, the less unhealthy fat they consume.

Not only that, but a healthy portion of fiber speeds cancer-causing compounds out of the digestive system more quickly — before they have a chance to make trouble.

Even if experts debate how all this really works, anyone who loads their plate with whole grains, legumes, fresh fruits, and vegetables will say there's no arguing with natural success.

Burkitt also considered fiber a protector against other conditions, like gallbladder disease, varicose veins, and hiatal hernia.

## How to fit more fiber into your day

Now that you have so many good reasons to eat fiber, consider these ways to get more into your diet. But don't overdo it. Adding too much fiber to your diet too quickly can cause unpleasant side effects, like gas, bloating, abdominal cramps, and diarrhea. Your best bet is to add fibrous foods gradually.

**Start the day with a whole-grain cereal.** Read food labels to find a cereal that contains at least 5 grams of fiber per serving. Top it off with raisins, sliced bananas, or chopped apple.

**Eat some vegetables raw.** Munch on carrot or celery sticks, and lunch on a crunchy garden salad. When you cook veggies, steam or sauté them just until tender.

**Snack on fresh and dried fruits.** And whenever possible, eat the skins of fruits and vegetables. That's where you'll find the most fiber.

**Substitute brown rice for white.** With that switch, you'll triple the fiber. Try some less-familiar unprocessed grains as well, like bulgur, couscous, or kasha.

**Add beans to soups and stews.** Replace meat a couple of times a week with dishes like bean burritos or red beans and rice. To prevent gas and bloating, don't cook dried beans in the same water you soak them in.

**Sip some psyllium.** Sometimes dental problems make chewing difficult, and you have to choose soft, low-fiber foods. At times like these, it may be helpful to supplement your diet with Metamucil — made from the fiber of ground psyllium seeds. This isn't a laxative, but it can help your bowels function normally if you take it daily, not just when you are constipated.

> ### Fiber in breakfast foods
>
> If you want to increase your fiber intake, start your day with a high-fiber breakfast. By making the right food choices, you are well on your way to meeting your fiber goal of 20 to 35 grams a day.
>
> **Low-fiber breakfast**
> 1 cup orange juice = less than 1 gram
> 1 cup cornflakes = 1 gram
> 1 slice white bread = 1 gram
> TOTAL = less than 3 grams of fiber
>
> **High-fiber breakfast**
> 1 whole orange = 3 grams
> 1 cup raisin bran = 8 grams
> 1 bran muffin = 4 grams
> TOTAL = 15 grams of fiber

# Minerals

· · · · · · · · · · · · · ·

When you think of precious minerals, you probably think of gold and silver. But where your health is concerned, others — like calcium and iron — are far more precious. Each of these dietary minerals is unique and carries out its own life-giving task.

Scientists have divided these nutrients into two groups — major and trace minerals — depending on how much of the mineral is in your body.

## 7 minerals you can't do without

The major minerals stand out from others simply because there are more of them in your body. If you could remove all your body's minerals and place them on a scale, they would weigh about 5 pounds. Almost 4 pounds of that would be calcium and phosphorus, the two most common major minerals. The five other major minerals would make up most of the remaining pound.

**Calcium.** By far the most abundant mineral in your body, calcium makes your bones and teeth strong and hard. Without it, they would be as floppy as your ears. Imagine trying to get around then.

Calcium doesn't just stay trapped in your skeleton, though. Small amounts of it travel into your blood. There, it's essential for steadying your blood pressure and helping your muscles contract. One rather important muscle — your heart — needs calcium to keep pumping.

Calcium is critical during childhood if you want to have strong bones as an adult. But no matter how old you are, it's never too late to get more of this important mineral.

**Phosphorus.** The second-most plentiful mineral in your body works hand-in-hand with calcium to build and maintain strong bones and teeth. Phosphorus is a crucial ingredient in DNA and cell membranes and helps make healthy new cells all over your body. To top it off, phosphorus helps turn your food into energy.

**Chloride.** Your stomach would be useless without this element. Chloride is a main ingredient in your digestive stomach acids. It also helps to assure that all of your body's cells get their fair share of nutrients — no small job at all.

**Magnesium.** This is the least common major mineral in your body, but that doesn't hold magnesium back. First, it helps keep your bones and teeth healthy, then it makes sure calcium, potassium, vitamin D, and proteins do their jobs. When you flex your muscles, you need magnesium to help them relax again.

Recently, experts even found a connection between magnesium and heart health. A deficiency of the mineral could increase your risk of heart attack and high blood pressure.

**Potassium.** Keeping your blood pressure steady, maintaining your heartbeat, balancing water in your cells, and assuring your muscles and nerves work properly are a few of potassium's many important jobs. Like magnesium, this mineral might be essential for heart health.

**Sodium.** This mineral usually gets a bad rap because it's the main element in salt. But your body needs sodium to maintain its balance of fluids. Nowadays, most people try to limit their salt, or sodium, intake for health reasons. Those who are "salt-sensitive" are especially at risk for heart disease. But it would benefit everyone to lower their daily sodium intake to 2,400 milligrams or less.

**Sulfur.** This mineral is a number one supporting actor. It doesn't do much on its own, but it's part of other star nutrients like thiamin and protein. Sulfur is especially important in proteins because it gives them shape and durability. Your body's toughest proteins — in your hair, nails, and skin — have the highest amounts of sulfur.

## Trace minerals — small but powerful protectors

By definition, each trace mineral makes up only a tiny percentage of your total body weight — less than one-twentieth of a percent, to be exact. But their small amounts only make them more valuable. They carry out enormous tasks that are as important as the jobs of any of the more common nutrients.

| Mineral | What It Does |
|---|---|
| **Major Minerals** ||
| **Calcium** | builds bones and teeth, contracts muscles and nerves, sends nerve messages, controls blood pressure |
| **Chloride** | makes stomach juices for digestion, balances levels of other minerals |
| **Magnesium** | builds bones and teeth, relaxes muscles, makes proteins, helps body use nutrients, steadies heart rhythm |
| **Phosphorus** | builds new cells, produces energy |
| **Potassium** | sends nerve messages, relaxes nerves, maintains chemical balances, steadies blood pressure |
| **Sodium** | balances fluid levels, sends nerve messages |
| **Sulfur** | builds vitamins and proteins, removes toxic chemicals |
| **Trace Minerals** ||
| **Boron** | helps body use calcium, builds bones and joints |
| **Chromium** | produces energy, balances blood sugar level |

| Signs of Deficiency | Good Sources | Dietary Reference Intakes* (DRI) | |
| --- | --- | --- | --- |
| | | Women Age 51+ | Men Age 51+ |
| **Major Minerals** | | | |
| bone loss (osteoporosis) | dairy foods, small bony fish, legumes | 1,200 mg | 1,200 mg |
| muscle cramps, trouble concentrating, loss of appetite | salt | 750 mg | 750 mg |
| tiredness, loss of appetite, muscle cramps and twitches, convulsions, depression, confusion | nuts, legumes, whole grains, dark leafy greens, seafood | 320 mg | 420 mg |
| loss of appetite tiredness, pain in bones | meats, dairy foods | 700 mg | 700 mg |
| dehydration, weakness, trouble concentrating | fresh fruits and vegetables, fish, legumes, dairy foods | 3,500 mg | 3,500 mg |
| muscle cramps, trouble concentrating, loss of appetite | salt, processed foods | 500 mg | 500 mg |
| n/a | all protein-packed foods | n/a | n/a |
| **Trace Minerals** | | | |
| bone loss (osteoporosis) | non-citrus fruits, nuts, legumes, dark leafy greens | n/a | n/a |
| high blood sugar level | meats, nuts, cheese | 50-200 mcg | 50-200 mcg |

*DRI are new tools for figuring out how much of a vitamin or mineral you should include in your daily diet. They replace and add to the older RDA (recommended dietary allowances).

| Mineral | What It Does |
| --- | --- |
| **Trace Minerals** | |
| **Copper** | makes red blood cells, produces energy, fights free radicals |
| **Fluoride** | protects bones and teeth |
| **Iodine** | makes thyroid hormones, steadies metabolism |
| **Iron** | carries oxygen throughout the body, produces energy |
| **Manganese** | produces energy, builds bones and joints |
| **Molybdenum** | fights free radicals |
| **Selenium** | makes thyroid hormones, fights free radicals, strengthens immune system |
| **Zinc** | produces energy, makes DNA, helps body use vitamin A, fights free radicals, heals wounds, boosts immune system |

| Signs of Deficiency | Good Sources | Dietary Reference Intakes* (DRI) | |
|---|---|---|---|
| | | Women Age 51+ | Men Age 51+ |
| **Trace Minerals** | | | |
| weakness, pale skin, unhealed wounds | organ meats, seafood, nuts, seeds | 900 mcg | 900 mcg |
| dental cavities | tea, seafood, tap water | 3 mg | 4 mg |
| goiter | seafood, salt, dairy foods | 150 mcg | 150 mcg |
| weakness, pale skin, trouble concentrating | meats, eggs, legumes, dried fruits | 8 mg | 8 mg |
| n/a | nuts, legumes, whole grains, tea | 2-11 mg | 2-11 mg |
| severe headache, rapid heartbeat, confusion | dairy foods, legumes, whole grains | 45 mcg | 45 mcg |
| muscle weakness and pain, cataracts, heart trouble | meats, seafood, whole grains | 55 mcg | 55 mcg |
| diarrhea, infections, loss of appetite, weight loss, unhealed wounds | meats, shellfish, legumes, whole grains | 8 mg | 11 mg |

*DRI are new tools for figuring out how much of a vitamin or mineral you should include in your daily diet. They replace and add to the older RDA (recommended dietary allowances).

**Iodine.** Your thyroid gland uses this nutrient to make its hormones. These compounds control your body temperature, regulating the metabolism of every major organ. A lack of iodine can wreak havoc with your body and cause a condition called goiter.

**Iron.** Without a teaspoon of this mineral in your body, you couldn't breathe. Iron makes up hemoglobin and myoglobin, two compounds that carry oxygen throughout your blood and your muscles. No wonder you feel weak and listless when you are iron deficient.

**Selenium.** Now famous for preventing cancer, selenium also carries out important daily tasks in your body. It helps your thyroid use iodine, for instance, and it's important for a healthy immune system. A deficiency in selenium can cause heart and thyroid disease.

**Zinc.** This mineral has many jobs. Cleaning up free radicals, building new cells, and producing energy from other nutrients are just three. A zinc deficiency can be dangerous, leading to digestion problems and deficiencies in other nutrients.

**The mighty five.** Chromium, copper, fluoride, manganese, and molybdenum are five trace minerals you'll find in common foods and drinks. They are responsible for everything from strong teeth (fluoride) to your blood-sugar level (chromium). They are so important that nutritionists have set daily requirements for each of them to make sure you get enough.

Experts are also investigating a handful of other minerals to see how essential they are to your body. Boron is one that seems promising as an important ingredient in bone and joint health.

## When too much is toxic

In larger amounts, minerals become more hazardous than healthy. So talk with your doctor before taking mineral supplements such as iron and selenium.

You also need to be careful with over-the-counter remedies like antacids. They contain magnesium, and an overdose can lead to diarrhea and even kidney damage. Zinc lozenges for cold therapy can also be dangerous if you take too many.

Even soft drinks and convenience foods can be a problem because of their high phosphorus content. Too much phosphorus can interfere with your body's ability to absorb and use calcium. Like everything else, follow moderation when trying to meet your daily mineral requirements. If you eat a balanced diet, you won't ever have to worry about getting too much.

# Phytochemicals

Natural chemicals in plants, called phytochemicals or phytonutrients, can have a powerful effect on the human body. Found in fruits, vegetables, herbs, and spices, these tens of thousands of substances have been used to treat and prevent diseases since ancient times.

Many cultures like the Chinese and American Indians have always looked to plants for healing. And even today, the World Health Organization says about 80 percent of the people on earth use natural medicine — mostly involving plants.

However, modern man's passion for science and advanced technology has inflated the market for pills and capsules, replacing whole sources of nutrition. That's why you'll find a host of supplements in stores and on the Internet offering an easy supply of phytochemicals.

But there is very little evidence these plant chemicals do the same job once you take them out of their original "package"— possibly because the chemicals need other parts of the plant to work properly. As always, the best way for you to get the most benefit from phytochemicals is to eat whole foods.

| Phytochemical | Type | Good sources |
|---|---|---|
| **Anthocyanins** | Flavonoid | blueberries, strawberries, raspberries, blackberries, currants |
| **Beta carotene** | Carotenoid | carrots, sweet potatoes, pumpkins, mango, cantaloupe, apricots, spinach, broccoli |
| **Capsaicin** | | chili peppers |
| **Catechin** | Polyphenol | green tea, red wine, red grape juice |
| **Curcumin** | Polyphenol | turmeric, ginger |
| **Daidzein** | Flavonoid | legumes, soybeans* |
| **Ellagic acid** | Polyphenol | strawberries, grapefruit, blackberries, blueberries, raspberries, walnuts, pomegranates |
| **Genistein** | Phytosterol | soybeans* |
| **Lignans** | Phytosterol | whole grains, flaxseed |
| **Limonene** | Monoterpene | orange and lemon peel, cherries |
| **Lutein** | Carotenoid | collard greens, spinach, kale, broccoli, turnip greens, zucchini, corn, kiwi, red seedless grapes |
| **Lycopene** | Carotenoid | guava, papaya, pink grapefruit, tomatoes, watermelon, cooked tomato products |
| **Phytic acid** | | wheat germ, soybeans* |

*Warning: New research claims that soy may accelerate brain aging. For more information, see the *Memory loss* chapter.

| Possible benefits |
|---|
| acts as antioxidant to fight heart disease, protects vision, and combats cancer |
| preserves eyesight; strengthens immune system; works as an antioxidant to fight heart disease, cancer, memory loss, rheumatoid arthritis, respiratory distress syndrome, liver disease, Parkinson's disease, and complications of diabetes |
| regulates blood clotting |
| protects against cancer, fights heart disease |
| protects against stomach, breast, lung, colon, and skin cancers; fights inflammation |
| protects against breast, colon, ovarian, and prostate cancers; guards against osteoporosis |
| works as an antioxidant to fight cancerous tumors, especially of the lung, liver, skin, and esophagus |
| protects against breast, colon, ovarian, and prostate cancers; strenghtens bones, fights menopause symptoms |
| protects against breast, colon, ovarian, and prostate cancers; fights heart disease |
| protects against cancer |
| preserves eyesight, protects against cancer |
| protects against esophageal, stomach, and prostate cancers; preserves eyesight |
| protects against cancer and heart disease |

| Phytochemical | Type | Good sources |
|---|---|---|
| **Quercetin** | Flavonoid | tea, red onions, buckwheat, citrus fruits |
| **Resveratrol** | Flavonoid | red grapes, red wine |
| **Sulforaphane** | Isothiocyanate | broccoli, cabbage, kale, cauliflower, brussels sprouts, ginger, onions, bok choy |
| **Tannins** | | tea, whole-grain cereals |
| **Zeaxanthin** | Carotenoid | broccoli, grapes, spinach, collard greens, kale, turnip greens, zucchini, orange peppers, kiwi, red seedless grapes, egg yolks |

*Warning: New research claims that soy may accelerate brain aging. For more information, see the *Memory loss* chapter.

Choose lots of fruit, double the amount of vegetables you normally eat, season your dishes with herbs and spices, and plan several meatless meals that contain legumes and whole grains. In addition, cook your vegetables lightly since heat destroys many of these natural substances.

Some foods contain literally hundreds of phytochemicals and some specific phytochemicals do more than one kind of job. Here are the most common types you might read about in the news.

**Carotenoids.** Carotenoids are a group of over 600 dyes found in plants that provide color ranging from light yellow to red. They include beta carotene, lycopene, lutein, and zeaxanthin. Studies show that carotenoids act as antioxidants in your body and boost your immune system. In addition, people who eat lots of carotene-rich foods have less risk of heart disease and cancer. Besides deeply colored fruits and vegetables, other sources of carotenoids are green, leafy herbs, rose hips, and spices like paprika and saffron.

| Possible benefits |
|---|
| fights inflammation, protects your arteries, fights allergies, protects against cancer, fights bacteria |
| fights heart disease, protects against cancer, fights inflammation |
| protects against cancer |
| protects against cancer |
| preserves eyesight |

**Flavonoids.** Flavonoids are another group of more than 4,000 plant pigments that give many flowers and herbs their yellow, orange, and red color. The most common flavonoids are called flavonols, flavones, and isoflavones. Large studies prove that people who regularly eat foods rich in flavonoids are much less likely to develop heart disease or have a stroke than those who avoid such foods. Also, the flavonoids in green tea have shown an amazing ability to reduce the risk of cancer.

**Organosulfur compounds.** Garlic, the best-known food containing these, makes your immune system stronger, destroys germs, and keeps cancer-causing substances from forming. Isothiocyanates are a type of organosulfur compound found in cruciferous vegetables. Animal and human studies show they can fight off cancers of the colon, breast, and digestive tract.

**Phytosterols.** Phytochemicals in this group are similar to the steroid hormones your own body makes. They act like estrogen or progesterone and are important for fighting breast, prostate, and ovarian cancers, osteoporosis, and heart disease. Lignans, an example of these friendly plant chemicals, can slow the growth of breast tumors.

**Polyphenols.** This category of phytochemicals contains phenolic acids. They work as antioxidants to protect against cancer, fight heart disease, and kill bacteria. Also found in green tea, these can protect cells in your colon and stomach from becoming cancerous. In addition, they kill bacteria, fungi, and viruses.

# Protein

. . . . . . . . . . . .

Protein is a part of every cell in your body, and no other nutrient plays as many different roles in keeping you alive and healthy. It is important for the growth and repair of your muscles, bones, skin, tendons, ligaments, hair, eyes, and other tissues. Without it, you would lack the enzymes and hormones you need for metabolism, digestion, and other important processes.

When you have an infection, you should eat more protein because it helps create the antibodies your immune system needs to fight disease. If you are injured, you may need more, as well, to help your blood clot and make repairs.

Your body can use protein for energy, if necessary, but it's best to eat plenty of carbohydrates for that purpose and save your protein for the important jobs other nutrients can't do.

**Pick your protein carefully.** Your body needs many different proteins for various purposes. It makes them from about 20 "building blocks" called amino acids. Nine of these are essential amino acids, which means you must get them from food. The others are nonessential. This doesn't mean you don't need them. You just don't have to eat them because your body can make them.

It's easiest to get protein from meat, chicken, turkey, fish, and dairy foods. Cooked meat is about 15 to 40 percent protein. Foods from animal sources provide complete protein, which means they contain all the essential amino acids.

Next to meat, legumes — beans, peas, and peanuts — have the most protein. But they are called incomplete proteins because they are lacking some essential amino acids. You can get complete protein if you combine them with plant foods from one of these categories — grains, seeds and nuts, and vegetables. Eat any two or more of these plant foods, with or without beans, and you get complete protein.

You don't have to eat these foods in the same dish, or even in the same meal. But many cultures have created combinations that work well — like corn and beans in Mexico, or rice and split peas in India. Many Americans enjoy legumes and grains in a peanut butter sandwich.

> ### Beware the dangers of a high-protein diet
>
> If you are looking for a quick way to lose weight, it's easy to get fired up about a high-protein diet. Unfortunately, the American Heart Association, the American Dietetic Association, and other health organizations advise against it.
>
> An initial drop in weight is common with a high-protein diet, but it's due primarily to water loss. These diets don't work very well in the long run — nor do they build muscles as they claim. Most important, they can be dangerous, increasing your risk of heart disease, kidney and artery damage, and bone loss.
>
> While most high-protein foods contain plenty of vitamin B12 and iron, they are low in other vitamins and minerals. Only a diet with lots of fruits, vegetables, and grains supplies the other nutrients that keep you healthy.

**Make digestion easier.** Your body can digest and use animal protein more easily than plant protein. But be sure to avoid excess fat by choosing lean meats and low-fat dairy products. Legumes are next easiest to digest, followed by grains and other plant sources.

Cooking protein foods with moist rather than dry heat, perhaps boiled in a stew rather than fried, or soaking meat in a marinade using wine, lemon juice, or vinegar makes it easier to digest.

**Set healthy limits.** Since protein is so important to your body's survival, you may think you need to eat a lot of it. Fortunately, your body actually recycles protein from tissues that break down and uses it to make new ones. So you don't need more than 10 to 15 percent of your total calories from protein.

Protein deficiencies are common in poor, undeveloped countries. Even in modern nations, they sometimes occur in certain groups. In fact, vegetarians need to be very careful about eating the right combinations of plant foods to get enough complete protein.

The chances are far greater that you eat too much protein, especially from meat sources. The typical Western diet includes about 100 grams of protein, while 50 grams is closer to what your body needs.

If you are healthy, with no liver or kidney problems, you can get rid of any excess with little trouble. Yet, meat protein can be expensive and high in fat, two good reasons not to eat more than your body can use.

# Vitamins

. . . . . . . . . . . . . . . . .

Simply put — you can't live without vitamins. Your body needs a certain amount each day. Missing your daily quota once in a while doesn't hurt. But if you shortchange yourself on vitamins on a regular basis, you put yourself in danger.

Luckily, you'll find plenty of vitamins in grains, legumes, fruits, seafood, lean meats, vegetables, and other healthy foods. Include these food groups in your daily diet, and you'll protect yourself from a long list of diseases, including cancer, heart disease, arthritis, cataracts, depression, pellagra, anemia, macular degeneration, thyroid disease, and memory loss — just to name a few.

Vitamins are critical for everyday bodily functions like digestion and thinking. Without enough of them, your body can't complete these tasks and starts to break down. Some vitamins also act as antioxidants. They're your body's tiny foot soldiers, tirelessly watching over you and fighting off harmful molecules called free radicals. A free radical has one or more extra electrons that make it unstable, so it goes off and steals an electron from another molecule to make itself stable again. This causes a chain reaction that eventually results in tissue damage and disease. Antioxidant vitamins come to your rescue by giving up electrons to stabilize free radicals and help keep your body healthy.

All vitamins are one of two types — fat-soluble or water-soluble. Both are equally important; your body just uses them in different ways.

## 4 fat-astic vitamins you can't afford to miss

Your body absorbs, transports, and stores fat-soluble vitamins with bile and fat. That explains their name. It also explains why you should avoid taking these vitamins in high doses, especially in supplement form. They naturally build up in your fatty tissues and liver, and their levels only go down gradually as your body uses them. If you take in too much at once, your body has no way of dumping the excess. That can leave you very sick.

Getting these four vitamins from food sources is the best way to get the amount that's just right.

**Vitamin A.** This fat-soluble vitamin is most famous for protecting your eyesight, but vitamin A carries out many other jobs, too. It keeps you healthy by assuring that your cells divide properly into new ones. It's especially important for your skin cells and the lining of your digestive track. Vitamin A is also famous for boosting your immune system.

**Vitamin D.** You don't have to worry about this bone-building nutrient if you live in Florida, southern Italy, or another sunny location. That's because your skin can turn sunlight into vitamin D. For most people, it doesn't take long in the sun to get the needed amount. Whether you get it from the sun or from food, vitamin D controls your body's levels of calcium and phosphorus. That's key for keeping your skeleton strong.

**Vitamin E.** Breathing is a dangerous proposition without this fat-soluble vitamin. Natural actions like this produce free radicals, unstable compounds that attack your body's cells and nutrients. In the process, they produce more free radicals, starting a chain reaction that can lead to cancer, heart disease, and other chronic illnesses. Vitamin E stops this snowball before it starts rolling.

**Vitamin K.** This vitamin isn't on any food's nutrition label, but it's still important. Without vitamin K, your blood couldn't clot. It also helps your body use calcium and ensures that your bones stay strong.

## Fight disease with Bs and C

In your body, water-soluble vitamins float freely in your blood or in the watery fluid between your cells. They don't stick around for long, though. Your body doesn't store them but instead uses them or flushes them out through your kidneys. This means you don't have to worry about overloading on water-soluble vitamins. But you do need to replace them often.

**B vitamins.** These nutrients generally help your body carry out its day-to-day chores, though each one is important for its own special reasons. Thiamin (B1) and riboflavin (B2), for instance, work to turn your food into energy. Folate gets its hands dirty building DNA, the genes in each one of your cells. With the help of B6 and B12, folate also makes red blood cells, your body's oxygen delivery boys. B vitamins make sure almost every part of your body runs smoothly, from your brain to your big toe. By keeping your body strong and healthy, these vitamins help you fight off sickness and disease.

**Vitamin C.** This is probably the most famous vitamin of all, renown as a cold cure, a cancer fighter, and the king of antioxidants. Vitamin C deserves all the attention. It safeguards you from free radicals, and it's also in charge of making collagen. This substance helps hold together all the cells and tissues of your body, including ligaments, tendons, and scar tissue. It also supports your bones and teeth.

## Understand your daily requirements

RDA, DRI, IU, RE — these are all ways of measuring vitamins. It can be confusing if you don't know what these terms stand for. Get them straight to make sure your diet is vitamin-complete.

DRI (dietary reference intakes) are new guidelines that replace the RDA (recommended dietary allowances) you're probably familiar with. The DRI include the RDA but also take into account new research on disease prevention, the upper limits you can safely take, and the average nutrients required by healthy people worldwide. The DRI are not minimum requirements, but rather are recommendations for the best and safest amounts for each age group. Experts believe the DRI more accurately show a person's daily nutrition requirements.

To understand DRI recommendations, keep in mind that anything ending in "grams" is a metric weight. Micrograms (mcg) are the smallest, and it takes 1,000 mcg to make 1 milligram (mg). Likewise, it takes 1,000 mg to add up to 1 gram. Fat-soluble vitamins are sometimes listed as IUs (international units). And you may see RE (retinal equivalent) or RAE (retinal activity equivalent) used to measure vitamin A. All these measures tell you how much of the vitamin you are getting. Just be sure they fall within the guidelines listed in the following chart.

| Vitamin | Dietary Reference Intakes* (DRI) | | What it does |
|---|---|---|---|
| | Women age 51+ | Men age 51+ | |
| Fat-soluble vitamins | | | |
| **A** (Retinol) | 800 RE or 4,000 IU | 1,000 RE or 5,000 IU | controls eyesight, builds new cells, protects skin and mucous membranes, fights infection and free radicals |
| **D** (Calciferol) | 10-15 mcg or 400 IU | 10-15 mcg or 400 IU | builds bones, controls calcium and phosphorus levels in your body |
| **E** (Tocopherol) | 15 mg or 22 IU | 15 mg or 22 IU | fights free radicals |
| **K** (Phylloquinone) | 65 mcg | 80 mcg | forms blood clots, controls calcium levels |
| Water-soluble vitamins | | | |
| **B1** (Thiamin) | 1.1 mg | 1.2 mg | produces energy, sends nerve messages, brings on healthy appetite |
| **B2** (Riboflavin) | 1.1 mg | 1.3 mg | produces energy, helps vision, builds new cells |
| **B3** (Niacin) | 14 mg | 16 mg | produces energy, builds DNA |
| Folate (Folic acid) | 400 mcg | 400 mcg | makes and repairs DNA, removes homocysteine from blood |
| **B12** (Cobalamin) | 2.4 mcg | 2.4 mcg | makes new cells (especially red blood cells), protects nerves |

*DRI are new tools for figuring out how much of a vitamin or mineral you should include in your daily diet. They replace and add to the older RDA (recommended dietary allowances).

| Good sources | Suggested daily servings |
|---|---|
| **Fat-soluble vitamins** ||
| liver, dairy, eggs | 1/3 oz. of beef liver *or* 6 cups of skim milk |
| fortified milk, eggs, liver, sardines | 4 cups of skim milk *or* 9 oz. of shrimp *or* 4 oz. of salmon |
| vegetable oils, dark leafy greens, nuts and seeds, wheat germ | 2-1/2 oz. of wheat germ *or* 5 tbs. of canola oil *or* 1 oz. of sunflower seeds |
| dark leafy greens, cruciferous veggies | 1/2 cup of broccoli *or* 1 cup of cabbage |
| **Water-soluble vitamins** ||
| whole grains, nuts, legumes, pork | 2-1/2 cups of cooked black beans or green peas *or* 5 slices of watermelon |
| dairy, dark leafy greens, whole grains | 2 cups of skim milk *or* 2 cups of raisin bran |
| protein-rich foods, dairy foods, fish, nuts, whole grains | 1 can (6 oz.) of light tuna *or* 4 oz. of chicken breast |
| dark leafy greens, legumes, seeds, enriched breads and cereals | 2 cups of cooked black beans or cooked frozen spinach *or* 1-1/4 cups of toasted wheat germ |
| meats, fish, dairy foods, eggs | 2 cups of low-fat cottage cheese *or* 1-1/2 oz. of salmon |

| B6 (Pyridoxine) | 1.5 mg | 1.7 mg | makes red blood cells, builds proteins, regulates blood sugar, makes brain chemicals, protects immune system |
|---|---|---|---|
| Biotin | 30 mcg | 30 mcg | produces energy, helps body use other B vitamins |
| B5 (Pantothenic acid) | 5 mg | 5 mg | produces energy |
| C (Ascorbic acid) | 75 mg | 90 mg | makes collagen for skeleton and skin, fights free radicals, bolsters immune system, helps body absorb iron |

*DRI are new tools for figuring out how much of a vitamin or mineral you should include in your daily diet. They replace and add to the older RDA (recommended dietary allowances).

# Water

• • • • • • • • • •

When you think about a healthy diet, it's easy to overlook the most important nutrient of all — water. It's the "juice" that keeps your body's chemical processes going. It dissolves minerals, vitamins, and other nutrients and carries them to where you need them. And it helps form the structure of your cells, tissues, and organs.

Before you were born, water cushioned your entire body against the shocks of the world. Today, it cushions your joints and spinal column. Water helps regulate your body temperature, lubricates your digestive tract, and maintains pressure in your eyes.

| | |
|---|---|
| dark leafy greens, seafood, legumes, whole grains, fruits and veggies | 3 bananas *or* 3 potatoes *or* 6 oz. of beef liver |
| liver, egg yolks, legumes, nuts, cauliflower | 3 oz. of peanut butter *or* 3-1/2 oz. of oatmeal |
| whole grains, organ meats, broccoli, avocados | 2 cups of wheat germ *or* 6 oz. of bran |
| citrus fruits, dark leafy greens, cruciferous veggies, bright-colored fruits and veggies | 1 cup of strawberries or raw broccoli *or* 1 orange or whole grapefruit |
| | |

**Replace what you've lost.** You need to drink as much liquid every day as you lose through perspiration and excretion. Otherwise, your body will become dehydrated. If you lose 5 percent of your body fluids and don't replace them, you may experience headache, fatigue, lack of concentration, and an elevated heart rate. Lose greater amounts, and you face the risk of confusion, shock, seizures, coma — even death.

**Sip water throughout the day.** Don't wait until you feel thirsty to drink a glass of water. Your thirst, especially as you get older, may not be a reliable gauge of your body's need. You could be two cups low before you feel it.

**Drink more when it's hot.** When the weather is hot and dry, or you get more exercise than usual, you'll need more water. If you eat a lot of soups or juicy fruits and vegetables, you may require less. Most people need between 8 and 12 cups of fluids a day.

Don't include alcohol or beverages with caffeine, like coffee, colas, or tea, in your count. These are diuretics, which cause you to lose water faster than usual. If you drink any of these, you need to drink more water to replace what you lose. Herbal teas and juices are good substitutes when you want something other than water.

# Food + technology = boon or bust?

Even before the first tractor rolled onto a cornfield, agriculture and technology have been partners — whether it involved a wooden hoe, an irrigation system, or computerized soil analysis. And with every modern advance, crops have gotten larger, fields have become more productive, and pantry shelves are better stocked. However, many people are now concerned that hi-tech tampering with the food supply is unhealthy.

Genetically modified (GM) foods or those containing genetically modified organisms (GMO) have been on the market for several years. You've probably eaten them without knowing it. Producers aren't required to identify these foods, although the Food and Drug Administration recently proposed voluntary labeling. Common GM food crops include soybeans, corn, potatoes, squash, canola, and papaya.

One of the goals of genetic modification is for scientists to change the DNA make-up of plants so they are more resistant to insects and weeds. This way, farmers can use fewer chemical insecticides or herbicides.

To change a food this way, a scientist first inserts an extra gene into a plant. This gene may come from an entirely different species. For example, a bacterium gene is often added to a corn plant so it can create its own insecticide. These modified plants are then bred with ordinary plants to create new varieties.

Many believe if you eat foods from these plants, those extra genes could remain in your body and trigger a virus or even cancer. Other experts argue that almost half the soybean crop and about one-fourth of the corn crop now consists of genetically modified plants. And people have been eating these foods for some time with no ill effects.

The debate over the safety of what some call "Frankenfoods" will undoubtedly continue, with many demanding laws to ban or regulate GM foods. If you're concerned, choose products with the label "GMO-free" whenever possible.

### New USDA labeling defines organic

The label says "organic," but does that mean it's healthy? Perhaps not in the past, but soon a new USDA ruling will end years of confusion about food products that claim to be natural.

These new national standards for organic foods give farmers clear production, handling, and processing guidelines and you, as a consumer, exact information about what you're buying.

For example, organic farmers can no longer use genetic engineering, radiation, sewage sludge for fertilizer, or any synthetic pesticide or fertilizer. In addition, animals used for meat, milk, eggs, etc., cannot receive hormones or antibiotics.

# Acerola

· · · · · · · · · · · · ·

**Benefits**

Protects your heart

Combats cancer

Supports immune
  system

Fights fungus

Smoothes skin

Barbados cherry, West Indian cherry, cereza, or acerola — whatever you call it, this tropical fruit is a rare treat. On the outside, it looks like a red cherry, but bite into it, and you're in for a surprise. Many people say it tastes like a tart apple, although its flesh is soft and juicy. And unlike an apple or a cherry, the acerola is bursting with vitamin C. Just one cup of this little fruit has almost 30 times the recommended dietary allowance. That's more than all other foods on the planet — except the even rarer camu-camu berry.

It's no wonder you'll find acerola in natural vitamin C supplements, beauty products, and juice drinks. Unfortunately, the whole fruit is harder to come by, mainly because it doesn't travel well. If you leave it out for only a few hours, it will begin to spoil.

The acerola grows in warm climates from southern Texas and California, through Mexico and the Caribbean, and down into South America. If you'd like to try an acerola and you live far away from these areas, just visit a nearby farmer's market and ask for it by name — "Ah-sah-roll-lah." It's worth a try. If you're lucky enough to find it, you'll be getting your hands on a fruit prized in Latin America for treating diarrhea, fever, and even hepatitis. Plus, you'll get a not-so-shabby antioxidant blast against cancer, heart disease, and skin problems.

## 3 ways acerola keeps you healthy

**Hinders heart disease.** Just one tiny acerola has over 80 milligrams of vitamin C. That's as much as a whole grapefruit. And according to the major medical studies, that's enough to cut your risk of heart disease, stroke, and high blood pressure. Vitamin C fights free radicals, makes your blood vessels more flexible, lowers your blood pressure, and re-energizes the other top antioxidant, vitamin E. All the things you need to keep your heart running smoothly.

**Cancels cancer.** If you want to lower your risk of cancer, eat foods rich in antioxidants. Once they are in your body, antioxidants stop free radicals dead in their tracks before they cause cell damage, while others fix the damage already done by these troublemakers. Either way, antioxidants work hard to keep cancer away. Since acerolas have two of the top free-radical scavengers in the business — vitamin C and beta carotene — you owe it to yourself to track down these tropical treasures.

**Tunes up your immune system.** Eating foods high in vitamin C may not cure the common cold, but it can help strengthen your defenses against pesky bacteria and viruses. Research shows vitamin C encourages your immune system to be all that it can be against the bad guys — just like the Army. With vitamin C's help, your body sends out white blood cells that hunt down and literally gobble up germs.

### Camu-camu — the vitamin C champion

Out of the deep, dark rainforests of South America's Amazon River, there comes a wild fruit that beats out the mighty acerola as vitamin C champion of the world. It's the camu-camu berry — a tiny, purplish, pulpy berry that food companies in Japan and France already squeeze into juices, jams, and other sweet treats.

In many other countries, you'll find powdered camu-camu in natural vitamin C supplements. The fruit is getting so popular that farmers are setting up camu-camu fields in the middle of the jungle. You'll probably be seeing and hearing more and more about them in the future.

## Pantry pointers

Your best bet for finding acerolas is at a farmer's market that carries exotic food. If that doesn't work, find a Chinese grocery store and ask if they sell a snack called "haw flakes." Haw flakes are candy wafers made from dried acerola. They're tart, delicious, and nutritious. Your local health food store might stock fruit drinks powered with acerola juice, as well as natural vitamin C supplements made with the fruit.

Before you buy supplements containing acerola, consider these facts:

◆ Supplements can be expensive, especially name brands.

◆ They may not do what they advertise. Doctors are unsure whether supplements work the same way as nutrients taken from fresh fruits and vegetables.

◆ Megadoses of vitamin C over 2 grams a day can cause side effects, like diarrhea, kidney stones, and problems digesting other nutrients.

◆ Many governments don't regulate supplements, so there's no way of knowing exactly how much and what grade of nutrients goes into them.

It's always a good idea to check with your doctor before taking any supplements.

---

### An age-old remedy for aging skin

In traditional Latin American medicine, the acerola is renown as an astringent and a powerful weapon against ringworm and other fungal infections. And now the American Academy of Dermatology suggests there's one more way the Barbados cherry may heal the skin. The abundant amount of vitamin C in the acerola may heal cuts, wipe away wrinkles, and clear up other blemishes caused by aging. In fact, many anti-aging skin creams tout that they have acerola in them. The next time you're shopping for a skin cream, look for acerola in the ingredients and try it for yourself.

| Eat | |
|---|---|
| Blueberries | Strawberries |
| Spinach | Eggs |
| Wheat germ | Broccoli |
| Beets | Tuna |
| Nuts | Milk |
| Flaxseed | Beans |

**Avoid**

Foods high in saturated fat, such as red meat and whole-milk dairy products

# Alzheimer's disease

• • • • • • • • • • • • • •

"I have recently been told that I am one of the millions of Americans who will be afflicted with Alzheimer's disease," Ronald Reagan, former president of the United States, announced in November 1994. "I intend to live the remainder of the years God gives me on this Earth doing the things I have always done," he declared. "Unfortunately, as Alzheimer's disease progresses, the family often bears a heavy burden. I only wish there was some way I could spare Nancy from this painful experience."

In his message, Reagan summed up the tragedy of Alzheimer's disease (AD). Those suffering from AD face the reality of losing touch with their old lives. Family and friends are forced to watch a loved one slowly fall victim to the dreadful condition.

Scientists aren't sure exactly what's behind AD. Some suspect a certain gene — apolipoprotein E 4 allele (Apo E4) — plays a major part in your brain's decline. Other experts believe years of oxidative stress also are at the root of the problem.

Whatever causes Alzheimer's disease attacks the part of your brain that controls speech, thoughts, and memory. You gradually lose the power to recall the past and the ability to carry out your daily life. AD usually hits around age 65 and older, and your risk goes up each year after that.

Through this dark cloud, however, there is a ray of hope. According to AD experts like Dr. Grace Petot, a professor at Case Western Reserve University, people can change their lifestyles to lower their risk. Boost your fruit and vegetable intake for a start.

From her research, Petot discovered that many AD sufferers ate fewer fruits and veggies as adults.

Science, she suggests, also points to a connection between heart disease and Alzheimer's. So eating a heart-healthy diet might protect you, too. That means a lot of high-fiber, low-fat foods. It's also a good idea to exercise both your mind and your muscles. "Keeping the brain active and the body active," Petot says, "is beneficial in many ways."

## Nutritional blockbusters that fight AD

**Antioxidants.** Thanks to cutting-edge research, experts now hope AD can one day be prevented. Antioxidants, those powerful substances that fend off cancer and heart disease, might also safeguard your brain against free radicals. Antioxidants appear to slow — and even reverse — the memory loss caused by free-radical damage.

Supplements usually only contain one antioxidant, so eat a variety of fruits and vegetables to get the most benefit. Fruits and vegetables are rich in many antioxidants — not just beta carotene or vitamin C, but flavonoids, too. Flavonoids make memory-saving marvels out of snacks like blueberries, strawberries, and spinach.

**B vitamins.** You also need foods rich in B vitamins to help protect your brain from AD. At least two studies show Alzheimer's sufferers have lower levels of folate and B12 than their non-AD peers. Low B-vitamin levels, according to several other studies, appear to lead to lower scores on IQ and memory tests.

Vitamin B12 helps your body make neurotransmitters, chemicals that help carry messages between your nerves and brain. Another B vitamin, thiamin, helps nerve signals travel from your brain to different parts of your body. These important tasks could be why a lack of B vitamins might affect your brain's health.

To get more folate into your diet, try dark leafy greens, broccoli, beets, beans, and okra. Meats, eggs, and dairy products are good sources of B12. For older adults, who might have trouble absorbing B12, experts suggest eating fortified breakfast cereals. Wheat germ, nuts, beans, and rice will give you your full day's supply of thiamin.

**Omega-3s.** Look to the sea to find help against Alzheimer's. Fish are the greatest source of omega-3 fatty acids. These fat molecules protect against heart disease and inflammation and may lead the attack against Alzheimer's as well. One of AD's possible causes is beta-amyloid plaque, clumps of protein that build up in the victim's brain. Experts believe beta amyloid might be connected with inflammation of the brain's blood vessels. So it makes sense that anti-inflammatory omega-3 fatty acids could help.

It's a good idea to eat as much fish as you can net. Experts recommend at least two servings of salmon, tuna, mackerel, or other cold-water fish per week. For you landlubbers who think fish are for the birds, get your omega-3 from flaxseed, walnuts, and dark leafy greens. And while you punch up omega-3, limit your intake of omega-6 fatty acids. They compete with omega-3 and can cause inflammation. Foods high in omega-6 include fried and fast foods, salad dressings, and baked goods.

---

### A word of caution

Just say no to foods loaded with saturated fat. That's what AD researcher Grace Petot discovered after examining the diet of more than 300 senior citizens. Eating a diet high in fat, the research suggested, greatly increased the risk of AD for people with the Apo E4 gene. Experts for some time have seen a connection between heart disease, fat, and Alzheimer's. They aren't sure exactly why, although they suspect fat attracts more harmful free radicals.

"Fats are subject to oxidation," Petot explains, "producing free radicals which then can cause damage to cell walls and DNA." Whether you have the AD gene or not, it's always a good idea to substitute whole grains, fish, fruits, and veggies for fatty snacks and fast food.

"It's never too late for people to improve their lifestyles," Petot affirms.

# Apples

**Benefits**

Protects your heart

Prevents constipation

Blocks diarrhea

Improves lung capacity

Slows aging process

Cushions joints

There's no easier way to add a dose of nutrition to your day than by crunching on a tasty apple. You probably first experienced its delightful flavor as a baby, when applesauce introduced you to real food. And now, whether it's a Granny Smith, a McIntosh, or a Red Delicious, you think of apples as old friends. Grown throughout the world, apples are high in fiber, vitamins, minerals, and antioxidants. They're fat-free, cholesterol-free, and low in sodium. In short, eating apples is a smart part of a healthy lifestyle.

## 6 ways apples keep you healthy

**Regulates your day.** You don't have to worry about staying regular anymore. Whether your problem is visiting the bathroom too often or not often enough, apples can help.

A British researcher, Dr. D.P. Burkitt, believes one of the easiest ways to prevent all sorts of illnesses, is to avoid constipation. He calls the diseases caused by chronic constipation "pressure diseases." Appendicitis, diverticular diseases, hemorrhoids, hiatal hernias, and even varicose veins can all be caused by straining to pass small, hard stools.

Just one apple with its skin contains 4 to 5 grams of fiber — the most important nutrient in keeping your bowels working like a well-oiled machine. Keeping yourself regular without relying on harmful laxatives could be as easy as replacing that afternoon snack of potato chips or cookies with a crisp, delicious apple. And think of the calories you'll save. The average apple has about 80 calories while a serving of chips weighs in at 150 calories and you'll get about 200 from just a few cookies.

But that's not all apples can do. They're also good for diarrhea, thanks to an ingredient called pectin. This carbohydrate has a congealing effect in your intestines that helps firm things up and return you to normal. Applesauce is actually the best apple product for diarrhea, since it's made without the high-fiber skin. But watch out for extra sugar. Some brands of applesauce dump a truckload of sweeteners into an otherwise healthy food, and too much refined sugar could make your diarrhea worse.

**Keeps your body young.** By now you know antioxidants can protect you from many of the diseases that seem to be a part of aging. In fact, so many people are taking supplements for antioxidant protection that it's become a multibillion-dollar industry. But the evidence is mounting that whole foods can do more for you than pills.

When scientists compared a 1,500-milligram vitamin C supplement to one small apple, the results were astounding — the antioxidant values were equal. That means a fresh apple has more than 15 times the antioxidant power of the recommended daily dose of vitamin C. And that's just for starters. The researchers also found an ordinary apple was able to stop the growth of colon and liver cancer cells in test tubes. Unpeeled apples were especially effective. The question you need to ask yourself: Why waste money on flavorless supplements when you can get better antioxidant firepower from a sweet, crunchy fruit?

**Cuts your risk of heart disease.** Sometimes it's hard to remember which food is good for which part of your body. The next time you pick up an apple, examine it carefully. It's shaped a bit like a heart — and that should help you remember apples are good for your heart.

It's the magnesium and potassium in apples that help regulate your blood pressure and keep your heart beating steadily, and it's the flavonoid quercetin, a naturally occurring antioxidant, that protects your artery walls from damage and keeps your blood flowing smoothly.

In fact adding flavonoid-rich foods like apples to your diet has been scientifically confirmed to lower your risk of heart disease. There's proof of this in a study of Japanese women who ate foods high in quercetin. They were less likely to get coronary heart disease than other women and they had lower levels of total and LDL, or bad, cholesterol.

**Strikes at the heart of strokes.** Apples are even a smart choice for helping avoid strokes. Scientists aren't sure which ingredient in this multi-talented fruit to credit, but the connection is clear — people who regularly eat apples are less likely to have strokes than people who don't.

**Protects your joints.** In areas of the world where fruits and vegetables make up a large part of the diet, very few people get arthritis. Compare this to modernized countries where fruits and vegetables have been replaced with fast, processed food and you'll find up to 70 percent of the population suffers from some form of arthritis. Just a coincidence? Not according to nutrition experts. They link this trend in part to boron, a trace mineral many plants, including apples, absorb from the soil.

If you eat like most people, you'll get about 1 to 2 milligrams (mg) of boron a day, mostly from non-citrus fruits, leafy vegetables, and nuts. Experts believe, however, you need anywhere from 3 to 10 mg a day to affect your risk of arthritis. To boost your boron intake to this level, you'd have to eat more than nine apples a day.

This is probably an unreasonable amount for most people, but don't despair. Pair an apple with other boron-rich foods like a few tablespoons of peanut butter and a large handful of raisins, and you'll not only have a delicious afternoon snack, but you'll make your joint-saving quota of boron at the same time.

**Helps you breathe deeply.** Your lungs are assaulted every day by cigarette smoke, air pollution, pollen, and other air-borne nasties.

On top of that perhaps you suffer from asthma, emphysema, or similar lung condition. If all you want to do is take a deep breath, then grab an apple.

A five-year study of more than 2,500 men from Wales found those who ate five or more apples per week were able to fill their lungs with more air than men who didn't eat apples. Experts believe you might be getting some special protection from the antioxidant quercetin. Unfortunately, eating apples can't reverse a lung condition you already have, but you just might add a new line of defense against further damage.

## Pantry pointers

Buy apples that are unbruised, firm, and have good color. Take them out of their plastic bag and store them in your refrigerator — loose in the produce bin or in a paper bag is best. And since they will absorb odors, keep them away from strong-smelling foods like garlic and onions.

### A word of caution

Before you take home a jug of cider from that orchard or roadside stand, listen to this. Unpasteurized apple juice or cider could contain harmful *E. coli* bacteria. You may think you're buying something natural and wholesome, but in this case modern processing means a healthier product.

On the other hand, try to buy organically grown apples — ones produced without chemicals. Since apple growers aren't required by law to tell you what they've sprayed on their fruit, you could be getting more than you bargained for. Some apples will still carry high amounts of pesticides that are especially harmful to children. If you can't find organically grown apples, either scrub your produce well or sacrifice that fiber-rich peel before eating.

# Apricots

• • • • • • • • • • • • • • •

**Benefits**

Combats cancer

Controls blood
pressure

Saves your eyesight

Slows aging process

Shields against
Alzheimer's

Alexander the Great fell in love with this surprisingly sweet fruit in Asia, where he found them growing wild. When he returned to Europe from his military expeditions, he brought some with him.

The ancient Romans gave the apricot its name — from the Latin word for "precocious" — because the apricot is the first fruit of the season to ripen. The name stuck, and the apricot spread all over, from Europe, to America, and all the way to Australia.

The apricot is a fantastic fruit — loaded with beta carotene, iron, fiber, vitamin C, and several B vitamins. If you dry an apricot, its nutrients get more concentrated, making dried apricots a great snack.

Whether fresh or dried, eating apricots will help you fight the effects of aging, protect your eyesight, ward off cancer, and prevent heart disease.

## 4 ways apricots keep you healthy

**Combats cancer.** If you get indigestion from eating tomato products — the prime source of lycopene — here's great news for you. Apricots, especially dried ones, are another source of lycopene, the amazing carotenoid that can help prevent prostate, breast, and several other cancers. Though apricots aren't nearly as good a source of lycopene — about 30 dried ones have the same amount as one tomato — munching on them throughout the day can boost your lycopene quicker than you think.

Apricots are also a good source of the most famous carotenoid of them all — beta carotene. This powerful antioxidant reduces your risk of some types of stomach and intestinal cancers. To get these benefits, experts suggest getting at least 5 milligrams of beta carotene each day. That's equal to about six fresh apricots.

**Halts heart disease.** Eating dried apricots as a snack can punch up your levels of iron, potassium, beta carotene, magnesium, and copper. These important nutrients help control your blood pressure and prevent heart disease. Plus, as few as five dried apricots can give you up to 3 grams of fiber, which sweeps cholesterol out of your system before it has a chance to clog your arteries.

**Chases away cataracts.** What you eat can affect your vision. Dr. Robert G. Cumming, the lead researcher for the Blue Mountains Eye Study, says, "Our study confirms the importance of vitamin A for cataract prevention." Cumming adds, "Our overall conclusion is that a well-balanced diet is needed for eye health."

Since apricots are a good source of beta carotene, which your body converts to vitamin A, and several other nutrients, they could be just what you're looking for.

**Adds to a long life.** Believe it or not, some people claim apricots are the secret to living to age 120. They get this idea from the Hunzas, a tribe living in the Himalayan Mountains of Asia. Common health problems, like cancer, heart disease, high blood pressure, and high cholesterol, do not exist in Hunza. And researchers are wondering if apricots, a main part of their diet, are partly responsible. The Hunzas eat fresh apricots in season and dry the rest to eat during their long, cold winter.

### A word of caution

Many dried apricots are preserved with sulfites. Though these preservatives don't affect most people, they can bring on a life-threatening allergic reaction in some asthma sufferers.

If you have asthma, watch out for sulfite warnings on packages of dried apricots. It's best to play it safe — buy the untreated kind or stick with fresh apricots.

Although eating apricots can't guarantee you'll live a long life, recent research suggests the little fruit may help you live a better life. The B vitamins in dried apricots may protect you from Alzheimer's and age-related mental problems, like memory loss.

## Pantry pointers

From June to August, the finest fresh apricots roll into your super-market from California and Washington state. Keep your eyes peeled for the tastiest of the bunch. They'll wear a beautiful, bright orange skin, and they'll look and feel plump. Avoid apricots with yellowish or greenish tinges and those that are hard, shrunken, or bruised.

Just like their cousin the peach, apricots can ripen on your kitchen counter at room temperature. When they feel and smell ripe, wrap them in a paper bag and store them in your refrigerator. They'll stay fresh for several days.

During the winter months, satisfy your apricot craving with fruits imported from South America, or enjoy canned apricots, jams, spreads, and nectars.

# Artichokes

● ● ● ● ● ● ● ● ● ● ● ● ● ● ● ● ● ● ●

| Benefits |
| --- |
| Aids digestion |
| Lowers cholesterol |
| Stabilizes blood sugar |
| Protects your heart |
| Guards against liver disease |

Artichokes have been around for a long time. Originally found around the Mediterranean Sea, they were used by the ancient Romans to treat poor digestion. Somewhere along the line, the Romans realized artichokes also made great appetizers, and they have been a traditional Italian food ever since.

The Latin name for this greenish-purple vegetable is *Cynara scolymus*. Sometimes called French or Globe artichoke, it's the flower of the plant that is sold in grocery stores. But don't confuse it with the Jerusalem artichoke, which is really a tuber that grows in North America.

One medium artichoke supplies 20 percent of the vitamin C you need for the day. With only 60 calories, it's also a good source of potassium and magnesium, both important for a healthy heart. And like most fruits and vegetables, it's packed with disease-fighting antioxidants that nutritionists rave about.

## 3 ways artichokes keep you healthy

**Steps up digestion.** As it turns out, the ancient Romans were onto something when it comes to artichokes and digestion. An ingredient in artichoke leaves helps your liver form bile — something necessary for good digestion. If your liver doesn't produce enough bile, your food doesn't get broken down properly, and you end up with stomach pains and indigestion.

If you feel sick to your stomach, overly full, and have abdominal pain after eating a normal-sized meal, you may suffer from dyspepsia — a fancy name for poor digestion.

Several scientific studies showed dramatic improvements in people with dyspepsia after being treated with artichoke extracts. You can also get help for your indigestion the way the ancient Romans did — by eating a delicious artichoke with your dinner.

**Chokes out heart disease.** Bile from your liver does more than help you digest food. It also helps break down cholesterol from the fat you eat. But a liver that doesn't produce enough bile lets too much cholesterol get by — kind of like the *I Love Lucy* episode where the chocolate assembly line starts moving too fast for her to keep up. People with liver problems can have high cholesterol even if they eat a low-fat diet.

That's where artichokes come in. Because they can help you make more bile, you might be able to lower your cholesterol by eating them. A study in Germany showed that taking artichoke extract for six weeks caused LDL cholesterol, the bad kind, to fall by more than 22 percent. As a bonus, artichokes might also be able to block some new cholesterol from forming in your liver.

**Lowers blood sugar.** Your liver is busier than you might think. In addition to breaking down fatty foods, it also stores extra glucose (sugar) in the form of glycogen and turns it back into glucose whenever it gets a phone call from your blood saying that supplies are too low. This is a great system in a perfectly working body. But some people have faulty phone lines, and their livers work day and night cranking out glucose their blood doesn't need. This overproduction of glucose can lead to diabetes and other health problems.

In animal studies, researchers found that substances in artichokes kept livers from making too much glucose. More studies need to be done, but scientists think artichokes might someday be useful to people with noninsulin-dependent diabetes. In the future, people might use plants, like artichokes, to keep their blood sugar production in check.

## Pantry pointers

Choose artichokes with even, green color. Don't buy any that look wilted, dried out, or moldy. Heavy, small heads are best.

Small artichokes are good for appetizers, and larger ones can be used for stuffing with a variety of fillings and served as an entree.

### A word of caution

Artichokes can cause skin rashes in some people. Although it's rare, a few people will develop a rash on their hands after touching artichokes. If this happens to you, don't worry. The rash should clear up in a few days, but you should probably avoid artichokes in the future.

Be sure to trim about an inch off the top with a sharp knife. And then trim about one-quarter inch from the tips of the leaves since this part is inedible and rough on your hands.

Artichokes can be steamed in a steamer basket or boiled in water. They should be tender and ready to eat in about 30 minutes. If you're in a hurry, you can microwave them more quickly. First, rinse them with water to add some moisture. Then wrap each one in microwave-able plastic wrap. For four artichokes, microwave on high for 10 to 15 minutes or until the meaty part at the base of the artichoke is tender.

You can serve these veggies hot or cold. Some people serve a dipping sauce with artichokes. It would be a shame to ruin a low-fat food with a rich sauce, so try a low-calorie, yogurt-based dip.

If you've never eaten an artichoke, you might be a little confused about what part is edible. The outer leaves are hard and a little bitter, but at the bottom of the leaf, where they pull away from the stem, there is a soft, velvety hunk of "meat" that you can eat by gently pulling the leaf through your teeth. After you've nibbled all the leaves this way, you're left with the best part of the artichoke — the heart. This is a soft, nutty-flavored center that can be eaten whole. Just scrape off the soft fuzz with a spoon before you dig in.

| Eat | |
| --- | --- |
| Oranges | Broccoli |
| Brussels | Wheat germ |
| sprouts | Almonds |
| Cottage | Tomatoes |
| cheese | Avocados |
| Oysters | Beans |
| Coffee | Water |

**Avoid**

Specific foods that trigger your asthma attacks

# Asthma

• • • • • • • • • • • • •

Asthma is often misdiagnosed in older adults because of the common belief that it is just a childhood disease. But according to the American Lung Association, experts now think about 10 percent of the people with asthma are over age 65.

Some adults with asthma have dealt with the disease all their lives. Others may have had asthma as a child and experienced it again after many symptom-free years. But if you've developed breathing problems as an adult, you have lots of company. Late-onset asthma is becoming more common and is often triggered by a serious respiratory infection.

Women are more likely to be affected than men, possibly because of their smaller airways. Researchers think hormones may also play a part. They've found that women who are on hormone replacement therapy (HRT) are 50 percent more likely to develop asthma than women who aren't on HRT.

Although asthma is a serious and potentially fatal disease, you can protect yourself by avoiding things that trigger an attack. Cigarette smoke, cold air, dust, and mold are a few examples of asthma triggers. And research shows that eating foods rich in certain nutrients may help reduce your asthma symptoms.

## Nutritional blockbusters that fight asthma

**Vitamin C.** Researchers say antioxidant vitamins could play an important role in preventing asthma or controlling its symptoms. Vitamin C is the perfect example. Studies have found that vitamin C not only improves asthma symptoms, it helps you avoid the disease altogether. For top-notch asthma protection, mix up a fruit salad with oranges, pineapple, strawberries, kiwifruit, and papaya. Then pile your dinner plate with high-C vegetables like broccoli, red and green peppers, brussels sprouts, cabbage, and peas.

**Vitamin E.** Another antioxidant powerhouse that may cut your risk of asthma is vitamin E. A study in Saudi Arabia found that children who had the least vitamin E in their diets were three times more likely to get asthma. Research also shows that vitamin E helps protect you from developing this condition as an adult. For extra lung protection, sprinkle some vitamin E-packed wheat germ, almonds, peanuts, or sunflower seeds on a salad or in baked goods.

**Vitamin A.** This vitamin completes the asthma-fighting trio of antioxidants. Studies find that people who eat vitamin A-rich foods tend to have clearer air passages, which makes breathing easier. You'll find vitamin A in meat and dairy products, especially beef and chicken livers, cottage cheese, ricotta cheese, and egg yolks.

**Lycopene.** Think pink — or red — to help avoid asthma symptoms. Lycopene, the carotenoid that gives foods their pink or red coloring, may protect against asthma, according to a recent small study. Researchers gave people with exercise-induced asthma 30 milligrams of lycopene each day for one week. At the end of the week, more than half the people showed significant protection against asthma symptoms.

It's always best to get your nutrients from foods, and in this case, it could earn you double protection. Many foods that contain lycopene, such as tomatoes, pink grapefruit, and watermelon, are also high in vitamin C.

**Magnesium and selenium.** These minerals may be the dynamic duo of asthma-fighting minerals. Magnesium acts as a bronchodilator, which means it helps open up your airways, making it easier to breathe. Selenium's power against asthma may come from its antioxidant abilities. Studies show that people with low levels of selenium are more likely to have asthma. You'll find selenium in meats and shellfish and in vegetables and grains grown in selenium-rich soil. Food sources of magnesium include avocados, oysters, and beans. Broccoli is a good source of both minerals.

**Water.** A tall glass of water could be your ally if you're asthmatic. Researchers at the University at Buffalo (UB) discovered that the symptoms of people with exercise-induced asthma got worse, both before and during exercise, when they didn't drink enough water.

Frank Cerny, Ph.D., stresses the importance of drinking water, especially if you have asthma. "The message continues to be, 'Drink fluids whenever you get the chance,'" says Cerny, chairman of the UB Department of Physical Therapy, Exercise, and Nutrition Sciences. "If you have asthma, dehydration may make it worse, particularly during exercise."

---

> **A word of caution**
>
> An important step in controlling your asthma is identifying and avoiding your triggers. While good nutrition may ease your symptoms, eating the wrong food can set off an attack. Almost any food can be an asthma trigger, but the most common ones are eggs, peanuts, milk, wheat, soy, and citrus fruits.

Your body needs water long before you feel thirst so don't wait until you're thirsty to wet your whistle. Make sure you drink at least six full glasses of water every day — more when you exercise.

**Caffeine.** Start your morning with a fragrant cup of coffee, and you may ease your asthma. Caffeine is chemically related to theophylline, a drug used to treat asthma. When you have an asthma attack, the muscles around your airways tighten up and your passages swell, making it difficult to breathe. Caffeine helps relax your bronchial tubes so your airways stay open. Research shows that caffeine can help improve symptoms for up to four hours.

# Atherosclerosis
• • • • • • • • • • • • • • • • • • • • • • •

| Eat | |
| --- | --- |
| Salmon | Tuna |
| Flaxseed | Garlic |
| Tea | Carrots |
| Sweet | Olive oil |
| potatoes | Wheat germ |
| **Avoid** | |
| Foods high in saturated fat, such as red meat and whole-milk dairy products | |

Imagine hundreds of cars zooming down an eight-lane highway. One lane disappears, and then another, until the same cars crawl bumper-to-bumper along a one-lane country road.

That's sort of what happens when you have atherosclerosis. Your arteries, the highways for your blood, harden and narrow, and the same amount of blood has to make its way through a much tighter space. This traffic jam in your arteries leads to all sorts of trouble, including heart attack and stroke.

Atherosclerosis occurs when cholesterol, fat, and other substances in your blood build up in the walls of your arteries. The process can begin when you're a child, but it may not become a problem until you're in your 50s or 60s. As this muck gathers in your arteries, it forms plaque. Plaque can clog or completely block arteries, cutting off blood flow to your heart or brain. That's when you have a heart attack or stroke.

Too much cholesterol and triglycerides — types of fat — in the blood, high blood pressure, and smoking cause the most damage to your arteries. Other risk factors for atherosclerosis include diabetes, a family history of the condition, stress, obesity, and an inactive lifestyle. Men, in general, are at greater risk, as are people who have an "apple" body shape — with the fat gathering at the belly rather than the hips and thighs.

You can fight atherosclerosis by making good food choices. Cut back on saturated fat and cholesterol from meat and whole-milk dairy products, and look for the following foods that lower cholesterol, bring down blood pressure, and keep your blood flowing smoothly.

## Nutritional blockbusters that fight atherosclerosis

**Fish.** Reel in a big, fat fish and wriggle off the hook of atherosclerosis. Omega-3 fatty acids, the polyunsaturated kinds found in fatty fish like tuna, mackerel, and salmon, protect your arteries from damage.

First, omega-3 takes out triglycerides, the fats that build up on your artery walls. It also stops your blood's platelets from clumping together. That way, your blood remains smooth instead of sticky. Sticky blood can clot and block blood flow. Lastly, omega-3 might lower blood pressure.

No wonder so many studies show that eating fish can reduce your risk of heart disease. The American Heart Association recommends eating at least two fish meals a week.

You can find a form of omega-3 called alpha-linolenic acid in walnuts, which lower cholesterol. Other sources of omega-3 include flaxseed, wheat germ, and some green, leafy vegetables, like kale, spinach, and arugula.

**Garlic.** Anything fish can do garlic does, too. The sulfur compounds in this amazing herb not only lower cholesterol and triglycerides, but they also go after only the LDL or "bad" cholesterol and leave the HDL or "good" cholesterol alone.

Garlic can also lower blood pressure so your arteries don't take as much of a pounding. Thanks to a substance called ajoene, garlic keeps your blood from clumping and clotting. One study even showed garlic helps your aorta, the body's main artery, remain elastic as you age.

Experts recommend getting 4 grams of garlic — about one clove — into your diet each day.

**Fiber.** During the course of a day, you should eat about 25 to 35 grams of fiber. If you do, you'll boost your general health and give atherosclerosis quite a battle.

Certain types of soluble fiber, such as the kind in oats, barley, apples, and other fruits, shrink your cholesterol levels. It works by slowing down your food as it passes through your stomach and small intestine so your "good" cholesterol has more time to take cholesterol to your liver and out of your body. Eating more than 25 grams of fiber every day might also cut your risk of developing high blood pressure by 25 percent.

Fiber comes with an added bonus — it fills you up. After a fiber-rich meal, you feel full, so you're less likely to overeat and put on unwanted pounds. Because being overweight increases your risk of atherosclerosis and other heart problems, eating fiber could be part of an effective strategy to guard your arteries.

You'll find fiber in fruits, vegetables, and whole-grain breads and cereals.

**Antioxidants.** An unarmed intruder poses less of a threat than one with a weapon. By stopping free radicals from oxidizing LDL cholesterol, antioxidants remove much of the danger. Once oxidized, LDL cholesterol makes a beeline for your artery walls much faster. In fact, some scientists believe LDL cholesterol only harms you once it has been oxidized.

Vitamin C, vitamin E, and beta carotene are antioxidants. Peppers, oranges, strawberries, cantaloupe, and broccoli give you vitamin C, while carrots, sweet potatoes, spinach, mangoes, and collard greens are full of beta carotene. Sources of vitamin E include wheat germ, nuts, seeds, and vegetable oils.

While you munch on those fruits and vegetables, you'll get the added benefit of antioxidant substances called flavonoids. Resveratrol in grapes, anthocyanins in cranberry juice, and quercetin in onions, apples, and tea are some of the flavonoids that help your heart and arteries.

> ### Mine these minerals for better circulation
>
> High blood pressure and atherosclerosis go hand in hand. When you have high blood pressure, the force of your blood against your artery walls causes damage that contributes to atherosclerosis. And when you have atherosclerosis, your heart has to work harder to pump blood through your arteries, leading to high blood pressure.
>
> So, if you're worried about atherosclerosis, start thinking about your blood pressure. Make sure to get plenty of potassium, magnesium, and calcium — minerals that may lower blood pressure. A diet rich in fruits, vegetables, whole grains, and low-fat dairy products should give you plenty of these minerals. Also, if you are salt sensitive, cut back on salt — or sodium — which could raise your blood pressure.

**Monounsaturated fat.** To keep your blood running smoothly, maybe you need an oil change. Olive oil, the main source of fat in the heart-healthy Mediterranean diet, has mostly monounsaturated fat. This type of fat slashes the "bad" cholesterol without harming the "good" cholesterol. It also prevents clotting, giving your arteries even more protection.

Like fiber, monounsaturated fat also fills you up so you're less likely to overeat.

Think about switching from soybean or corn oil to olive oil. After all, the Greeks — even while enjoying a rather high-fat diet — rarely develop atherosclerosis.

Besides olive oil, sources of monounsaturated fat include avocados, nuts, and canola oil.

**Ginger.** Make your dinner a little bit tastier and your arteries a little bit healthier with this ancient spice. Ginger contains phytochemicals called gingerol and shogaol, which give it its antioxidant power.

Animal studies show ginger not only lowers LDL cholesterol and triglycerides, it also prevents LDL oxidation. On top of that, ginger also keeps your blood from clotting by reducing the stickiness of your platelets.

# Avocados

. . . . . . . . . . . . . . . . .

According to legend, a Mayan princess ate the first avocado in 291 B.C. Fortunately, you don't have to be royalty to reap the rewards of this tasty tropical fruit.

**Benefits**

Lowers cholesterol

Controls blood pressure

Helps stop strokes

Battles diabetes

Combats cancer

Smoothes skin

Avocados, nicknamed "alligator pears" because of their bumpy exteriors, come in several varieties. Some have a green covering. Others are dark purple or almost black. Some are smooth, while others are bumpy. Some are small, and others weigh as much as 4 pounds. Yet, when you slice them open, they all have the same delicious light green, nutty-flavored flesh inside.

The avocado got its name from the ancient Aztec word for "testicle." Maybe that's why men once thought eating avocados would boost their virility.

In earlier times, avocado pulp was used as a hair pomade to stimulate hair growth and to help heal wounds. Native Americans treated dysentery and diarrhea with its seeds. Even today, its oil can be found in many cosmetics.

But the avocado probably should have been named after the Aztec word for "heart," considering how it can help this vital organ. Loaded with monounsaturated fat, potassium, fiber, and antioxidants, the avocado fights high cholesterol, high blood pressure, heart disease, and stroke.

But that's not all. The "alligator pear" also snaps its mighty jaws at diabetes and cancer.

## 6 ways avocados keep you healthy

**Crushes cholesterol.** The avocado is high in fat — 30 grams per fruit, but it's mostly monounsaturated fat. This fat helps protect good HDL cholesterol, while wiping out the bad LDL cholesterol that clogs your arteries. That means you not only lower your bad cholesterol, you also improve your ratio of good HDL to total cholesterol.

But there's more than just monounsaturated fat at work. An avocado contains 10 grams of fiber, as well as a plant chemical called beta-sitosterol. These both help lower cholesterol. Throw in vitamins C and E — powerful antioxidants that prevent dangerous free radicals from reacting with the cholesterol in your blood — and it all adds up to a healthier you.

In fact, one study from Australia demonstrated how eating half to one-and-a-half avocados a day for three weeks could lower your total cholesterol by more than 8 percent without lowering your HDL cholesterol.

During the same study, a low-fat, high-carbohydrate diet also lowered the participants' total cholesterol — but slashed the "good" cholesterol by almost 14 percent.

**Bashes high blood pressure.** You've probably heard that bananas are a good source of potassium. What you probably don't know is that avocados, with over 1,200 milligrams of potassium per fruit, contain more than two-and-a-half times as much potassium as a banana. This is important because many studies show that potassium helps lower your blood pressure.

Magnesium, another important mineral found in avocados, could help lower your blood pressure, too. Some researchers think magnesium relaxes blood vessels and allows them to open wider. This gives blood more room to flow freely, reducing blood pressure. But results have been mixed. Some studies show magnesium lowers blood pressure, while others show no effect.

**Strikes out stroke.** When it comes to taking on a deadly killer like stroke, who wants to fight fair? Gang up on stroke with avocado's three heavy hitters — potassium, magnesium, and fiber.

In the Health Professionals Follow-Up Study, which included more than 43,000 men, researchers found that the men who got the most potassium in their diet were 38 percent less likely to have a stroke as those who got the least. Results were lower for fiber (30 percent) and magnesium (30 percent).

**Hammers heart disease.** By controlling your cholesterol and blood pressure, avocados can help reduce your risk of heart disease.

But avocados offer more protection. If you increase your daily fiber intake by 10 grams, the amount in one avocado, you decrease your risk of heart disease by 19 percent. Vitamin C, potassium, and folate, part of the B-vitamin family, have also been linked to a reduced risk of heart disease.

Folate also helps your heart by keeping homocysteine from building up to dangerous levels. Homocysteine, a by-product of protein metabolism, can harm your arteries and increase your chances of a heart attack or stroke.

According to the California Avocado Commission, avocados have more folate per ounce than any other fruit.

**Defends against diabetes.** If you have diabetes, you're probably looking for ways to replace the saturated fat in your diet with more carbohydrates.

Instead, consider substituting some of those carbohydrates with monounsaturated fat, the kind you get from avocados. Not only do avocados lower your LDL cholesterol without lowering HDL cholesterol, they also can reduce the amount of triglycerides, another type of fat, in your blood. A high triglyceride level can be a warning sign of heart disease.

Eating high-fiber foods, like avocados, can benefit people with type 2 diabetes in several ways. One study published in *The New England Journal of Medicine* found that a high-fiber diet (50 grams per day) lowered cholesterol, triglyceride, glucose, and insulin levels.

Avocados have earned the backing of the American Diabetes Association, which has included avocados in its collection of suggested recipes.

> ### Treat yourself to an avocado facial
>
> Beauty, they say, is only skin deep. Luckily, avocado has moisturizing power to help make your skin more beautiful.
>
> For years, people have used avocado as a natural facial treatment, especially for dry skin. It's easy to do in your own home. Just remove your makeup and wash your face with warm water and soap or your favorite cleanser. Mash some avocado and mix it with a little milk or oatmeal and apply it to your face. Leave it there for 10 minutes, then rinse it off with lots of water.
>
> If you have dry skin, or just want to pamper yourself, reach for an avocado — the bumpy fruit that smooths your skin.

**Curbs cancer.** Another reason to eat a lot of fiber is its possible protective effect against certain cancers, particularly colon and breast cancer.

Researchers looking at data from The Seven Countries Study recently concluded that adding 10 grams of fiber to your daily diet could cut your risk of dying from colon cancer by 33 percent over 25 years.

Although a few studies have found fiber ineffective in preventing cancer, many experts still recommend eating plenty of high-fiber foods.

Avocado's arsenal of powerful antioxidants — glutathione and vitamin C — also help fight cancer by neutralizing harmful free radicals that can damage your cells. Glutathione may ward off oral and throat cancers, and vitamin C has been linked to lower rates of oral, breast, lung, stomach, and cervical cancers.

And don't forget about beta-sitosterol and folate. They may protect you from colon and breast cancer, too.

## Pantry pointers

Ripe avocados should be soft enough to "give way" to gentle pressure. If you can't find a ripe avocado in the store, choose a heavy, unblemished one and let it ripen in a paper bag for a few days at room temperature.

To get at the good stuff, cut an avocado lengthways around the seed and rotate the halves to separate. Using a spoon, remove the seed, then scoop out the flesh.

When exposed to air, an avocado discolors quickly, so use it as soon as possible. Squeezing lemon or lime juice on the cut avocado will help prevent discoloration.

Karen Duester, a spokesperson for The Food Consulting Company in Del Mar, Calif., says, "The avocado provides more of several nutrients than 20 of the most commonly eaten fruits. Including avocado in an otherwise healthful diet can be considered a healthy and tasty way to add variety to your meals."

If you'd like to take advantage of this nutritional powerhouse, try Duester's healthy suggestions:

◆ Mash the soft fruit and mix with salsa.

◆ Float avocado cubes in a bowl of hot tomato soup.

◆ Spread avocado with jam on a bagel.

◆ Toast a tortilla-wrapped avocado wedge.

◆ Mash potatoes with a peeled and seeded avocado.

◆ Crown crackers with chunks of avocado.

◆ Fill egg white halves with guacamole for a new twist on deviled eggs.

You can also add avocado slices to salads or sandwiches or just eat the fruit plain. For a healthy alternative to mayonnaise, butter, or cream cheese, try mashed avocado.

### Benefits

Protects your heart

Controls blood
  pressure

Strengthens bones

Blocks diarrhea

Quiets a cough

# Bananas

● ● ● ● ● ● ● ● ● ● ● ● ● ● ●

Before you peel that banana, take a moment to appreciate all its wonderfully healthy qualities. Each one is full of potassium, folate, and vitamin B6 for your heart and bones, and vitamins A and C for antioxidant protection. It's packed with fiber for regularity and melatonin for adjusting your internal clock. In fact, bananas are one of the foods selected to display the American Heart Association's stamp of approval — meaning they meet the AHA's standard for saturated fat and cholesterol.

Bananas are most likely the cheapest fruit in your grocery store and come in an astounding 500 varieties. You might run across the Cuban Red, Ice Cream, Lady Finger, Horse or actually an Apple banana. Botanists believe the banana is originally from Asia and probably had seeds at one time. But somewhere along the line a seedless variety sprang up, much to the delight of monkeys and humans everywhere.

What you've got is an inexpensive, wholesome fruit that comes in its own germ-proof package. With only 100 calories each, bananas are one food you can eat without guilt.

## 5 ways bananas keep you healthy

**Hits heart disease hard**. The next time you see your doctor, check the homocysteine levels in your blood. If they're high, you're at risk for heart disease. While this might be a hereditary condition, you could also be vitamin deficient. It's easy enough to cut your homocysteine and reduce your chances of developing heart disease by getting extra folate.

Eat a banana and you've just gotten 22 micrograms of this important nutrient. Of course you'd have to eat more than a bunch to get enough folate solely from bananas. But by simply making them part of a well-rounded diet, you could give heart disease the heave-ho.

**Bottoms out blood pressure.** If you have heart disease, chances are you're limiting salt and fat to keep your blood pressure down. But that's only half the story. You may be able to send those bp numbers into a nose-dive by eating plenty of fruits and vegetables. It's the calcium in green leafy vegetables and the potassium in fruits like bananas that seem to make the difference.

Frank M. Sacks, M.D., professor of nutrition at Harvard School of Public Health, thinks the potassium connection is important. "Individuals should eat more fruits such as bananas, oranges, and green leafy vegetables to help prevent high blood pressure," he says. "If you already have high blood pressure, then you should eat a diet high in potassium or take supplements." Most experts will tell you, however, to talk to your own doctor before you begin taking any supplements.

**Builds better bones.** You might not think a soft, curved fruit could keep your bones straight and strong. But bananas can do just that thanks to their high potassium content — a mineral your body needs in order to absorb calcium.

Here's how it works. Calcium needs potassium, just like Fred Astaire needed Ginger Rogers. If you don't have enough potassium, calcium gets lonely and leaves the dance floor. Even if you're drinking plenty of milk and eating lots of dairy products, without enough potassium, you might not be getting all the calcium you need.

Researchers have found that elderly men and women who get lots of potassium — on average 3,000 milligrams a day — have higher bone mineral density, a measure of bone strength. This means they are less likely to develop osteoporosis, a disease that makes healthy bones look like Swiss cheese. If you can get about five servings of potassium-rich foods every day, you'll be well on your way to stronger bones. Eat potatoes, milk, orange juice, and bananas and let the dance begin.

---

### Pick a peck of plantains

For another healthy treat, try out banana's exotic relative, the plantain. This large, reddish-brown fruit looks like a banana, but claims to treat and even prevent ulcers.

In animal studies, plantains caused the stomach lining to grow. It thickened, actually preventing new ulcers from forming, and covered over existing ulcers, allowing them to heal — kind of like putting salve on a cut.

You can buy plantains at most grocery stores, but don't eat them like a banana — they have to be cooked. They'll turn dark in about three or four days and that means they're ready to prepare. Many people fry plantains in oil, but why ruin a fat-free food? Try boiling, baking, or mashing them like potatoes.

**Combats diarrhea.** When you suffer from diarrhea, your body loses vital fluids and minerals. If you become weak and dizzy, it's a sign you've lost enough to become dehydrated. Severe diarrhea can even affect your heart. Simply drinking a couple glasses of water, however, won't get your system back to normal — you need something more. According to the American College of Gastroenterology, bananas are the perfect food after an attack of diarrhea. The potassium gets right to work helping control the balance of water in your cells.

**Quiets a cough.** If you have a cough that just won't quit and a burning sensation in your throat after meals, you may suffer from heartburn and acid reflux. For a soothing natural solution, eat a banana or take banana powder — a dried, ground form of the fruit you can find in health food stores.

## Pantry pointers

Buy your bananas green since some growers in South America use chemicals to help ripen the fruit. Just keep them on the counter for a few days until they're a happy shade of yellow.

---

### A word of caution

If you have kidney disease, your doctor may have told you not to eat too many bananas. Some people with damaged kidneys develop a condition called hyperkalemia — too much potassium in your blood. Potassium build-up is serious and can cause weakness and paralysis and can lead to heart failure.

| Benefits |
| --- |
| Lowers cholesterol |
| Controls blood pressure |
| Combats cancer |
| Battles diabetes |
| Prevents constipation |

# Barley

● ● ● ● ● ● ● ● ● ● ●

What do Spartacus and Budweiser have in common? Barley — the hearty grain that gladiators ate to give them strength and that breweries use to make beer.

Barley's popularity and status as a health food goes back thousands of years. Greeks cultivated it as long ago as 7000 B.C., and ancient Chinese, Egyptians, and Romans made it an important part of their diet. People also used barley to treat boils, stomach disorders, and urinary tract infections.

Today, barley crops up mostly in soups, cereal, beer, and animal feed. But its ability to fight heart disease, cancer, and diabetes should earn it a more prominent place in your diet. After all, barley practically overflows with fiber and contains key minerals like potassium, phosphorus, magnesium, and iron.

Loading up on soups and cereal made with barley isn't the only way to get more of this great grain. Next time you're baking, try sifting some barley flour into the mixing bowl. Or add some barley to your rice to create a more fiber-rich meal.

Think of it as entering the arena to battle the enemies of good health.

## 5 ways barley keeps you healthy

**Conquers cholesterol.** Behind every healthy food, there's a healthy ingredient. In the case of barley, the behind-the-scenes dynamo is a form of soluble fiber called beta-glucan. Powered by beta-glucan, barley has shown time and time again it can lower

70

cholesterol. And remember, when you cut artery-clogging cholesterol, you also cut your risk of heart disease. Even in forms as various as barley flour, oil, muesli, or pasta, the results are the same.

As food travels through your body, low-density lipoprotein
(LDL) particles carry cholesterol to cells, where it can do damage.
High-density lipoprotein (HDL) particles pick up the cholesterol
and whisk it to your liver, which converts it to bile and gets rid of
it. This process is called "reverse cholesterol transport."

Dr. Barbara Schneeman, a researcher with the USDA's
Agricultural Research Service and professor of agricultural and environmental sciences at the University of California-Davis, believes
barley affects cholesterol levels through its viscosity, or stickiness.

Because beta-glucan is sticky, it slows down the movement of
food through your stomach and small intestine. That gives the
HDL particles more time to pick up cholesterol, reducing the
chances it will be absorbed later. "It's slowing lipid absorption and
giving more time for reverse cholesterol transport to happen,"
Schneeman explains.

**Balances out blood pressure.** This healthy grain contains
potassium, a mineral that keeps your blood pressure in control.
Along with fiber and magnesium — also in barley — potassium
may lower your chance of stroke. In fact, the Food and Drug
Administration (FDA) recently decided to allow foods meeting
specific requirements for potassium, sodium, fat, and cholesterol
to advertise they reduce the risk of high blood pressure and stroke.
You may see a claim like this on your next package of barley.

**Manages weight.** Obesity seriously raises your risk for a variety of health problems, including heart disease. But the fiber in
barley can help you lose weight. Here's how.

A certain hormone in your gut, cholecystokinin (CCK), is associated with feelings of fullness. When people eat a low-fat diet,
their CCK levels go up, then back down to normal, or fasting,
level. When they eat barley, their CCK still goes up after the meal,
but it never makes it all the way back down to fasting level. That

means you'll probably feel more full after a barley meal. And if you feel full, you're less likely to overeat and put on unwanted pounds.

"Fiber intake doesn't cause weight loss. Energy restriction causes weight loss," Schneeman stresses. "The challenge for most people is to stay in control between meals. If something like fiber promotes a little bit of a feeling of fullness, it can help in that phase."

**Curbs colon cancer.** When it comes to roller-coasters, bigger and faster means better. If you want to protect yourself against colon cancer, start thinking this way about your stool.

It's the fiber in barley that may give you this protection. It adds bulk to your stool and hurries it through your large intestine. In fact, a study headed by Dr. Joanne Lupton of Texas A&M University showed that eating barley bran flour increased stool weight by almost 50 grams and slashed transit time by 8 hours.

Don't get confused, however. Barley does slow food down in your stomach and small intestine — which helps out with cholesterol levels. But foods normally spend 10 times longer in your large intestine, which absorbs cancer-causing agents. That means a bulkier, faster-moving stool is less likely to hang around and cause trouble.

Barley might also battle colon cancer by changing the tiny organisms in your large bowel. When these organisms react with beta-glucan, they might produce compounds that protect your colon tissue.

---

### Few cheers for beers

If you're looking to reap the benefits of barley by drinking beer, look elsewhere. It's true breweries use barley, but they remove most of the beta-glucan so the sticky stuff doesn't gum up the machines. Therefore, you're not going to get fiber from a frosty mug.

You might gain some health benefits, though. One recent study in the British Medical Journal states that men who drink a moderate amount of beer daily are less likely to have a heart attack than those who never drink. However, the heart attack odds skyrocketed if they drink twice a day or more.

Bottom line: If you don't drink beer, it's not worth taking up the habit. But if you already drink, limit yourself to about one beer a day.

"Take any one of these proposed mechanisms," Schneeman says. "By itself, it's not enough to prove a relation between fiber and cancer. It could be, in fact, multiple factors coming together. But you need this stuff for a healthy gut. Don't forget in trying to prevent disease, you're trying to keep your gut healthy as well."

**Defeats diabetes.** Because of barley's effect on cholesterol and other heart concerns, you might have guessed it would be a good food for diabetics. Experts specifically recommend a high-fiber diet with both soluble and cereal fiber. Barley fits the bill.

Schneeman again points to viscosity as a possible factor. Instead of glucose rushing through the blood, demanding insulin all at once, it oozes through at a snail's pace. This affects the demand for insulin by "slowing it down; spreading it out a bit," she says.

## Pantry pointers

Barley may be a great source of fiber, but not all forms have the same amount. With over 31 grams of fiber per cup, whole-grain barley offers you the most protection. Pearl barley, the most common form, is more refined — meaning some of the nutrients are removed. One cup of cooked pearl barley contains around 5 grams

### A word of caution

If you have celiac sprue disease, stay away from barley. Like most grains, barley contains gluten, a mixture of proteins that can damage the lining of your intestines. Beware, too, if you suffer from a gluten food allergy, in which case barley could cause cramps, diarrhea, and other problems.

New research also suggests that barley and other foods rich in lectins, a type of plant protein, could increase the risk for rheumatoid arthritis (RA) in people whose genes make them susceptible to this disease. The theory is the lectins spur your immune system to attack your body's own joints, leading to inflammation. If you already suffer from RA, try eliminating cereal grains like barley, oats, and wheat from your diet. Your symptoms may improve.

of fiber. That's almost one-fifth the amount experts say you need every day. Barley flour or meal, on the other hand, contain almost 15 grams of fiber per cup.

Other varieties include coarsely ground Scotch barley and barley grits. Like whole-grain barley, you'll find these in most health food stores.

| Benefits |
| --- |
| Prevents constipation |
| Helps hemorrhoids |
| Lowers cholesterol |
| Combats cancer |
| Preserves sexual function |
| Stabilizes blood sugar |

# Beans

· · · · · · · · · · ·

Beans, a well-known member of the legume family, are sometimes called the "poor man's meat" because they're a cheap way to get protein.

Besides being high in protein, they have almost no fat. And here's another great benefit — they are packed with fiber to keep you regular and to keep your cholesterol and blood sugar down. They even have lots of phytochemicals — antioxidants that can help prevent cancer.

Despite their star quality, many people shun beans. In fact, the more modern a country is, the less likely its people are to eat beans. Bean consumption is often directly related to income, with richer people eating less. And as you probably know from the rhyme you chanted as a child, legumes are famous for their ability to cause gas. Between their image as a food for poor people, and the gas issue, beans have a serious public relations problem.

But nutritionists are trying to get the word out that you can eat beans and have friends, too. You can easily reduce the amount of gas legumes produce by changing the water a few times while you're boiling them. Another alternative is to add a product called Beano to legumes after cooking. A few drops is all it takes to make them "wind free."

## 4 ways beans keep you healthy

**Conquers constipation and heals hemorrhoids.** Constipation is not only uncomfortable, it can cause hemorrhoids and diverticulosis, a weakening of the walls of the intestines caused by compact stools and straining. Eventually the weak walls form little pouches that can trap digested food and become infected. This can cause terrible pain and leave scar tissue that leads to even more constipation.

Hemorrhoids form when pressure causes your veins to stretch out of shape. Varicose veins are also linked to constipation, since straining to pass dry stools can put enough pressure on your leg veins to make them leak. In modern societies, all of these problems are common. Many people live with chronic constipation, never realizing that a change in diet could rid them of the problem for good.

But in parts of the world where people eat lots of plant food, like legumes, constipation and the diseases it causes are very rare. That's because the cell walls of plants can't be digested, which means lots of fiber to keep stools ready for a quick, painless exit. Adding a delicious meal of rice and beans or black bean soup to your weekly menu could help keep you far from constipation and the diseases it causes.

**Flushes out cholesterol.** Beans are good for your heart. If you eat them instead of a fatty meat, you've put a good dent in your daily glob of cholesterol. And they fill you up without lots of calories —

### Serve vitamin C with beans

Beans are a good source of iron, but the type of iron — nonheme — is not easily absorbed by people. Eating foods high in vitamin C, like citrus fruits, dark green leafy vegetables, and tomatoes, can help you absorb more of the iron. Plus, it's a great way to squeeze more fruits and vegetables into your diet.

only 225 calories in a one-cup serving. A study of healthy men showed that when they ate about two and a half cups of beans each day they ate significantly less fat and lowered their total cholesterol levels. Another study found that the more canned beans men with high cholesterol ate, the lower their cholesterol. And even though the men were eating as many calories as usual, they lost weight.

But the heart-smart work of beans doesn't stop there. The fiber in legumes is like a bouncer for some big, bad cholesterol particles. Some of these thugs get shown to the door before they can do any damage to your arteries or heart.

**Resurrects erections.** If you're a man who's been thinking about trying Viagra, you might want to give beans a try first. Beans contain a protein called L-arginine that can increase blood flow to your penis for better erections. In a recent, small study, 27 men who had erectile dysfunction for at least six months were given 5 grams of L-arginine daily — equal to about 5 cups of cooked beans. After six weeks, nearly a third of them were able to have erections again. You might not be able to eat five cups of beans each day, but why not add a few servings and see if you notice a difference.

### Black bean salad

1 15-ounce can black beans

1 15-ounce can corn

1/4 cup green pepper, chopped

3 green onions, chopped

1 teaspoon garlic, minced

3 tablespoons olive oil

1/4 cup balsamic vinegar

Drain and rinse beans and corn. Mix with other ingredients.

Chill for at least an hour. Makes 4 to 6 servings.

**Cuts your cancer risk.** What you eat could be a life or death decision. That's because diet is linked to more than 30 percent of cancers in North America. But diet is something you can control. Research shows that people who eat red meat can lower their risk of colon cancer by eating legumes three times a week or more. More research needs to be done, but scientists are focusing on substances in legumes called lignans and phytochemicals — natural cancer fighters.

Dr. Richard Rivlin of Memorial Sloan-Kettering Cancer Center in New York thinks that phytochemicals will be the key to preventing cancers in the future.

"The end-product of this research into phytochemicals will be powerful and precise tools for reducing incidence of cancer," said Rivlin at a conference in 1999. "Faced with an individual at risk for a specific kind of cancer, we will be able to prescribe specific foods and perhaps supplements that, consumed together, will significantly reduce that risk."

## Pantry pointers

Uncooked beans are easy to find at the grocery store and simple cooking directions are on the bag. Just remember to change the water you boil them in a few times. Canned beans are just as nutritious, and you only have to warm them up. But there is one drawback — the added salt. You can get rid of some salt by rinsing the beans in a colander before heating.

Try combining different types of beans for a cold salad. Black beans mix nicely with Great Northern and kidney beans. Add a low calorie vinaigrette dressing for a cool summer salad.

### A word of caution

Several varieties of beans, especially red kidney beans, are poisonous in their raw state. The beans contain phytohaemagglutinin, which is toxic to people and animals. But soaking beans in water for at least five hours and cooking them in fresh water for at least 10 minutes will destroy the toxins.

Beware of cooking beans in crockpots that don't get hot enough to boil water. Some beans are actually more toxic if they are heated to about 175 degrees, but not boiled.

Symptoms of poisoning include vomiting, diarrhea, and stomach pain within one to three hours after eating. Although most people recover within a day, some might need to be hospitalized to replace lost fluids.

| Benefits |
| --- |
| Combats cancer |
| Protects your heart |
| Controls blood pressure |
| Aids weight loss |
| Strengthens bones |

# Beets

• • • • • • • • • • •

The next time you're craving a sugary treat try beets. They have the highest sugar content of any vegetable. In fact, 40 percent of the world's refined sugar comes from beets. Yet, unlike sugary desserts, this brightly colored root is low in calories and high in nutrients.

Believe it or not, people from ancient Greece to Renaissance Italy tossed the beautiful beet root away. Instead, they only ate the beet's green leaves. It wasn't until the end of the 1700s that people started munching on the root and reaping the benefits.

Beets are loaded with potassium, magnesium, beta carotene, and folate, one of the B-vitamins. The most nutritious part of the plant — the leaves — are a good source of potassium, magnesium, calcium, folate, and beta carotene. These nutrients can help keep your heart healthy and your bones strong. They may even prevent cancer.

## 5 ways beets keep you healthy

**Halts cancer.** If you are a woman who drinks alcohol every day — even small amounts — you are more likely to get breast cancer. But, according to a recent study of almost 90,000 women, a high daily intake of folate (600 micrograms) may lower your risk. The women in the study who seemed to get the most benefit were those who drank only a little more than one alcoholic drink a day — like a large glass of wine or a mug of beer. The researchers say alcohol interferes with the transport and metabolism of folate. This means less folate reaches your body's tissues.

And don't forget the beta carotene. Several studies suggest that a diet rich in carotenoids, like beta carotene, may prevent lung cancer and prostate cancer.

**Heads off heart disease.** Folate is also known as a heart-healthy nutrient because it lowers the level of homocysteine in your blood. Homocysteine, a by-product of protein metabolism, can damage and narrow your arteries, which leads to heart attacks and strokes.

**Clobbers high blood pressure.** Eating a few beets — and other foods high in potassium, like dried apricots and avocados — may help control your blood pressure. Keeping your potassium levels up, experts say, helps to keep your blood pressure down.

**Helps you lose weight.** High-fiber foods control your appetite by absorbing water and slowing down your digestion. This makes you feel full longer and helps you eat less. Just one cup of beet slices has almost as much fiber as a cup of cooked oatmeal and yet adds only 75 calories to your daily lineup.

**Strengthens your bones.** If you're concerned about osteoporosis, ease your mind by eating beets. The red roots are rich in three nutrients — potassium, magnesium, and beta carotene — that experts say keep your bones strong.

> **The under-appreciated, often-ignored leaves**
>
> Beet leaves — especially when small, crisp, and fresh — are delicious and nutritious. Instead of tossing them in the garbage, trim off the tough part of the stem that hangs below the leaf. Then heat up some olive oil in a frying pan, add your favorite seasonings, and throw in your washed beet leaves. After you've sautéed them until they're soft, dig in and enjoy.

## Pantry pointers

Now that you're ready to buy some beets, you have a choice to make — canned or fresh? Canned beets are easier to prepare, and they taste almost as good as fresh ones. But consider this — fresh beets have twice as much potassium and folate as canned beets.

Don't let fresh beets intimidate you. They are easy to cook. Try baking them like a potato. Here's how:

◆ Clip off all but one inch of their stem. This will keep all of the nutrients and moisture in the root.

◆ Scrub beet gently under water, being careful not to tear the skin.

◆ Wrap each beet in aluminum foil and bake at 375 degrees for about an hour or until tender.

Short on time? Cook them in your microwave. Zap four or five medium-sized beets in a covered dish with one-quarter cup water for about 10 minutes. Keep them covered and let stand for another 5 minutes.

---

| Benefits |
|---|
| Combats cancer |
| Protects your heart |
| Stabilizes blood sugar |
| Boosts memory |
| Fights urinary tract infections |
| Prevents constipation |

# Blueberries

• • • • • • • • • • • • • • • • • •

Every now and then, a great food comes along that not only tastes good but is good for you, too. Blueberries are sweet, juicy, cute, delicious, and they're packed full of all sorts of amazing health benefits — like vitamin C, fiber, calcium, and iron. And as far as getting antioxidant protection, you can't do better than a serving of blueberries.

No matter how healthy you may be, molecules called free radicals are created in your body whenever cells turn oxygen into energy. And these molecules are out to destroy healthy cells. Given enough time and opportunity, free radicals cause all kinds of sickness — even heart disease and cancer. Luckily, nature provides a delicious antidote in blueberries.

Each little fruit contains the pigment anthocyanin, which gives the berry its blue color — kind of like dye you can eat. But anthocyanin is also a potent antioxidant that hunts down and destroys free radicals. Scientists at the USDA-ARS Human Nutrition Research Center on Aging recently came up with a way to measure the total amount of antioxidants in foods. Blueberries scored near the top of their list. They discovered blueberries are so full of goodness that a half cup serving has the same amount of antioxidants as five servings of foods like peas, carrots, apples, squash, or broccoli.

"Blueberries provide a relatively concentrated source of antioxidants," says Dr. Ronald L. Prior, one of the researchers. "With other fruits and vegetables, blueberries provide a way to increase antioxidant intake, which may have long term health benefits."

You'll find members of the blueberry family throughout Europe and Asia, including England where they grow a distant cousin called bilberries. But more than 40 varieties are also native to North America. Don't confuse them with huckleberries, however, which look similar, but have large seeds.

## 6 ways blueberries keep you healthy

**Puts the crunch on cancer.** Cancer is often the end result of free radicals gone haywire. But you can short-circuit these killers with powerful antioxidants like the ones found in blueberries. Recent studies in Germany found foods high in antioxidants like anthocyanin seemed to protect people from cancer. The more of these types of antioxidants people ate, the less likely they were to develop cancer.

**Beats heart disease.** For years doctors have known free radicals attack your arteries, leaving them scarred and more easily clogged by fatty deposits. The longer this goes on, the higher your risk for heart attacks and strokes. But they also know certain antioxidants fight free radical damage and keep your blood from getting too sticky.

German researchers discovered people who ate the most antioxidant-rich foods, like blueberries, were the least likely to die of a heart attack. If heart disease runs in your family, blueberries, which help keep your arteries open and strong, could be one delicious way to protect yourself.

**Stabilizes blood sugar.** Blueberries are a favorite folk remedy for high blood sugar, but scientists only recently found their own proof. Animal studies in Italy showed blueberries lowered blood sugar levels by about 26 percent. Although diabetes is a serious illness that requires professional care, it certainly couldn't hurt to sprinkle a handful of these healthy berries on your cereal or whip some into an energy-boosting smoothie. If you have diabetes, talk to your doctor about any changes in your diet.

**Gives UTIs the slip.** Researchers know *E. coli* bacteria cause a lot of urinary tract infections (UTIs). For years doctors thought the acid in certain fruits, especially cranberries, worked to get rid of UTIs by chasing away these bacteria. Now they know blueberries, like cranberries, contain antioxidants that actually change the structure of the bacteria — they become powerless to attach themselves to your cells and start multiplying. The secret to fewer UTIs: Eat more blueberries.

**Keeps your mind sharp.** Exciting new studies at Tufts University in Boston suggest blueberry extract may improve memory, coordination, and speed tests. You just might be able to reverse some of the symptoms of aging by adding blueberries to your daily menu.

**Restores regularity.** People in Sweden have used blueberries for hundreds of years as a cure for diarrhea. It may be blueberries counteract the bacteria causing diarrhea or it could be their soluble fiber keeps your bowels humming along regularly. A single cup of blueberries contains about 15 percent of your daily recommended intake of fiber. Just think, you might be able to throw away both your diarrhea and laxative medications simply by adding blueberries to your diet.

## Pantry pointers

Look for plump, dark blueberries without any mold, and use or freeze them within five days. Since heating destroys some vitamins in the berry, it's best to eat them uncooked. Freezing, however, does not affect the nutritional benefits. Don't wash the berries before freezing, though, since they'll end up clumping together. Toss some blueberries in your next fruit salad, in your morning muffins or pancakes, or on ice cream, and enjoy.

# Broccoli

• • • • • • • • • • • • •

| Benefits |
| --- |
| Strengthens bones |
| Saves your eyesight |
| Combats cancer |
| Protects your heart |
| Controls blood pressure |

Today, people are eating 900 times more broccoli than they did 25 years ago. Perhaps it's because this "crown jewel of nutrition" is one of the healthiest foods you can buy. Ounce for ounce, broccoli has more than twice as much vitamin C as oranges. It's also a good source of folate, vitamin A, potassium, and calcium. And this member of the cabbage family contains several phytochemicals that may help prevent disease.

## 8 ways broccoli keeps you healthy

**Builds better bones.** You probably never imagined broccoli could battle osteoporosis, but it's got plenty of calcium, potassium, and magnesium — nutrients that may help prevent or slow this bone-breaking disease. It's also one of the few nondairy foods full of calcium that your body can absorb easily. Vegetarians and people who are lactose intolerant may find broccoli an important addition to their daily menu.

**Keeps vision keen.** You want to keep the world around you sharp and clear for as long as possible. That's why you should start protecting yourself against cataracts and age-related macular degeneration right now. One way is to make sure broccoli is on your shopping list. This cruciferous vegetable is loaded with lutein and zeaxanthin, two carotenoids that may lower your risk of developing both these vision thieves. According to research, broccoli and spinach are the best foods for the job and the more you eat, the higher your protection.

**Closes down prostate cancer.** Tomatoes aren't the only food to protect your prostate. Cruciferous vegetables like broccoli, cauliflower, and brussels sprouts can swing the odds in your favor. Eat three servings of these veggies every week and research shows you could just about cut your risk of prostate cancer in half.

**Battles breast cancer.** If you're a woman, you really only need one reason to add broccoli to your diet — breast cancer. Researchers at the University of California at Berkeley claim a natural element in broccoli, called indole-3-carbinol, can stop the growth of breast cancer cells. Leonard F. Bjeldanes, professor of toxicology in the College of Natural Resources at UC Berkeley says, "Indole-3-carbinol hits the cancer from a different angle than other anticancer drugs, which makes it a very powerful and interesting chemical." Not only is broccoli a fresh and tasty addition to your menu, but it looks like a true healing food as well.

**Improves heart health.** Vegetables are good for your heart because they're low in fat and have no cholesterol. But broccoli, in particular, is one of the superstar heart protectors because of its well-rounded nutritional qualities. It's rich in folate, a B vitamin that fights the artery-damaging amino acid homocysteine, and it's also jampacked with those natural chemicals called flavonoids. These protect your blood and arteries from clotting, oxidation, and inflammation.

A 10-year study of over 34,000 post-menopausal women found those who ate foods high in flavonoids reduced their risk of fatal heart attack by one-third. You need to eat broccoli or other brightly colored vegetables several times a week to get this heart-saving benefit.

**Balances out blood pressure.** Think sodium and think high blood pressure. Think broccoli and think potassium, calcium, vitamin C, and magnesium, four of the "good guy" nutrients that help control blood pressure. The famous DASH diet, sponsored by the National Heart, Lung, and Blood Institute and the National Institutes of Health, is designed to bring blood pressure — and the risk of heart disease and stroke — down. It recommends eating whole foods chock-full of these good guys.

> ### 'Sprout' a little cancer protection
>
> Fresh sprouts have gotten a lot of bad press lately, but if you miss that healthy crunch on your favorite sandwich, reach for broccoli sprouts. Developed by researchers at Johns Hopkins University School of Medicine, these little cancer-fighters are loaded with a natural compound that boosts your body's antioxidant defenses. They are also a good source of fiber, vitamin C, and calcium. And now the sprout industry is confident of their safety since the Food and Drug Administration (FDA) issued strict guidelines for sprout production.

**Lowers lung cancer risk.** Certain chemicals in broccoli, cabbage, and bok choy, called isothiocyanates, limit DNA damage and urge your body to produce cancer-fighting antioxidants. If you smoke, you are, of course, more likely to develop lung cancer and eating broccoli may only make a small difference. But if you are truly ready to launch an attack on lung cancer, put out the cigarettes and dish up the vegetables.

**Crushes colon cancer.** Antioxidants are probably the most powerful natural weapon you have against cancer. And lutein, an antioxidant in broccoli and other vegetables, means business when it comes to colon cancer. Researchers can't say exactly why, but if you eat foods high in lutein, you're less likely to develop colon cancer.

## Pantry pointers

When buying fresh broccoli, look for a deep green color — sometimes tinged with purple — and crisp leaves. Refrigerate it for up to four days, but don't wash it until you're ready to eat.

If you steam or microwave your broccoli, you'll save more of the nutrients. But it's also great boiled, stir-fried, or added to any casserole.

| Eat | |
|---|---|
| Strawberries | Kiwi |
| Oranges | Papaya |
| Red peppers | Spinach |
| Cabbage | Carrots |
| Avocados | Tomatoes |
| Olive oil | Cucumbers |

# Bruising

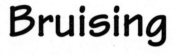

When you got a bruise as a child, it was considered a badge of honor. As an adult, bruises can be ugly and even embarrassing. Thank goodness they usually aren't a serious problem. Most of them heal completely by themselves within a week or so. But if you are bruising a lot, even from bumps you hardly notice, you might have a vitamin deficiency.

## Nutritional blockbusters that fight bruising

**Vitamin C.** Every time you damage your body, you can break arteries, veins, and tiny capillaries. Blood seeps under your skin from these breaks and forms the familiar black and blue bruise. Vitamin C can strengthen your blood vessels by helping form collagen, a protein found in all your connective tissues, including skin. Even a minor deficiency of Vitamin C can make you bruise more easily.

---

> ### A word of caution
>
> If you take certain medications regularly, including aspirin, you just might bruise more easily — perhaps due to internal bleeding. See your doctor if you get a lot of bruises for no apparent reason or they don't heal within a few days. She may change your prescription or run some tests to rule out any serious disorders.

To protect yourself from bruises, eat lots of fruits and vegetables rich in vitamin C — like oranges, strawberries, kiwi, papaya, red peppers, broccoli, and brussels sprouts. And if you feast on these foods fresh and uncooked, you'll get more of this important vitamin.

**Vitamin K.** A bruise that seems to appear from nowhere or a cut that won't stop bleeding could be a sign of a vitamin K deficiency. You'll find this vitamin, which helps your blood clot, in spinach, cabbage, carrots, avocados, cucumbers, tomatoes, dairy products, and olive and canola oil. So fill your plate but, again, keep it fresh. Heating these foods doesn't seem to affect their amount of vitamin K, but freezing them may destroy it.

# Bulgur

· · · · · · · · · · ·

### Benefits

Combats cancer

Protects your heart

Battles diabetes

Promotes weight loss

Helps stop strokes

Bulgur, bulghur, or burghul — however you spell it, it's all the same, and it's all good. This deliciously healthy grain is made from whole wheat berries or kernels that have been steamed, dried, and cracked. Some people confuse bulgur with cracked wheat, but bulgur is different since it's been pre-cooked.

This form of wheat is popular in Middle Eastern countries as the main ingredient in tabbouleh, a traditional salad of bulgur, parsley, cucumbers, tomatoes, olive oil, and lemon juice. It's also one of the oldest recorded types of foods — the Chinese may have eaten it as early as 2800 B.C. Lucky for us bulgur is still around, because it has a hearty, nutty flavor, and is easy to cook. Don't forget how nutritious it is, either. Bulgur is a good source of insoluble fiber, protein, magnesium, iron, manganese, and B vitamins.

## 4 ways bulgur keeps you healthy

**Stops stroke.** Try some tabbouleh or a side of bulgur pilaf instead of potatoes and you'll add more than just variety to your diet. Recent research says eating whole grains like bulgur can reduce your risk of stroke.

Researchers at Brigham and Women's Hospital in Boston analyzed information on more than 75,000 women participating in the Nurses' Health Study. They found those who ate the highest amount of whole grains cut their risk of an ischemic stroke — the kind caused by a blood clot to your brain — almost in half. Replacing refined grains like white rice and bread, cakes, biscuits, or pizza made from white flour, with whole grains like oatmeal, brown rice, bran, dark bread, and bulgur can mean a longer, healthier life.

**Curtails cancer.** The scientific community may not agree on how whole grains discourage cancer, but no one is arguing with the proof. If you were to look at all the research done on whole grains and cancer, you'd find positive results in 95 percent of the studies.

It may be the amount of fiber, antioxidants, or phytoestrogens in whole grains that do the trick. Or perhaps it's the way unprocessed grains help regulate your body's glucose levels. In any event, bulgur battles digestive system cancers, like colon cancer, and hormone-related cancers, such as breast and prostate cancer.

Remember, though, refining foods destroys many of the healthy components. Whenever possible, you should choose whole grains that are unprocessed.

**Holds up heart disease.** In most Middle Eastern or Asian countries people get plenty of whole grains. But if you live in a western country, you are probably getting much less than nutrition experts recommend. Because of this, heart disease is widespread.

Whole grains like bulgur are good for your heart because they help control your weight, lower your blood pressure, and reduce bad LDL cholesterol levels while keeping your good HDL cholesterol steady. All this happens through a healthy combination of fiber, carbohydrates, essential fatty acids, and vitamins.

Study after study reports the more whole grains you eat, the lower your risk of developing heart disease. Louis Sullivan, M.D., former Secretary of the U.S. Department of Health and Human Services, takes the research seriously. "Increasing whole grain consumption could have a profound impact on the health of the nation," he says. "We could reduce the incidences of heart disease and cancer substantially."

Look for FDA-approved labels on certain products that say: "Diets rich in whole grain foods and other plant foods and low in total fat, saturated fat, and cholesterol may reduce the risk of heart disease and certain cancers."

---

### Cooking bulgur with ease

If you know how to cook rice, preparing bulgur will be a snap. Just don't remove the lid or stir while your bulgur is absorbing the water. Here are cooking instructions from the Wheat Foods Council:

For one serving (or one-half cup cooked bulgur), combine 3 tablespoons of dry bulgur in a saucepan with 1/3 cup plus 1 tablespoon water. Boil. Cover; simmer 15 minutes. Let stand 5 minutes.

To prepare in the microwave, combine 3 tablespoons bulgur, 3/4 cup water, 1/4 teaspoon oil, and a dash of salt in a 1 1/2-quart microwave safe container. Cook on high 12 minutes, turning container every two minutes. Let stand five minutes.

**Drop-kicks diabetes.** Bulgur is a good bet for battling diabetes, whether you want to avoid the disease, or already have diabetes and need sensible food choices.

It's no secret, people who eat whole grain foods on a regular basis are less likely to develop diabetes. The more fiber you eat, the better your chances — more than three servings a day will make a difference. And since whole grain products tend to have a low glycemic index, bulgur is a good food to include in your diet if you're diabetic. (See the *Diabetes* chapter for an explanation of the glycemic index.)

## Pantry pointers

Look for boxes or bags of bulgur in your grocery or health food store. It comes in three grades — coarse, medium, and fine — although you may only find the medium variety in your supermarket. Coarse cooks up like rice, medium is delicious as a morning cereal, and fine is most often used in tabbouleh. Store bulgur in an airtight container at room temperature for up to a month. For longer storage, keep it in your refrigerator or freezer.

---

**Benefits**

Combats cancer

Prevents constipation

Protects your heart

Promotes weight loss

Helps hemorrhoids

---

# Cabbage

• • • • • • • • • • • • •

Cabbage is a descendant of wild sea plants that grow along the coast of England and other parts of Europe. This head-shaped vegetable is an important food in both Europe and Asia.

The Irish are well-known for corned beef and cabbage, and the Germans contributed sauerkraut. Koreans have been making a cabbage meal called kimchi (pronounced kimCHEE) for 3,000 years. Made of fermented cabbage, radishes, hot peppers, lettuce, and garlic, some people even eat it for breakfast.

The cabbage family is part of the *brassica* group and covers several vegetables, including broccoli and cauliflower. The plants are classified by the arrangement of their parts. If the leaves are tightly folded to form a ball, it's head cabbage. Kale and collards have leaves that are loose and open. Plants that resemble miniature heads are called brussels sprouts. Chinese cabbage, also called Napa, is light green or white and looks a lot like romaine lettuce. Bok choy is a vegetable that looks more like thick, white celery with leaves, but it's still cabbage. Even stranger is kohlrabi, which looks like a turnip but, like your odd uncle Marvin, is still part of the family.

*Brassica* vegetables are super hero foods in the war against cancer. They're also good sources of fiber and vitamin C. And at only 17 calories per half cup of cooked cabbage, you won't have to worry about your waistline expanding.

## 2 ways cabbage keeps you healthy

**Karate-chops cancer.** One of the most exciting new studies about *brassica* vegetables came from the University of Massachusetts. A group of 34 postmenopausal women were asked by researchers to eat more *brassica* vegetables — about two servings a day. The women only lightly cooked the vegetables by steaming or stir-frying during the month-long study. Amazingly, just by eating more of these vegetables, the women were able to raise their levels of an enzyme that can protect against breast cancer.

Melanie Polk, Director of Nutrition Education at the American Institute for Cancer Research in Washington tells people how to eat to avoid getting cancer. She says that cabbage has two particular phytochemicals — isothiocyanates and indoles — that protect against cancer.

"One of these famous isothiocyanates is called sulforaphane, and it seems to stimulate the production of anti-cancer enzymes," she says. "So that means it would increase the body's natural ability to ward off cancer. The indoles seem to stimulate enzymes that make estrogen less effective, which might possibly decrease the risk of breast cancer."

Studies from all over the world prove that the cabbage family can protect you from many types of cancer.

Korean researchers found that eating lots of cabbage decreases your risk of stomach cancer. Other studies showed that brussels sprouts can protect you from colon cancer. And in a Chinese hospital study, doctors found that if you eat Chinese cabbage regularly, you're less likely to get brain cancer.

Harvard nutritionists studied 47,000 men over a 10-year period and found that the more cabbage the men ate, the less likely they were to get bladder cancer. Yet, coleslaw did not seem to offer protection from bladder cancer, and researchers aren't sure why.

But that's not all the cancer-fighting cabbage family can do. Scientists at the Jiangsu Institute of Cancer Research in Japan made a startling discovery when they studied more than 500 male smokers with and without cancer. They found that smokers who ate cabbage at least three times a week had only half the risk of developing lung cancer as other smokers.

**Chases away constipation.** Cabbage is an excellent source of fiber, and it helps bulk up your bowel movements for easy elimination. Adding this crunchy vegetable to your diet a few times a week could help prevent constipation and the problems that come with it, like hemorrhoids and diverticular disease — little pouches that form in your colon. Some researchers think that straining to have a bowel movement can even cause varicose veins and hiatal hernias.

You might have a little trouble digesting cabbage if your body isn't used to *brassica* vegetables. But that's normal. Just add some to your diet a little at a time. Polk suggests sprinkling a bit of shredded cabbage on a salad filled with colorful vegetables.

"If raw cabbage causes a problem," she says, "then cooked cabbage may be tolerated better."

## Pantry pointers

When buying cabbage, choose a head that is firm, not soft or spongy.

To cook cabbage, cut the head into quarters and gently boil it for 15 minutes, or stir-fry in canola oil until it's tender. Pair it with cooked egg noodles for an Eastern European treat. Season to taste with salt, pepper, and paprika.

If you make coleslaw, hold the mayo. Cabbage is a low-fat food but not if you drown it in a fatty dressing. Try a low-calorie dressing or a vinaigrette instead.

Brussels sprouts should be steamed until tender — about 10 to 15 minutes. Try stir-frying them in a bit of olive oil and garlic for a super-healthy side dish.

### A word of caution

If you've had surgery for stomach cancer or a peptic ulcer, you might not be producing enough stomach acid to break down certain vegetables, like brussels sprouts.

If you don't have the right amount of acid, your stomach and small intestine can form vegetable masses, called phytobezoars. These masses of undigested food sometimes have to be removed by surgery.

To be safe, you're better off avoiding brussels sprouts if you've had stomach surgery.

| Eat | |
| --- | --- |
| Garlic | Tomatoes |
| Onions | Broccoli |
| Spinach | Collard |
| Mushrooms | greens |
| Brown rice | Tuna |

**Avoid**

Foods high in saturated fat, such as red meat

Foods high in refined sugar, such as pastries

# Cancer

. . . . . . . . . . . . .

With the right tools, your body might be able to protect itself from cancer. Experts believe now, more than ever, you have the power to live a cancer-free life. Choose to eat a balanced diet, to exercise, to avoid smoking and drinking, and you'll be choosing a lifestyle for cancer prevention.

Start by eating mostly plant-based foods. According to the American Cancer Society, balancing your diet this way could cut your cancer risk by one-third. Limit meats, fatty and sugary foods, and other empty calorie snacks. Punch up your intake of fruits, vegetables, legumes, and whole-grain breads and cereal. The nutrients, antioxidants, and fiber in these foods can help your body work smoothly, down to the last cell. And that's where it matters, because cancer starts when just one cell stops working properly.

With your new daily menu in place, cut your risk even more by exercising. Healthy eating combined with exercise will help control your weight. If you are 20 to 30 percent over the average weight for your age, sex, and height, you are considered obese and that carries its own risks. Obese women are more likely to get cancer of the breast, uterus, ovary, and gallbladder. For obese men, it's colon and prostate cancer.

In addition to watching your diet and exercising, if you cut out smoking and drinking, you could prevent up to 70 percent of all cancers. No wonder experts say cancer prevention is in your hands.

# Nutritional blockbusters that fight cancer

**Antioxidants.** Fruits, vegetables, and other plant-based foods are powerful weapons in the war against cancer. They're loaded with antioxidants, natural chemicals that reinforce your own anti-cancer defenses by fighting free radicals. Since free radicals invade your cells and create cancer, all antioxidants are essential ammo.

Many fruits and vegetables contain the big three — vitamin C, E, and beta carotene. Then again, some come armed to the teeth with even more antioxidants like flavonoids. These compounds give color, flavor, and taste to plants. Your best bet is to load your plate with these seven super sources.

◆ **Cruciferous vegetables.** Also known as *brassicas,* this food group includes broccoli, cauliflower, cabbage, kale, bok choy, kohlrabi, rutabaga, turnips, and brussels sprouts. They're famous for containing phytochemicals with long names like isothiocyanates, indoles, and glucosinolates. These natural substances appear to safeguard your DNA from cancer-causing mutations. They might even stop the growth of tumors. You'll get the most cancer protection if you eat these veggies raw or only lightly cooked.

◆ **Onions and garlic.** These fragrant bulb vegetables, called alliums, also include scallions and chives. Mince or crush them to release their full anti-cancer powers, and don't overcook them. Follow these tips and you'll benefit from their flavonoids and sulfur compounds, which get free radicals before they get you.

◆ **Citrus fruits.** Oranges, lemons, limes, grapefruits — these flavorful fruits are a two-for-one deal against cancer. Their pulp and juice are loaded with vitamin C. This antioxidant superhero might prevent more than eight different kinds of cancer in one fell swoop: cancers of the bladder, breast, cervix, colon and rectum, esophagus, lung, pancreas, and stomach. Plus, citrus fruits have antioxidants called monoterpenes in their peels. Shave off some of the fruit's outer skin — the zest — and add it to drinks or dishes for the benefit of these chemicals.

◆ **Berries.** According to the USDA-ARS Human Nutrition Research Center on Aging, these little morsels pack one of the biggest antioxidant punches. Natural chemicals like anthocyanin and ellagic acid deliver blows to cancer-causing pollutants. So eat strawberries, blueberries, cranberries, and other fruits that are so "berry" good for you.

◆ **Green leafies.** Most vegetables with big floppy leaves and a dark green color — like romaine lettuce, collards, beet leaves, and spinach — contain carotenoids. These hi-powered antioxidants take out toxins and free radicals before they can harm your cells. Carotenoids are especially powerful against lung cancer. So passive smokers take note — green leafies, as well as carrots and sweet potatoes, might be the protection you need from those pollutants you inhale.

◆ **Tomatoes.** Lycopene is an antioxidant that sets tomatoes and other red fruits apart. This carotenoid appears to protect against cancers of the colon, stomach, lung, esophagus, prostate, and throat. Get as much lycopene as possible by sautéing tomatoes in olive oil, or by eating red pasta sauces and pizza. Snacking on red grapefruits, guavas, and watermelon will also lift your lycopene levels.

◆ **Herbs and spices.** Use these cancer-fighters instead of salt to zest up your meals. Basil, rosemary, turmeric, ginger, and parsley all contain flavonoids and other compounds that send your antioxidant levels through the roof. Fresh herbs are generally more potent cancer fighters than dried.

This list is not complete. Dozens of foods contain antioxidants that ward off cancer. Don't forget green tea's polyphenols.

Or olive oil's vitamin E. And there's the alpha and beta carotene in carrots. Load up your grocery cart with antioxidant power and start challenging cancer.

**Selenium.** This trace mineral is also an antioxidant, in that it protects your cells and tissues from oxidation. For nearly 30 years, scientists have believed low selenium levels lead to a greater risk of cancer. Selenium is different from other antioxidants, however, because a normal diet of mostly unprocessed foods easily provides the suggested 55 micrograms a day.

Now, Dr. Mark A. Nelson, a professor and researcher at the Arizona Cancer Center, says, "The Nutritional Prevention of Cancer (NPC) Trial tripled the intake and suggests that higher levels of selenium may be necessary for cancer prevention." Until nutritionists conduct more research, though, no one can recommend the best, safest amount you should get. Experts warn selenium is a toxic mineral, which means too much of it, especially from supplements, is unsafe.

For now, Nelson's advice: "Eat a well-balanced diet." Foods especially high in selenium include mushrooms, seafood, chicken, and wheat.

**Folate.** Folate is an essential ingredient in making DNA. Without enough of this B vitamin, you could end up with broken chromosomes, one risk factor for cancer. No wonder, then, a folate deficiency appears to increase the risk for cancers of the cervix, lung, esophagus, brain, pancreas, breast, and especially the colon and rectum.

Munch on fresh, leafy green vegetables for a full-size serving of folate. Fortified cereals, beets, squash, and melon all provide a healthy amount, too. Eat these foods raw or lightly cooked since heat destroys the folate. Even microwaving will foil your folate intake.

**Fiber.** Dr. Denis Burkitt, author of *Eat Right — To Stay Healthy and Enjoy Life More,* first stated over 20 years ago that fiber might prevent colorectal cancer. "When diets are rich in dietary fiber," Burkitt said, "the stools passed are usually large. If carcinogens (the substances which produce cancer) are diluted in a large volume of stool and also if they are discarded out of the bowel fairly quickly (as happens with fiber-rich diets) rather than hanging around, they will be less dangerous."

Choose foods rich in insoluble fiber, the kind that won't dissolve in water — brown rice, fruits, beans, vegetables, wheat bran, and whole grains. These are also rich in nutrients and phytochemicals, making them complete anti-cancer packages.

**Omega-3.** Your body needs two fatty acids that it can't make on its own — linolenic or omega-3 and linoleic or omega-6. They're called essential nutrients and you must get them from foods. But you must get them in correct amounts. When one type of fatty acid drastically outnumbers the other, things can go haywire.

Most people get more than enough omega-6 fatty acids from a typical diet loaded with vegetable oils, and not enough omega-3s found in cold-water fish and other foods. Some experts believe this imbalance is linked to cancerous tumors. Too many omega-6 fatty acids may promote tumor growth, while getting more omega-3 fatty acids could prevent — even shrink — tumors.

---

### Grilling 101

"Grilling meats, poultry or, to a lesser degree, seafood, has been linked to the risk of breast, stomach, and colorectal cancer," warns Melanie Polk, the Director of Nutrition Education at the American Institute for Cancer Research. But if you can't bear to give up that flame-broiled steak or burger, at least reduce your risk by marinating meats for a minimum of 40 minutes.

Mix together three ingredients — an acidic liquid (like orange juice, wine, or vinegar), a flavoring (such as turmeric, or garlic), and something to hold everything together (like honey or olive oil). All these contain antioxidants and, combined, they help prevent the cancer-causing compounds, called heterocyclic amines (HCAs), formed during grilling.

And by the way, hamburger lore is wrong. Lower the flame and flip your burgers more than once. Turning them every minute will cook your burgers faster, kill any bacteria in the meat, and possibly reduce the HCAs.

Win the battle between the omega-3s and the omega-6s. Every week eat at least two servings of salmon, tuna, mackerel, herring, or other omega-3-packed fish. Include flaxseed oil, walnuts, and green leafy vegetables in your diet to boost your good fat intake even more.

And just as important — cut back on eggs, milk, processed grains, and anything that contains corn or soy oils. That includes almost all fried, fast foods and margarine. These foods are all high in omega-6s.

Trim down on red meats, too. They're high in fats — omega-6s and saturated fats. According to the American Cancer Society, a high-fat diet increases your risk of colon, rectum, prostate, and endometrium (uterine lining) cancers.

# Cantaloupe
· · · · · · · · · · · · · · · · · ·

| Benefits |
|---|
| Saves your eyesight |
| Controls blood pressure |
| Lowers cholesterol |
| Combats cancer |
| Supports immune system |

Chances are you've never eaten a cantaloupe.

Sure, you think you have. You've brought home that big melon with the gray, netted rind and the sweet, orange pulp. You've sliced it up on those still-warm days of late summer for breakfast or dessert. You've wiped the juice off your chin and maybe even appreciated its measure of potassium, fiber, folate, beta carotene, and vitamin C.

You just don't know its real name.

What you may call a cantaloupe is really a muskmelon. Like squash and pumpkins, people have been enjoying this member of the gourd family for its pleasant scent and delicious taste since at least 2400 B.C. But the muskmelon does more than merely smell and taste good. It also helps protect you from eye problems, cancer, and heart disease.

So bite into a nice, juicy muskmelon. You'll get a mouthful of flavor and a wealth of health benefits — even if you call it a cantaloupe.

## 3 ways cantaloupe keeps you healthy

**Looks out for eye problems.** Cantaloupes are full of beta carotene, a carotenoid your body converts into vitamin A. This natural chemical not only gives the melon its brilliant orange color but also acts as an antioxidant in your body, protecting your eyes from cataracts and macular degeneration. These two serious eye problems most often strike seniors. Cataracts blind over 1 million people worldwide every year and age-related macular degeneration (AMD) is the leading cause of blindness in people over 65. But you can guard against both by eating the right foods. Check out the evidence.

Australian researchers conducting the Blue Mountains Eye Study found people who took in at least 3,000 retinol equivalents (RE) of vitamin A a day cut their risk of developing nuclear cataracts — the kind that affects the central area of your lens — in half. Although this amount of vitamin A is more than the government normally recommends, it's still a safe level as long as you're getting the vitamin from whole foods, not supplements. Eat one small cantaloupe and you're halfway to this sight-saving goal.

Antioxidants like beta carotene may safeguard your retina from free radical damage and keep the blood vessels surrounding your eye working properly — all factors that protect against AMD. According to studies out of five major ophthalmology centers, the more carotenoids like beta carotene you eat, the lower your risk of developing this disease. Vitamin C — plentiful in cantaloupe — is an antioxidant superpower. Eat one small cantaloupe, containing over 180 milligrams of vitamin C, every day and you could cut your risk of developing macular degeneration by one-third.

**Pumps out heart disease.** There's safety in numbers. Especially when you're facing a number of dangers. High blood pressure, cholesterol, and homocysteine all contribute to heart disease. Fortunately, cantaloupe has enough nutrients to counter all of these threats.

◆ Potassium keeps your blood pressure under wraps, particularly when you watch your sodium intake, too. And cantaloupes contain plenty of potassium. One cup of cubed cantaloupe provides about one-fourth of the recommended daily allowance (RDA) of this key mineral. But potassium might not be acting alone.

◆ That same cup of cubed cantaloupe gives you more than 100 percent of the RDA for vitamin C. That's good because according to researchers from the Boston Univer-sity School of Medicine, vitamin C works to lower blood pressure, is linked to reduced risk for heart disease and stroke, and may improve blood flow in people with chronic heart failure.

◆ Folate, part of the B vitamin family found in cantaloupe, can control homocysteine, a substance that's known to trigger strokes and heart attacks. Even though one cantaloupe won't give you all the folate you need to make a heart-healthy difference, it can be an important and delicious part of your daily menu.

◆ Cantaloupe contains soluble fiber, which can dramatically lower your cholesterol. Experts even recommend this type of fiber for people with diabetes because of its heart-friendly effects. One cantaloupe can give you five of the 25 grams of fiber you need every day.

**Keeps cancer at bay.** Any pirate worth his eye patch knows the best treasure is always buried. Beneath a cantaloupe's outer layer you'll find not only tasty fruit but also a treasure chest of anti-cancer weapons including folate and fiber.

Vitamin C, however, is the big gun that acts as an antioxidant, capturing free radicals that can damage your cells. It also boosts your immune system so you can fight off disease. Vitamin C is particularly powerful against breast, lung, throat, stomach, bladder, pancreas, and colon cancers.

## Pantry pointers

When shopping for a cantaloupe, choose a melon that is heavy for its size with a sweet but not overpowering smell and no soft spots. If it's ripe, store it in the refrigerator — just be sure to seal it tightly since cantaloupes can take on the odors of nearby foods. After all, you don't want your cantaloupe to smell like beef stew. If it's a bit hard or green, store it at room temperature until it's ripe.

| Benefits |
| --- |
| Combats cancer |
| Protects your heart |
| Saves your eyesight |
| Prevents constipation |
| Promotes weight loss |

# Carrots

• • • • • • • • • • • • • •

Try to remember your first carrot. If you're like most people, you probably ate your first carrot when you were very young. That's because mothers are smart. They know growing children need lots of vitamin A to have healthy eyes. And that's where carrots come in. This brightly colored vegetable is loaded with beta carotene, which your body converts to vitamin A.

Carrots are important for many other reasons, too. Take fiber, for instance. Carrots contain enough fiber to put you on the path to regularity and maybe even lower your risk of heart disease.

Then there are the carotenoids — beta carotene and alpha carotene — which might safeguard you against cancer and heart disease. Plus, carrots have few calories, no fat, and the highest sugar content of any vegetable besides beets. That's why they're so tasty.

No wonder people have been eating them for thousands of years. Believe it or not, the first carrots were actually purple and yellow. It wasn't until the 1600s that Dutch traders hit upon the idea of growing bright orange carrots. Now millions of people all over the world eat this variety — except in places like India, where they enjoy red carrots.

No matter what color carrots you eat, you'll be doing your body a favor.

## 5 ways carrots keep you healthy

**Battles breast cancer.** Eating carrots may reduce your risk of breast cancer by nearly 40 percent, according to a study of 13,000 women from the National Institute of Environmental Health Sciences. For the people in the study, snacking on cooked carrots twice a week did the trick. But the more carrots you eat, the researchers say, the more beta carotene you get and the stronger your protection.

Munch on some raw spinach every week, too, and you'll cut your risk of breast cancer even more.

**Foils lung cancer.** It isn't enough to be a nonsmoker. To protect yourself from second-hand smoke and air pollution, crunch on some carrots. That's right — doctors at the Harvard School of Public Health found that this popular orange root might lower your risk of lung cancer if you don't smoke. This time, carrots can thank their other carotenoid, alpha carotene, for this power. One carrot provides 3.5 milligrams of alpha carotene. And according to the Harvard study, that's more than enough for a daily dose.

Experts say carrots and their carotenoids may work by scavenging free radicals before they attack your cells, causing damage that can lead to cancer. The more carrots you eat, the fewer free radicals you'll have. This could mean a lower cancer risk.

**Prevents constipation.** One medium-sized carrot can give you a quick 2 grams of fiber. The fiber in carrots, according to a study from Germany, works as well as cereal grains at adding bulk to your stools. This makes them softer and easier to pass, which means regularity and less straining without taking harmful laxatives. To get the most fiber out of your carrots, stick with fresh or frozen ones. Canned carrots lose some of their fiber in the canning process.

**Fends off heart disease.** It's never too late to start fighting heart disease, especially when you've got carrots on your side. According to scientists at the Scottish Heart Health Study, if you have a high daily intake of fiber — 25 to 40 grams in a 2,000 to 3,000 calorie diet — you could lower your risk of heart disease by 30 percent. The same fiber in carrots that keeps you regular might also guard your ticker by lowering your cholesterol level.

**Watches out for cataracts.** Most people living in developed countries don't have to worry about going blind because of vitamin A deficiency. But cataracts are another story. If you want to reduce your risk of cataracts, eat plenty of carrots. Vitamin A is a powerful antioxidant that guards your eyes against cataract-causing free radicals.

---

### Focus on a rainbow of carrots

To give you another choice besides the usual orange kind, carrot experts with the USDA want to unveil a rainbow of carrots — red, yellow, white, and purple roots — in your grocery store. All the colors would have the same great taste. But because they contain different pigments, they each would offer different health benefits.

For instance, purple carrots get their color from anthocyanins, which could thin your blood and reduce your risk of heart disease. The red carrots, on the other hand, contain the carotenoid lycopene, famous for preventing prostate and other cancers.

So keep your eyes peeled. One day soon, these colorful carrots may be in a supermarket near you.

# Pantry pointers

When shopping for carrots, look for the ones that have a regular shape and the deepest orange color. Avoid carrots with black or dark-colored tops, cracks, mushiness, or root-like hairs growing out of their bodies. You can buy whole carrots or "baby" carrots already wrapped in bags. And there's a very good chance they will be fresh, even fresher than the carrots that still have their tops. Just make sure to inspect the carrots in the bag before buying them.

Keeping carrots at home is easy, but there is one catch. When you stick them in your refrigerator — wrapped in the bag you bought them in or in another loosely wrapped plastic bag — just make sure to separate them from fruits that give off ethylene gas, like apples and pears. This gas ripens fruit, but it makes carrots taste bitter.

To get the most nutrients from your carrots, shred them, and then stir-fry. The added heat breaks down the carrot's hard, crunchy cells, releasing beta carotene and other antioxidants.

### A word of caution

Research shows that the beta carotene in carrots may fight disease by fending off free radicals. And yet, beta carotene supplements have not done as well in scientific studies.

As Dr. I-Min Lee, researcher with the Women's Health Study at Harvard University, says, "I think consuming beta carotene supplements is different from eating fruits and vegetables rich in beta carotene that are also rich in other antioxidants." Beta-carotene pills, Lee points out, failed to lower the risk of cancer or heart disease.

Bottom line — stick with the beta carotene in fruits and vegetables. And don't take supplements without checking with your doctor first.

| Eat | |
| --- | --- |
| Carrots | Spinach |
| Wheat germ | Brown rice |
| Apricots | Sweet |
| Sunflower | potatoes |
| seeds | Tuna |

**Avoid**

Foods high in saturated fat, such as red meat

Salt and alcohol in large amounts

# Cataracts

· · · · · · · · · · · · · · · · ·

If you're a senior citizen, chances are you have cataracts. According to the American Academy of Ophthalmology, by age 75, just about everyone suffers from this painless but distressing condition. You may not even be aware of the changes in your vision at first, since cataracts develop gradually over the years. But eventually you'll notice things becoming blurry and colors turning dull as the lens in one or both of your eyes clouds over. You may experience double vision and become more sensitive to light. In time, your lens even begins to look yellowish or milky-white. The worst news: If your cataracts are left untreated, you could become blind.

Fortunately, cataract surgery is generally successful. But who wouldn't rather avoid getting them in the first place? Protect your eyes from overexposure to the sun, don't smoke, limit your alcohol, and make sure your diet has plenty of the foods that keep your "windows to the world" healthy.

## Nutritional blockbusters that fight cataracts

**Vitamin E.** If you are ready to launch an attack on cataracts, then load up on the antioxidants that guard your eyes against free radical damage. And here's a picture-perfect reason to get more of the powerful antioxidant vitamin E — you could reduce your risk of cataracts by up to 50 percent. Since experts recommend getting the nutrients you need from whole foods, snack on E-rich sunflower seeds, cook with canola oil, sprinkle some wheat germ on your cereal, substitute whole-grain flours for white flour, and eat brown rather than white rice.

**Vitamin C.** You'll delight your eyes in more ways than one with colorful foods that are chock-full of another protective antioxidant, vitamin C. At breakfast, include some luscious red strawberries or drink sparkling orange or tomato juice. For lunch, chop bright red and green peppers into a salad. And at dinner enjoy a rich green feast for your eyes with foods like broccoli, brussels sprouts, or bok choy.

**Vitamin A.** Vitamin A is a third antioxidant that helps keep cataracts from clouding your vision. It's found mainly in meats and dairy products, but your body can convert the plant carotenoids, beta carotene, lutein, and zeaxanthin, into vitamin A. Pick bright yellow fruits and vegetables like apricots, carrots, and sweet potatoes, for a hefty helping of beta carotene. Broccoli and Popeye's favorite, spinach, are great sources of lutein and zeaxanthin.

All these fruits and vegetables are super smart choices for another reason, too. They're packed full of fiber, one more weapon in your battle against cataracts.

**B vitamins.** Without just the right amount of several nutrients, experts say you might be at greater risk of developing cataracts. The Blue Mountains Eye Study discovered people deficient in protein, vitamin A, niacin, thiamin, and riboflavin were more likely to get nuclear cataracts, the kind that affects the central part of your lens.

Fill your breakfast bowl with enriched cereal and you'll get a good helping of niacin, thiamin, and riboflavin. This trio of B vitamins is important not just to your eyes, but also to every cell in your body. You can also get all three by spreading tuna on a whole-wheat bagel and washing it down with a glass of milk. Round your day off with a baked potato for niacin and thiamin and a helping of mushrooms full of niacin and riboflavin.

**Protein.** You probably get plenty of protein from the meat, fish, and dairy foods in your diet. But a protein deficiency could mean a greater risk of developing nuclear cataracts. If you are a vegetarian, pay careful attention to your proteins. Legumes, like kidney beans, black-eyed peas, and peanuts, are incomplete proteins. They'll protect your eyes best if you pair them with grains or vegetables that contain other proteins. Try combination dishes like beans and rice, or have peanut butter on whole grain bread for a healthy mix.

**Low-fat foods.** There's still no good news about a diet high in fat. In addition to numerous other health dangers, extra fat on your plate can increase your risk of getting cataracts.

Stick to lean meats and low-fat dairy products, and avoid cooking with saturated fats like lard, butter, and coconut oil. If you load up on lots of those sight-friendly fruits, vegetables, and grains, your taste buds will find it easier to say no to fats.

**Seasonings.** Before you reach for that saltshaker, listen to this. Australian researchers conducting The Blue Mountains Eye Study examined diet and the development of cataracts in almost 3,000 people between the ages of 49 and 97. They found those with the highest intake of salt, averaging about 3,000 milligrams (mg) a day, were twice as likely to develop cataracts as those getting only about 1,000 mg a day.

The best advice — try herbs instead of salt to spice up your favorite foods. Treat yourself to a spicy Indian curry dish with turmeric, and you might also curry favor with your lenses. This spice contains curcumin, another antioxidant that, based on animal studies, might help you keep clear of cataracts.

---

### A word of caution

Selenium is a mineral you may not hear much about. That's because thanks to the soil throughout the United States and Canada, if you eat plant foods you're probably getting enough. But since it's another important antioxidant, don't take chances. If you overcook your vegetables, you're likely to boil this mineral away. Steaming, sautéing, and microwaving are all quick-cooking methods that will lock in nature's goodness.

# Cauliflower

• • • • • • • • • • • • • • • • •

**Benefits**

Protects against prostate cancer

Combats breast cancer

Strengthens bones

Banishes bruises

Guards against heart disease

"Cauliflower," Mark Twain once said, "is nothing but cabbage with a college education." He's right in many ways. Along with other cruciferous vegetables — like brussels sprouts, broccoli, and kale — cauliflower and cabbage both add a powerful nutritional punch to your diet. But while the humble cabbage has fed the masses for centuries, many people may view cauliflower as a more elegant vegetable.

With its unique colors and neat appearance, cauliflower does stand out from other plain vegetables in the supermarket produce section. First there's your typical cauliflower with its fancy cream-colored florets. Then you have the hard-to-find types — the violet-colored variety that turns green when cooked and the kind that grows the shade of broccoli. Perhaps the most exotic cauliflower is the Romanesca. Its lime-green stalks spiral upward into points, like the spires of a castle.

Remember though, not only is cauliflower an interesting addition to your plate, it's loaded with vitamin C, folate, vitamin K, and fiber — nutrients that can protect you against osteoporosis, bruises, and heart disease. And like the other cruciferous vegetables, cauliflower stands up to cancer with the best of them. In over 21 studies, cauliflower's arsenal of nutrients seemed to protect against lung, stomach, and colon cancers.

## 4 ways cauliflower keeps you healthy

**Protects your prostate.** As simple as it may seem, eating a cruciferous vegetable like cauliflower just three or more times a week could reduce your risk of getting prostate cancer by a whopping 41 percent.

"It's not clear from case-control studies of cruciferous vegetables which component leads to this reduced risk of prostate cancer," says Dr. Jennifer Cohen, one of the researchers on this study from the Fred Hutchinson Cancer Research Center. But experts suspect that phytonutrients in cauliflower, called glucosinolates, deserve the credit. These chemicals may sound a call to arms in your body, causing the release of enzymes that take the bite out of cancer-causing substances. Your body then flushes them out before they can harm your DNA.

**Turns the tables on tumors.** There's good news for post-menopausal women. Eating cauliflower just might discourage breast cancer. According to a cutting-edge study by the University of Massachusetts, those fabulous glucosinolates in cruciferous vegetables like cauliflower, cabbage, and broccoli, may help your body safely use estrogen, a hormone that otherwise could cause breast cancer. A couple of servings or about one-half cup of cauliflower a day could give you all the protection you need.

You'll get the most health benefit if you eat your vegetables raw or only lightly cooked. Try steaming or stir-frying for a great taste treat.

**Banishes bruises.** If you're over 50, you're likely to be vitamin K deficient. That's because as you age, your stomach becomes less able to absorb the vitamin K you need to thicken your blood. Take this warning seriously if you bruise or bleed easily.

Cauliflower is a smart solution for this problem. It doles out a solid dose of vitamin K — between 10 and 20 micrograms per cup. For a 120-pound woman, that's almost one-third her daily requirement. And for a 160-pound man, it's about one-fourth.

**Beefs up your bones.** It may surprise you to discover that cauliflower can keep your bones healthy. Doctors aren't sure why, but it's probably the special combination of vitamins K and C that do the trick.

Research shows getting more than 100 micrograms of vitamin K a day can begin lowering your risk of hip fracture. You'd get about a third of that amount in just two cups of cooked cauliflower.

And Vitamin C may slow down the advance of osteoporosis by helping your body make collagen, a bone building block. One-half cup of cauliflower has about 50 percent of your recommended daily amount of vitamin C. That's more C than in a whole cup of pineapple.

For a double dose of bone-saving nutrition, treat yourself to cauliflower soup made with skim milk. You'll not only get cauliflower's bone-strengthening benefits, but some much needed calcium and vitamin D, as well.

## Pantry pointers

Cauliflower is easy to find in your local supermarket since it's available year-round, but you'll still have to shop carefully for the best selection. Keep your eyes peeled for tightly closed clusters and green, fresh-looking leaves. Avoid cauliflower with brown spots or loose florets. When you bring the pick of the litter home, it will do just fine in the crisper bin of your fridge.

### A word of caution

Before you dish up a serving of cauliflower, check your pillbox. The clotting action of the vitamin K could work against any blood-thinning medication you take, like warfarin.

Also avoid this veggie if you suffer from gout, a form of arthritis where uric acid crystals sit in your joints and cause terrible pain and swelling. Cauliflower contains purines, substances your body turns into uric acid. One way to lessen the painful symptoms of gout is to keep purine-rich foods out of your diet.

Cooking it, however, may not be as easy as buying it. Cauliflower is well known for its strong cabbage-like odor. But if you microwave, boil, or steam it just until it's slightly tender, you'll cut down on the smell while locking in all those important nutrients.

## Eat

| | |
|---|---|
| Rice | Corn |
| Soybeans | Potatoes |
| Liver | Squash |
| Spinach | Sardines |
| Yogurt | Broccoli |
| Oranges | Nuts |

### Avoid

All foods containing gluten, such as wheat

# Celiac disease

• • • • • • • • • • • • • •

Celiac disease, also called celiac sprue, causes the hair-like villi of the small intestine to become inflamed and flattened. And since nutrients from food are absorbed through these tiny villi, the disease often leads to symptoms of malnutrition — even if you are eating healthy meals.

The culprit in celiac disease is gluten, and it's found in some of the most commonly eaten foods on earth — wheat, barley, rye, and oats. If you have celiac disease, you can't eat foods made from these grains without damaging your small intestine. And the stakes are high. Up to 15 percent of people with the disease develop gastrointestinal cancer or lymphoma. Yet, if you eat a gluten-free diet, you can usually recover completely, and your chances of getting cancer can return to normal.

Possible symptoms of celiac disease are weakness, anemia, bone pain, weight loss, stomach bloating, and diarrhea or bulky stools that float. All of these symptoms are a result of not getting nutrition from the foods you eat. In addition, celiac disease often leads to lactose intolerance — the inability to digest milk. Other conditions that sometimes show up with celiac disease are dermatitis herpeti-formis (burning, itching rashes that last for weeks or months), liver disease, juvenile diabetes, thyroid disease, lupus, rheumatoid arthritis, Sjogren's syndrome (very dry eyes and mouth), and ulcers of the mouth. But sometimes celiac disease has no symptoms at all, just the harmful changes in your small intestine.

Celiac disease affects one in every 300 people in Europe. It's especially prevalent in Italy and Ireland but very rare in Africa, Japan, and China. Doctors in the United States don't test for celiac disease very often, and people with these symptoms are often told they have irritable bowel syndrome or a nervous disorder.

Children who have untreated celiac disease are often small for their age, but normal-sized adults can develop it after severe stress, a viral infection, or pregnancy. Researchers aren't sure if it's present from birth and then triggered, or if you can develop it later in life. For some reason, breast-fed children seem to have some protection against developing the disease at a young age.

At this time, the only certain test for celiac disease is removal of a tiny piece of the small intestine to check for damage to the villi. If your doctor finds changes in your small intestine, and a totally gluten-free diet relieves your symptoms, chances are good you have the disease.

If you are diagnosed with celiac disease, you'll have to follow a strict, gluten-free diet for the rest of your life. Besides the obvious sources, like breads, you'll find that gluten is in all kinds of foods — sauces, gravies, candies, and many alcoholic drinks, like beer, gin, and whiskey. Ask questions in restaurants, and read labels in the grocery store. And if you're not sure, don't eat it.

People with celiac disease often have difficulty absorbing fat soluble vitamins, like A, D, and K, and can be deficient in these and other nutrients. But once you cut all gluten foods out of your diet, your small intestine should begin to heal, and food can again be your ally instead of your enemy. If you have severe malnutrition, your doctor might prescribe supplements.

## Nutritional blockbusters that fight celiac disease

**Gluten-free flours.** You'll have to completely avoid all breads and cereals containing wheat, rye, oats, barley, bran, graham, wheat germ, durum, kaska, bulgar, buckwheat, millet, triticale, amaranth, spelt, teff, quinoa, and kamut. Also off limits are malt and wheat starch, often used to thicken sauces.

You can replace these with breads and cereals made from rice, corn, soy, potato, and bean flour. Look for breads that are labeled "gluten-free" or make your own.

**Vitamin A.** Symptoms of a vitamin A deficiency are night blindness, inflammation of the eyes, reduced ability to fight infection, weight loss, loss of appetite, reduced saliva, and improper tooth and bone formation. You can counteract these symptoms with whole milk (if you aren't lactose intolerant — a problem for many celiacs), yellow and dark green vegetables, oranges, and liver.

**Vitamin D.** If you don't get enough vitamin D, your body can't use calcium to make strong bones. Good sources are fatty fish, like salmon, herring, and sardines, and their oils. Eggs, butter, and liver are also good foods to eat to restore levels of vitamin D.

Your body can also make vitamin D with the help of sunlight. But as you get older, the process doesn't work as well.

**Vitamin K.** This vitamin is important for proper blood clotting, and a lack of vitamin K can lead to anemia. Green leafy vegetables and liver are good sources.

**Magnesium.** If you have trouble absorbing nutrients, you could be deficient in magnesium, especially if you've had diarrhea for a long time. Not having enough magnesium can cause muscle tremors, personality changes, nausea, vomiting, and even convulsions. Fill up on nuts, legumes, soybeans, seafood, and green, leafy vegetables.

**Yogurt.** Everyone needs calcium for healthy bones. If you are lactose intolerant, you can get calcium from yogurt, which is easier to

---

**A word of caution**

You'll have to be a food detective to avoid all sources of gluten in your diet. For example, some herbal teas and nondairy creamers contain gluten, as does tuna in vegetable broth and any hydrolyzed vegetable protein. Avoid creamed vegetables, raisins and dried dates that have been dusted with flour, most canned soups, and sauces. Some types of cheeses, like blue, Roquefort, and Gorgonzola, are hidden sources of gluten. Even ketchup and soy sauce can contain gluten.

To help you make the right food choices for your health, find a good dietitian and contact a support group for celiacs.

digest than milk. Once you've been on a gluten-free diet for several months, you might be able to tolerate more and more milk products. Many celiacs find that lactose intolerance clears up as they get better.

# Cherries

• • • • • • • • • • • • • •

**Benefits**

Eases arthritis

Combats cancer

Protects your heart

Ends insomnia

Shields against Alzheimer's

Slows aging process

George Washington said, "I cannot tell a lie" when he confessed to chopping down the cherry tree. Like our country's first president, cherries are rather noble.

These seed fruits, which come in either sweet or tart varieties, hark back to 300 B.C. and have been enjoyed for centuries. European settlers brought cherry trees to America, and in 1852, the first cherry orchard was planted near Traverse City, Michigan, which has been dubbed the "cherry capital of the world."

But you don't have to hail from Traverse City to enjoy the many varieties of cherries. Some tart kinds are great for pies, juice, and jams, while sweet ones can be eaten right off the stem. You can even find dried cherries, which are similar to raisins.

Cherries boast not only great taste but also potential health benefits. With flavonoids, fiber, potassium, and traces of vitamins A and C, cherries have plenty of lookouts to guard your health. They're known to fight inflammation and, possibly, cancer.

Try some cherries, and when someone asks if you're enjoying a delicious and healthy food, you won't have to tell a lie. You can easily say "yes."

## 4 ways cherries keep you healthy

**Soothes arthritis and gout.** Life might not always be a bowl of cherries — but if it were, it might not be quite as painful.

That's because cherries can relieve pain. Long used as a folk remedy for gout, cherries now carry the clout of scientific evidence.

A recent study by researchers at Michigan State University found that anthocyanins, the same compounds that give cherries their red color, also help squash inflammation. These compounds stop the enzymes that make prostaglandins, hormone-like substances that cause inflammation and pain. Prostaglandins are the bad guys that aggravate conditions like headaches, arthritis, and gout.

Eating cherries every day may help relieve those conditions, says Dr. Muralee Nair, one of the MSU researchers. "If you have pain from chronic arthritis, and aspirin bothers your stomach, eating a bowl of cherries may reduce that pain," he says.

In fact, laboratory tests showed that 20 tart cherries were at least as effective as other pain-killing remedies, including aspirin, ibuprofen, and other nonsteroidal anti-inflammatory drugs. In some cases, they were much better.

"Cherry compounds are about 10 times more effective than aspirin," Nair affirms.

If you don't feel up to eating a whole bowl of cherries, you can get the same benefit from much fewer dried cherries. One dried cherry equals about eight fresh ones.

**Sidesteps cancer.** Research is still in progress, but cherries look promising as a protector against cancer.

Cherries contain a mighty anti-cancer chemical called perillyl alcohol that has been shown to inhibit tumors in rodents. They're also overflowing with antioxidants, which mop up the free radicals that can cause cell damage and cancer. Cherry's antioxidants include its anthocyanins as well as quercetin, a powerful flavonoid also found in apples and onions.

German studies of large numbers of fruits and vegetables found even more evidence. In one study, sweet cherries had some ability to counter two known clastogens, substances that can damage your chromosomes and potentially cause cancer. In another, both sweet and sour cherries were found to protect genes from mutations that can lead to cancer.

Even though the anti-cancer powers of the cherry haven't been conclusively proven, it never hurts to add potentially helpful foods to your diet. At the very least, you'll enjoy a sweet burst of goodness with every bite.

**Protects your heart.** Antioxidants are like guests at a party — the more the merrier. If such is the case, cherries are having one wild affair.

Cherries boast 17 compounds that combine for more antioxidant activity than vitamin C or E supplements. Located in the anthocyanins that give cherries their red color, these antioxidants may protect against atherosclerosis and heart disease by preventing the buildup of plaque in your arteries.

Like many fruits, cherries also provide fiber and potassium, both good soldiers in the war against heart disease. Fiber has been shown to lower cholesterol and reduce the risk of heart disease and stroke. Potassium fights heart disease by controlling your blood pressure so your heart doesn't have to work overtime. It also shields you from stroke.

**Puts insomnia to bed.** Have trouble sleeping? Cherries might be your key to dreamland.

Dr. Russel Reiter of the University of Texas Health Science Center recently discovered that cherries contain large amounts of melatonin, a hormone that helps you sleep.

"Certainly, cherries to this point have the highest concentration of melatonin we've measured in any fruit," Reiter says.

Melatonin works either as a direct sleep-inducing substance or by opening what Reiter calls "the sleep gate," which puts you in the right frame of mind to sleep. Eating cherries just before bedtime would give you the most benefit.

> ### Cherry burgers chase cancer away
>
> Next time you fire up the grill for a family cookout, don't forget the cherries. Unless you want a large helping of cancer to go with your burger and potato salad.
>
> Dr. J. Ian Gray of Michigan State University discovered that adding cherries to your meat helps protect it from cancer-causing substances that can crop up when you grill it. Called heterocyclic amines (HCAs), these substances are impossible to detect without sending your meat to a lab.
>
> "Cherries counteract the formation of HCAs," Gray says. "How, we do not fully understand."

Because it's an antioxidant, melatonin can also neutralize free radicals that contribute to cancer, Alzheimer's disease, and signs of aging, like crow's feet around your eyes.

Although research is still in the early stages, scientists think you may get all the melatonin you need by eating just a handful of cherries a day. Eating cherries might be especially important if you're older because as you age, your body doesn't produce as much melatonin on its own.

## Pantry pointers

Like a Chinese restaurant, cherries offer sweet and sour. When shopping for either variety, look for brightly colored and plump fruit. Sweet cherries should be firmer than sour cherries. You can buy cherries with or without stems; those with stems last longer, but those without are cheaper. You can store cherries in a plastic bag in the refrigerator.

Varieties of sweet cherries include Bing, Lambert, Tartarian, and Royal Ann, which are often used to make maraschino cherries. Early Richmond, Montmorency, and Morello are among the varieties of sour cherries. A typical cherry tree has about 7,000 tart cherries, enough to make 28 pies.

# Chestnuts

• • • • • • • • • • • • • • • • • • •

| Benefits |
|---|
| Promotes weight loss |
| Protects your heart |
| Lowers cholesterol |
| Combats cancer |
| Controls blood pressure |

Like a wacky cousin at your family reunion, chestnuts are a little different. Even for a nut, the chestnut is nutty.

First of all, the chestnut hardly has any fat. Most nuts, like almonds or walnuts, contain around 50 percent fat. True, it's mostly monounsaturated — the "good" fat — but it's still fattening. Chestnuts, on the other hand, usually have less than 5 percent fat.

They also have less protein and minerals than other nuts. But the protein they have is very high quality. Compared to other nuts, they have more complex carbohydrates and vitamin C. About half the chestnut is made up of water (which makes it go rancid quickly). Fiber, potassium and folate are found in smaller amounts.

The ancient Chinese prized chestnuts as far back as 1600 B.C., and chestnuts were enjoyed in Japan and Europe for centuries. Up until the early 20th century, chestnuts flourished and were popular in America, too. Then a blight virtually wiped out the American chestnut, so today most of the chestnuts you see are imported.

It's easy to see why this particular nut has been so popular. Beneath its smooth, hard shell and bitter skin, the chestnut reveals delicious sweet meat with a taste similar to corn. Chestnuts also offer help for your heart and weight and may even fight cancer.

## 3 ways chestnuts keep you healthy

**Keeps your weight in check.** If you like to snack — and who doesn't — you might want to chomp on some chestnuts.

Watching your calories and fat intake, along with exercising, are key strategies in the battle to lose weight. Because chestnuts have only a fraction of the fat and calories of other nuts, they make a great alternative to almonds, walnuts, or cashews. Not to mention potato chips or sweets.

You not only get a more nutritious snack, you get a more substantial one, says Dr. Dennis Fulbright, a botany professor at Michigan State University.

"A cup full of chestnuts is about 300 calories. I suspect that someone who just sat down and ate a cup of warm, naturally sweet chestnuts will feel better and more satisfied than someone who sat down and ate a donut, which has more like 400 to 500 calories with a lot more fat," he explains.

Chestnuts don't magically make you lose weight, but evidence suggests they can help as part of a healthy diet. Fulbright notes that chestnuts are most likely to be eaten in areas where obesity is less frequent.

"Countries like Italy, France, Korea, China, and Japan, where obesity is rare, are places that still grow and eat chestnuts," he says, adding, "I wouldn't suggest they are less obese because they eat chestnuts, but it follows that if they eat natural foods like chestnuts, they are following other good dietary habits."

**Guides you to a healthier heart.** Since obesity is a major risk factor for heart disease, chestnuts can help your heart by narrowing your waistline.

But chestnuts can help your heart in other ways, too. The scant fat chestnuts contain includes monounsaturated fat, the kind that lowers cholesterol. Not only does it lower your total cholesterol, but it slashes the LDL, or "bad" cholesterol that clogs your arteries without harming the HDL, or "good" cholesterol.

Fiber also can lower cholesterol, while potassium and vitamin C help control your blood pressure. High blood pressure means higher risk for heart attack because your heart has to work harder than it should to pump blood through your body.

The whole package adds up to a healthier heart. Studies have shown that eating nuts lowers your risk for heart disease.

**Contributes to cancer prevention.** Chestnuts won't exactly make cancer quake in its boots, but they do contain some nutrients that have been linked to reduced rates of the dreaded disease.

Fiber and folate have mainly been credited with stopping colon cancer, while vitamin C may help prevent cancer at several sites, including the bladder, breast, and stomach.

## Pantry pointers

"Chestnuts roasting on an open fire ..." BOOM! Chestnuts can explode if you don't slit or poke holes in them. That's one good way to tell when a batch of roasting chestnuts is done — leave one unslit or unpoked to serve as a timer.

Of course, you don't have to roast chestnuts on an open fire. You can roast them in the oven or microwave, boil them, puree them, or even eat them raw. They can be used in desserts, side dishes, or main courses, including many traditional Italian meals.

You can find fresh chestnuts from September through February. Look for firm nuts, and store them in a cool, dry place.

| Benefits |
| --- |
| Aids digestion |
| Soothes a sore throat |
| Tames pain |
| Combats cancer |
| Clears sinuses |
| Boosts your immune system |

# Chili peppers
· · · · · · · · · · · · · · · · · · · · · ·

Eating a bowl of fiery chili or dipping into a spicy salsa is an experience you won't soon forget. Your mouth begins to burn and your nose starts to run. Then, just when it seems it couldn't get any hotter, it does, and you start to sweat.

Not only do many people enjoy this sizzling adventure, but if you have a taste for the tongue-tingling, you're actually doing your body good — chili peppers, for all their bite, are quite healthy. A whole pepper provides you with one and a half times the amount of vitamin C in an orange. And the red, yellow, and orange varieties are also great sources of beta carotene.

What makes all chili, or cayenne, peppers especially nutritious is the same ingredient that makes them hot — a chemical called capsaicin. According to experts, the hotter the pepper, the better it is for you, because that burning sensation on your tongue means you just got a good dose of capsaicin. Since capsaicin may ease stomach problems, prevent cancer, soothe a sore throat, and provide relief from other aches and pains, maybe you should let a pepper punch up your next pot roast.

# 4 ways chili peppers keep you healthy

**Improves indigestion.** Add a little cayenne to your next meal and your digestive system will certainly sit up and take notice. First the capsaicin gets the juices flowing and the muscles moving in your stomach — this speeds up the whole digestive process. Then it takes the air out of gas and bloating, so you won't feel so uncomfortable. Next, you may not know it, but it increases blood flow to your digestive tract, making it easier for your body to absorb nutrients from your food. Experts say spice up your life with chili peppers and you'll give poor digestion a powerful triple punch.

**Soothes that sore throat.** When your throat is sore and scratchy, the last thing you'd think to eat is spicy cayenne. But actually, it might be exactly what you should add to your plate. According to a recent study from Germany, a little chili pepper can numb a sore throat and help you swallow without pain in only a couple of days.

While commercially prepared drops and tablets were used in the research, a spicy dinner at home may get you the same results. Don't get carried away, though — try only a moderate amount of hot food at first, and only for minor sore throats. Serious sore throats that last more than a couple of days still need a look by your doctor.

The healing power of cayenne doesn't stop in your throat, either. One green or red pepper contains almost twice the Recommended Dietary Allowance (RDA) of vitamin C. That much could give your immune system a real boost. Ward off colds and other bad bugs by tossing together a fresh salsa. Combine a ripe tomato, a crisp onion, some tasty cilantro, a little lime juice, and, last but not least, hot peppers.

**Burns away pain.** If you suffer from chronic aches and pains, an over-the-counter cream containing capsaicin may be the miraculous medicine you're looking for. In dozens of studies, it numbed pain from common discomforts like neck ache, cluster headaches, and psoriasis to more serious ailments such as rheumatoid arthritis, diabetic neuropathy, osteoarthritis, shingles, post-surgery pain, skin tumors, and even amputation.

You must apply the cream four or five times a day for at least four weeks. Then the capsaicin causes your body to run out of substance P, the chemical that carries pain messages from your skin's nerves to your brain. Even though the painful condition still exists, your brain won't know about it and you won't feel it.

Capsaicin cream is serious stuff, however. At first it will burn on your skin, so make sure to use gloves when you apply it and keep it away from your eyes. Although it's available without a prescription, talk to your doctor before trying it — especially if you're wanting to treat a serious condition.

**Stands up to cancer.** It's a debate with no final decision — do chili peppers guard against or cause stomach cancer? You can find research to support both sides. Some say capsaicin may stop cancer-causing chemicals in their tracks before they damage your DNA. And other experts believe eating too many chili peppers may actually raise your risk of stomach cancer.

The safest bet, according to Melanie Polk, Director of Nutrition Education at the American Institute for Cancer Research, is moderation. "Chili peppers may be protective in moderate amounts," she says, "but using them in excess appears to increase cancer risk." While there are no exact recommendations yet, let your taste buds and your doctor be your guide.

## Pantry pointers

Picking just the right chili pepper can mean the difference between a zesty dish and a four-alarm fire. So beginners need to take it slow. Start with a mildly hot pepper, like the jalapeño. You'll recognize it by its thin green body and pointed end. The serrano, a plump, green or red pepper, is a bit hotter, so try it after you have some experience under your belt. For the truly adventurous, there's the habanero, a small bell-shaped pepper that comes in yellow, orange, red, or green. Don't let its pretty appearance fool you, though — it's the hottest of the hot.

---

## A word of caution

Capsaicin, experts stress, is very potent stuff. Whether in a cream, in a pepper, or in a powder, take care with it. If you don't wear gloves when handling it, make sure to wash your hands immediately with soap and warm water or, preferably, vinegar. And never, ever touch your eyes when capsaicin is around.

If you suffer from ulcers or chronic heartburn, chili peppers can irritate your stomach. Even people without these ailments can get indigestion from eating hot peppers. The key for everyone — know your limits when it comes to spicy foods.

---

If you can't handle even a jalapeño, don't give up. Try removing the pepper's seeds and pulp, where most of the capsaicin is stored. Or soak it in salt water for an hour before eating. If the pepper still burns your mouth, reach for a banana or milk instead of water to put out the fire.

# Chronic pain
• • • • • • • • • • • • • • • • • • •

| Eat | |
| --- | --- |
| Tuna | Salmon |
| Mackerel | Halibut |
| Flaxseed | Water |
| Turmeric | Walnuts |
| Chestnuts | Wheat germ |
| Olive oil | Canola oil |
| **Avoid** | |
| Foods containing omega-6 fatty acids, such as corn and soybean oils | |

You smash your finger with a hammer and, for a moment, the pain is almost unbearable. But this acute pain serves a purpose. It tells you something is wrong.

On the other hand, if you suffer with a chronic condition, like arthritis, fibromyalgia, or constant back pain, you may keep on hurting long past the time an injury should have healed.

Fortunately, recent scientific breakthroughs are helping to explain pain — both acute and chronic — and what you can do about it.

Take the example of your smashed finger. It was probably warm, red, and swollen for a while, which meant it was healing. During the healing process, different chemicals from your nervous and immune systems went rushing around, sending pain messages to your brain and directing the processes that would make your finger like new again. When the acute pain ended in a day or two, you probably forgot all about it.

With chronic suffering, the systems involved don't realize that there should be an end to your pain. Let's say you trip and fall. In the process, you tear a disk in your spinal column or damage the cartilage in your knee. It could heal as smoothly as your thumb did, but instead, you get caught in a cycle. The pain stimulates chemicals that cause inflammation, leading to other chemicals causing more pain — and on it goes.

"Unless we interrupt it," says nutritionist Carl Germano, co-author of the book *Nature's Pain Killers,* "this continuous feedback loop between the nervous and immune systems repeatedly generates inflammation and pain. This is how we end up suffering from chronic pain."

If hurting has become a way of life for you, keeping a positive mental outlook will give you some relief. And eating a balanced diet with lots of fruits, vegetables, and grains will prevent your body from getting run-down. You might want to take a daily multivitamin, too.

Germano says specific substances in the foods you eat can increase or decrease pain and inflammation. They can influence your tolerance to pain, as well. "We make these chemicals — the pain causers as well as the pain killers — in our bodies," he says. "Therefore, we can influence how much of which kinds of these chemicals we make by changing what we eat, and the supplements we take."

And here's another thing that can cause pain — allergic reactions to food. "Beware of food allergies that trigger inflammation and pain," says Germano. "It would be wise to try an elimination diet to determine the worst offenders for you." Wheat, corn, eggs, nuts, soy, citrus fruits and juices, and dairy products are the foods most likely to give you problems.

## Nutritional blockbusters that fight chronic pain

**Omega-3.** Your body needs omega-3 (linolenic acid) and omega-6 (linoleic acid), two essential fatty acids. They are called "essential" because your body can't make them. They must be supplied by the foods you eat.

Most people find it easier to get omega-6 than omega-3 in their diet. In fact, some people eat as much as 25 times more omega-6 than omega-3. But with that 25-to-1 ratio, you are just asking for pain. That's because omega-6 promotes inflammation and pain, while omega-3 does just the opposite.

"For people suffering from inflammation, the *amount* of essential fatty acids in the diet may not be as important as the *ratio* of the two," says Germano. In general, Germano suggests a ratio of between 4-to-1 and 10-to-1. But if you are fighting inflammation, he thinks a 2-to-1 to 4-to-1 ratio may be better.

Getting this ratio right is like adjusting the hot and cold water when you take a bath. If you run too much hot water in your tub, you have to turn it off and add some cold water to get it to the ideal temperature.

"Consuming a diet rich in omega-3 fatty acids decreases the amount of omega-6 fatty acids your cells absorb," explains Germano. And "long-term intake of omega-3 fatty acids may even decrease your long-term need for anti-inflammatory drugs."

So how do you get a ratio that will ease your agony? First, get rid of those vegetable oils — especially safflower, corn, soybean, and cottonseed. Use olive or canola oil instead. Go easy on meats, eggs, and milk. And get in the habit of eating more cold water fish, like Atlantic cod, Atlantic salmon, sockeye salmon, flounder, halibut, mackerel, tuna, bluefish, herring, and striped bass. It's your very best source of omega-3. "Fish are not only brain food, they're also 'anti-pain' food," says Germano. If you're not a fish lover, you can also get some omega-3 from nuts, seeds, and wheat germ.

When you eat less meat, you'll also reduce arachidonic acid, another substance that increases inflammation. Duck, the lean meat in particular, and the visible fat in pork are especially high in this pain-provoking acid.

**Tryptophan.** Foods like turkey and dairy products contain a lot of tryptophan, an essential amino acid that helps your brain make serotonin, a natural pain buffer.

But these high-protein foods also contain a lot of other amino acids. And the tryptophan has to compete with them for access to the brain. Germano compares it to a lot of people trying to get on an elevator at the same time, and "Mr. Tryptophan" is at the end of the line.

Fortunately, there's help for the tryptophan as it struggles to get inside the brain. By combining these proteins in moderate amounts with carbohydrates, like vegetables, fruits, and grains, you help it move to the head of the line. A combination dish — like cheese and pasta — can help push it through the door. Then it's just a matter of time before the serotonin can come to your rescue.

**Water.** The water in the disks of your spinal column supports as much as 75 percent of the weight of the upper part of your body. As a matter of fact, water is an important element in all your cartilage. This protective material helps keep your bones from scraping painfully against each other when you move.

You need at least eight 6-ounce glasses of water a day. Drinks containing alcohol or caffeine draw water out of your body. And sugary drinks can cause you to put on weight, which can put pressure on painful joints.

> ### A word of caution
>
> If you wake up with an aching back, think twice before reaching for a cup of coffee. At least one study connects caffeine with chronic back pain.
>
> Researchers aren't absolutely sure the caffeine is to blame because many coffee drinkers also smoke. And studies show smoking is connected not only to back pain but to other types of muscle and joint pain as well.
>
> If you are a heavy coffee, tea, or cola drinker, try cutting back to see if it helps.

**Turmeric.** If you are hungry for relief from your aching joints, sit down to a dish of curry-flavored stew. The curcuminoids in the spice turmeric, the ingredient that gives curry powder its yellow color, can be as powerful as nonsteroidal anti-inflammatory drugs (NSAIDs) in fighting inflammation. Talk to your doctor if you are interested in taking daily doses in the form of supplements.

# Cinnamon

· · · · · · · · · · · · · · · · · · · ·

| Benefits |
| --- |
| Kills bacteria |
| Aids digestion |
| Stabilizes blood sugar |
| Blocks diarrhea |
| Fights food poisoning |

Historians will tell you that in the ancient world, people were dying for cinnamon — literally. Considered more precious than gold, cinnamon was used in Egypt to preserve bodies after death.

This fragrant spice, wildly popular for its ability to perk up a pie, has a new role. Recent evidence shows that cinnamon can also make mincemeat out of germs.

Cinnamon comes from a bushy evergreen tree that grows in Sri Lanka, India, Indonesia, South America, and the West Indies. The inner bark of this tree is dried and used as a spice, while the oil is distilled and used in food, liqueurs, perfumes, and drugs.

## 3 ways cinnamon keeps you healthy

**Kills germs dead.** Cinnamon can kill *E. coli* , a dangerous bacteria that can cause severe diarrhea and flu-like symptoms. *E. coli* likes to hide in partially cooked meats and unpasteurized foods, like fresh apple cider.

When scientists added cinnamon to apple juice infected with a large amount of *E. coli,* the cinnamon destroyed more than 99 percent of the bacteria after three days at room temperature.

Dr. Daniel Y.C. Fung, who supervised the apple juice research, thinks cinnamon has a bright future in germ fighting. "If cinnamon can knock out *E. coli* 0157:H7," he says, "one of the most virulent foodborne microorganisms that exists today, it will certainly have antimicrobial effects on other common foodborne bacteria, such as *Salmonella* and *Campylobacter."*

**Peps up digestion.** For hundreds of years, the ancient Greeks and Romans used cinnamon for better digestion. Although scientists can't tell you how it works, it might have to do with the way cinnamon heats up your stomach. Whatever the reason, adding some cinnamon to your meal could help relieve your discomfort if you have trouble with frequent indigestion.

**Stabilizes blood sugar.** If you have adult-onset diabetes, talk with your doctor about using cinnamon in your diet. Test tube studies showed that a pinch of cinnamon can make insulin work better. While scientists are busy trying to figure out how cinnamon does this, you could be reaping the rewards of this ancient spice. Start sprinkling it on meats and vegetables or add it to fruit drinks. In the future, you're likely to see more research about cinnamon and diabetes.

---

> ## A word of caution
>
> Remember the old joke about the patient who complained to his doctor that "it hurts when I do this?" Well, the advice from the doctor is still good advice — "don't do that."
>
> Chewing cinnamon gum might cause a burning sensation in your mouth or even make ulcers form. That's a clue from your body to stop chewing the gum. If you experience a reaction like this, you should avoid cinnamon gums and candies.

## Pantry pointers

Be creative. Use ground cinnamon to spice up more than your apple cobbler and pumpkin pie. Try adding it to cooked carrots, winter squash, and sweet potatoes. You can also buy cinnamon sticks to swizzle in hot cider, coffee drinks, and juices. But be careful not to eat cinnamon oil. It can be toxic even in small amounts.

# Colds and flu

• • • • • • • • • • • • • • • • • • • • • • •

| Eat | |
| --- | --- |
| Chicken soup | Garlic |
| Water | Orange juice |
| Guava | Cantaloupe |
| Strawberries | Oysters |
| Carrots | Apricots |

| Avoid |
| --- |
| Dairy products when you have a cold because they increase and thicken mucus |

The old saying, "Feed a cold and starve a fever," may not be good advice. Eating certain foods can be great therapy for colds and flu, even if you have a fever.

In fact, research indicates that chicken soup — the world-famous cold remedy created with love by mothers everywhere — can help you feel better. The hot liquid moistens and clears your nasal passages and soothes your sore throat. And a recent study found that chicken soup can relieve symptoms of an upper respiratory tract infection by reducing inflammation.

Don't underestimate the emotional healing associated with chicken soup, either. When you're feeling miserable, a warm cup of soup can be very comforting.

And there's more. Some foods boost your immune system so you won't "come down" with the flu or "catch" a cold in the first place.

So go ahead and look through your cupboards. You're sure to find a variety of foods that can help speed your recovery and keep you healthy.

> ### Home remedies soothe and heal
>
> Almost everyone has a home remedy for cold and flu symptoms. You may sniff an onion to clear your nose; sip tea with ginger, mint, or chamomile; or gargle with salt water. And while there may not be scientific evidence to prove it, some of these home remedies may actually help.

## Nutritional blockbusters that fight colds and flu

**Garlic.** Garlic won't do much for your breath, but it helps prevent cold and flu viruses from invading and damaging your tissues. This powerful herb may also bolster your immune system. And if you toss some garlic into your chicken soup, you'll be getting two natural infection fighters at the same time.

**Water.** To prevent dehydration, drink plenty of water, especially when you have a cold or the flu. Dr. Mary L. Hardy, director of the Integrative Medicine Medical Group at Cedars-Sinai Medical Center in Los Angeles, believes in the healing power of water.

"The first defense system in the body consists of the mucous membranes lining the upper respiratory tract," she says. "And those work better when they're moist. Drink plenty of water and use steam treatments to provide internal and external hydration."

**Vitamin C.** Some people drink more orange juice the instant they feel the first sniffle or body ache — and it's probably a good idea. While vitamin C may not prevent colds, research shows it might shorten the length of time you suffer from cold symptoms. Guava, sweet red peppers, green peppers, strawberries, grapefruit, lemons, limes, and cantaloupe are good sources of vitamin C.

**Zinc.** Getting enough of this mineral in your diet may help reduce your risk of infection caused by bacteria and viruses. Oysters are a great source of zinc, but if you're not a shellfish fan, you can also find it in chicken, beef, lamb, turkey, beans, barley, and wheat.

**Beta carotene.** If you don't get enough beta carotene in your diet, you might be more likely to get a cold or the flu. Beta carotene, which is converted into vitamin A by your body, helps you fight infections. To get plenty of beta carotene, eat brightly colored fruits and vegetables. Good sources include carrots, pumpkin, sweet potatoes, kale, spinach, apricots, cantaloupe, mangoes, and broccoli.

# Constipation

| Eat | |
| --- | --- |
| Prunes | Apricots |
| Raisins | Pinto beans |
| Brown rice | Water |
| High-fiber cereal | Broccoli |
| Pasta | Apples |
| Oat bran | Avocados |

| Avoid |
| --- |
| Foods that have little or no fiber |

The next time you feel irritable and bloated from irregularity, don't reach for a laxative. Overusing laxatives could cause chronic constipation. Other culprits include medication you are taking, irritable bowel syndrome, or specific diseases. If you suspect your constipation is caused by one of these, see your doctor.

Fortunately, the solution for most constipation is as simple as getting more exercise, responding promptly when nature calls, and changing your diet.

---

### A word of caution

If you haven't been eating a lot of fiber, go slowly until your body is accustomed to it. Unpleasant side effects — like excessive gas, abdominal cramps, bloating, and diarrhea — won't be a problem if you add fiber gradually.

Unfortunately, eating an extremely high-fiber diet can cause you to lose important minerals. To replace these minerals, choose a variety of fiber-rich foods. Taking fiber supplements, which don't contain any nutrients, could lead to a deficiency.

---

## Nutritional blockbusters that fight constipation

**Fiber.** When your bowel movements don't happen easily, look at what you are putting on your plate. Chances are, you are piling it high with processed foods that have very little fiber. Or maybe you are filling it with meat, eggs, and dairy products. These foods don't have any fiber.

For better results, dish up lots of fresh fruits and vegetables. Add plenty of dried beans, like navy, kidney, or pinto, and include whole grains, like brown rice and barley. Choose whole-grain breads instead of white bread or toast, which has only one-fourth the fiber of the whole-grain kind. Toast also has a high "glycemic index," meaning that its carbohydrates are absorbed quickly, causing spikes in blood sugar which can lead to diabetes.

When you're grocery shopping, take time to read labels and pick cereals with a high-fiber content. General Mills' Fiber One, for example, has 13 grams of fiber in half a cup. Kellogg's All-Bran has 10 grams in the same size serving.

The fiber in these foods acts as a natural laxative. Like a sponge, it swells with water, making the stool soft enough to pass quickly and smoothly through your system.

The best way to get more fiber is to eat fiber-rich foods, which will also give you lots of nutrients. On the other hand, fiber pills don't have any nutrients and can even cause you to lose important minerals, like iron and calcium.

**Water.** Drink at least eight 6-ounce glasses of water and other liquids each day. It keeps food moving through your digestive tract, and it helps the fiber soften the stool for easy elimination. But watch out if you drink a lot of milk. It can cause constipation in some people.

And here's another reason to drink more water. Without enough liquid, all that fiber can cause an intestinal blockage.

# Cranberries

• • • • • • • • • • • • • • • • • • • • •

| Benefits |
| --- |
| Fights urinary tract infections |
| Protects your heart |
| Combats cancer |
| Guards against ulcers |
| Kills bacteria |

Cranberries were an important part of the Native American diet. To fortify themselves on long journeys, they ate a mixture of dried meat, animal fat, grains, and cranberries. Cranberries were also used for sauces, dyes, and medicine by the Pilgrims, and they have been an important commodity in New England ever since.

This native North American fruit grows in sandy bogs from the Carolinas to Canada. Most often, you find cranberries in cranberry sauce or cranberry juice cocktail. But they can also be used in chutney, pies, or cobblers, often combined with other fruit to counteract the cranberries' sourness.

Fortunately, there's nothing sour about this tiny red berry's health benefits. With powerful flavonoids, vitamin C, potassium, and fiber, cranberries can protect you from urinary tract infections, heart disease, and cancer. They might even fight ulcers and gum disease.

# 4 ways cranberries keep you healthy

**Attacks urinary tract infections.** Sometimes folk remedies are the best remedies. That's certainly the case with drinking cranberry juice to prevent painful urinary tract infections (UTIs). But, unlike many folk remedies, this one has scientific proof to back it up.

Dr. Jerry Avorn of Harvard Medical School led a study that showed cranberry juice reduced the risk of bacteriuria, or bacteria in the urine, in elderly women. Women who drank cranberry juice were only 42 percent as likely to have bacteriuria as those who were given a placebo beverage. If they did have bacteriuria, they were only about 25 percent as likely to have it again the following month. This means cranberry juice not only helps prevent UTIs, it might also help treat them.

Scientists once thought cranberry juice worked by making your urine too acidic for the bacteria to live, but it turns out a different process is at work. Flavonoids in the cranberry defend your urinary tract from unwanted intruders.

"What those compounds do in your body is keep the bacteria from being able to stick to the cells that line your urinary tract. If bacteria can't stay inside of you or stick to you, it can't colonize your urinary tract and you won't get an infection," says Dr. Ted Wilson, a professor at the University of Wisconsin – La Crosse.

These nonstick flavonoids can be especially helpful to elderly women because many women older than 65 can expect to get at least one urinary tract infection per year.

"Around here, in the Midwest, there are actually quite a few retirement homes that give people cranberry juice every day to help prevent UTIs," Wilson says.

Just one glass of cranberry juice a day might be enough to keep the infection-causing bacteria away.

**Guards your heart.** You've probably heard that drinking red wine or grape juice is good for your heart. But did you know cranberry juice might be even better?

Wilson discovered that cranberry juice prevents low-density lipoprotein (LDL) cholesterol, also called "bad" cholesterol, from becoming oxidized.

"What LDL cholesterol does is deliver cholesterol into the arterial wall," Wilson says. "And when LDL gets oxidized, LDL is delivered to the arterial wall much, much, much more rapidly. Once it's oxidized, it gets taken up and forms a plaque. And those plaques are what obstruct blood flow to your heart and your brain."

When you stop LDL oxidation, you slow down the process. That gives the LDL cholesterol less of a chance to stick to your arteries and clog them. Once again, the cranberry flavonoids are the heroes.

"The particular flavonoids in cranberry juice are particularly good at providing antioxidants and opening up or dilating blood vessels," Wilson says. He also speculates that, because of this, cranberry juice might be able to prevent blood clotting.

What's more, flavonoids are only the beginning. Cranberries are also high in fiber, which lowers cholesterol and helps reduce your risk of heart disease and stroke.

And don't forget about potassium, which keeps your blood pressure under control, and vitamin C, the powerful antioxidant that fights atherosclerosis, high blood pressure, and stroke.

So, how effective is cranberry juice when it comes to protecting your heart?

"In comparison to red wine or grape juice, very comparable or better," Wilson says. And here's the best part — one glass a day might do the trick.

**Wards off cancer.** Cranberries might give you an edge in your battle against cancer. At least that's what two studies show.

A Canadian study suggests that cranberry juice might prevent or treat breast cancer. And a study from the University of Illinois indicates that cranberries contain certain compounds with anti-cancer powers.

Vitamin C, which is found in cranberries, also has been linked to reduced risks of certain cancers, including bladder, breast, colon, throat, lung, and stomach cancers.

**Halts ulcers.** Cranberries might also prevent ulcers. According to Wilson, ulcers are often caused by a bacterial infection in your stomach lining, not acidity. If flavonoids can stop the bacteria from sticking to your stomach lining, they might stop ulcers from forming.

## Pantry pointers

Cranberry juice cocktails can differ greatly in the amount of actual cranberry juice. Some have as much as 27 percent, while others as little as 5 to 10 percent. The rest is mostly water and sugar to counteract the tartness. For the best health benefits, look for products with as much cranberry juice and as little sugar as possible.

Fresh cranberries usually show up in stores from October to December and come in 12-ounce plastic bags. You can refrigerate them for two months and freeze them for a year. You can also buy canned cranberry sauce or dried cranberries, which can be used like raisins.

---

### Tiny berry busts bacteria

The same cranberry compounds that stop bacteria from sticking to the lining of your urinary tract may protect your gums.

An Israeli study found that something in cranberries prevents different types of bacteria from clumping together and forming plaque in your mouth. This means cranberries might be a natural way to fight gum disease.

Unfortunately, researchers say most commercial cranberry juice cocktails have too much sugar to be a practical part of fighting plaque.

But they aren't giving up. They'll continue to study the cranberry to see if it could be used to make dental care products.

# Currents

· · · · · · · · · · · · · · · · ·

**Benefits**

Combats cancer

Protects your heart

Supports immune
 system

Helps stop strokes

Aids digestion

Controls blood pressure

Will the real currant please stand up? More than one fruit goes by that name. There's the red, white, or black berry that grows on shrubs and the tiny dried and seedless Zante grape, similar to a raisin. Whichever version of the currant you choose, you're sure to reap healthy benefits.

If you go with the Zante grape, which came to be called "currant" because it hails from Corinth, Greece, you get a boatload of fiber. A cup of these dried fruits gives you 9 grams.

Red and white currants are merely different colors of the same variety. A cup of these sweet berries provides nearly 5 grams of fiber.

But the healthiest currant of all might be the black currant, which is loaded with vitamin C. It's also a good source of potassium and ellagic acid, a substance that fights cancer.

Try any one of these currants, and you'll see an improvement in your current health.

## 3 ways currants keep you healthy

**Grapples cancer.** If you eat currants, you don't have to worry about getting enough vitamin C. Half a cup of black currants contains more than 100 milligrams (mg) of vitamin C — well over the recommended dietary allowance (RDA). That means plenty of punch in your fight against cancer.

Vitamin C gobbles up free radicals that can damage your cells and cause cancer. It also boosts your immune system so your body can fight the disease. Studies have linked vitamin C to lower risks of cancer at several sites, including the bladder, breast, colon, throat, lungs, prostate, and stomach.

But vitamin C isn't the only substance that can shield you from cancer. Black currants also contain ellagic acid. This polyphenol has been shown to stop cancer in the lung, liver, skin, and esophagus of lab animals.

Of course, the dried Zante currant's high fiber content makes it a worthy cancer opponent, too. According to some research, fiber is strongly associated with fighting colon cancer. Many health experts recommend eating more fruits and vegetables to avoid this dreaded disease.

**Stymies heart disease.** Dried fruits represent a more concentrated source of nutrients. That means dried Zante currants represent a concentrated assault on heart disease.

For example, a cup of these dried currants has almost three times as much potassium as a banana. Potassium, especially in conjunction with a low sodium intake, helps keep your blood pressure under control. It also lessens your chances of having a stroke. Add all that fiber, which lowers your cholesterol and reduces your risk of heart disease and stroke, and you have a tiny but potent heart helper.

Other kinds of currants are no slouches, either, when it comes to protecting your heart. Black currant seeds contain a form of omega-6 essential fatty acid called gamma-linolenic acid, which battles high blood pressure, clotting, and stroke. Vitamin C may also lower your blood pressure and risk of stroke.

**Toughens your immune system.** Scandinavians sometimes drink hot red or black currant juice as a treatment for colds and flu. They might be onto something.

With so much vitamin C, currants offer plenty of protection. Experts say there's not enough evidence to conclude that vitamin C prevents colds, but it does cut down on how long you're sick. It can also help you recover from more serious respiratory problems, like pneumonia and bronchitis. Just 200 mg a day — about the amount in a cup of black currants — was enough to show some improvement. That's because this mighty antioxidant vitamin helps boost your body's natural defenses.

More specifically, black currant seed oil — which has both gamma-linolenic and alpha-linolenic acids — has been shown to help the immune system in elderly people by cutting down on the production of inflammatory prostaglandins. These prostaglandins normally increase as you age, and they cause your immune system to break down. Currants, on the other hand, might help to rebuild it.

## Pantry pointers

Fresh currants can be hard to find. Their season lasts only from June to August, and some states still have a ban on growing currants because of a fungus from the early part of the 20th century.

Different currants have different uses. Black currants are used for making preserves and liquers, while the sweeter red and white kind can be eaten plain. Try baking with dried Zante currants or just snacking on them like raisins. You can sprinkle them with sugar and eat them out of a bowl, or use them in jams, jellies, and sauces. Currants stay fresh in the refrigerator for four days.

# Depression
. . . . . . . . . . . . . . . . . . .

| Eat | |
| --- | --- |
| Sweet | Spinach |
| potatoes | Chicken |
| Whole-wheat | Mushrooms |
| bread | Salmon |
| Tuna | Mackerel |
| Flaxseed | Walnuts |

| Avoid |
| --- |
| Foods containing omega-6 fatty acids, such as corn and soybean oils |

"It's very hard to explain how low you can get," says Lawrence Black. Over 10 years ago, Black, a native of Pennsylvania, began to suffer from depression. The illness came on gradually over time, and Black tried at first to deal with it on his own. Then one night, he woke up and realized he wasn't getting better. "I just couldn't take it anymore," he explains. "It was like I hit a wall."

Black is not alone. Every day depression and other mental illnesses darken the lives of over 340 million people worldwide. Depression brings with it feelings of sadness, pessimism, tiredness, and worthlessness that last two weeks, two months, or a lifetime.

Everyday activities you once enjoyed and did easily become impossible and joyless. "You get so low, you look for an escape," Black says. For Black, his escape was sleeping and being alone. For others, it might be never sleeping, overeating, alcohol abuse, or even suicide.

Experts aren't sure what's exactly at the root of this tragic mental illness. Problems with the brain's chemistry, genetics, seasonal changes, a recent bout with serious illness, a stressful life situation like divorce or pregnancy — these all can bring on depression, by themselves or in combination. For Black, it was the death of his father and the illness of his friend and business partner. "They were the two main events that brought the depression on," he believes.

Whatever the cause of deep sadness, you can't just "snap out of it" — just like a diabetic can't snap his fingers and get better. If you are depressed, you need help. Without it, severe depression will continue to cause psychological and even physical damage.

Black turned to his wife for support. Together they saw a psychiatrist. It was a tough road to recovery at first. But after trying three medications, he and his doctor found one that worked. "It makes me feel," he says, "like I did before — normal."

You can learn a lesson from Black's story — get help. It can work if you are seriously depressed or even if you just have the everyday "blues." Talk with your spouse or other loved ones, join a support group, meditate, start a hobby, pray, exercise — all these activities might help you feel better.

And surprisingly, eating the right foods and nutrients, experts believe, can lift your spirits and brighten your day, too.

## Nutritional blockbusters that fight depression

**B vitamins.** Believe it or not, a sweet potato or a spinach salad might help you beat the blues. Both are rich in folate and vitamin B6 or pyridoxine. Deficiencies in these two B vitamins, experts believe, can actually bring on the symptoms of depression. Vitamin B6 works by keeping your brain's neurotransmitters in balance. These chemicals control whether you feel depressed, anxious, or on a steady keel.

Experts aren't sure why folate fights the "blahs." But they do know low folate levels in your body can deepen depression, and high folate levels can help defeat it. You can find folate in most fruits and vegetables, especially spinach, asparagus, and avocados.

Eat chicken, liver, and other meats to feed your brain vitamin B6. Plant sources of the vitamin include navy beans, sweet potatoes, spinach, and bananas.

Depression can also signal a deficiency in thiamin, also known as vitamin B1. Stick with whole-wheat breads, meats, black beans, and watermelon to punch up your thiamin levels. These foods might help you feel more clearheaded and energetic.

**Iron.** Beating the blues might be as easy as eating iron-rich foods if you have iron-deficiency anemia. Over two billion people suffer from this condition and even more live with less-serious iron deficiency. A sour mood is a major symptom of a lack of iron. Other symptoms include pale skin, sluggishness, and trouble concentrating.

Iron-deficiency anemia often attacks pre-menopausal women, people who regularly take nonsteroidal anti-inflammatory drugs (NSAIDs), and others at risk for chronic blood loss. It's a good idea to visit your doctor if you suspect you're anemic.

To get more iron in your diet, try meat for starters. The darker the cut, the more iron it has. If you're a vegetarian, stick with legumes, fortified cereals, quinoa, kale, and other green leafy vegetables. And it's a good idea to top these foods with a rich source of vitamin C, like lemon juice. The vitamin C will help your body absorb the iron.

**Selenium.** You probably heard selenium fights cancer, but you might not know the mineral banishes bad moods, too. People who don't eat enough selenium-rich foods tend to be grumpier than people with a high dietary intake, according to recent research. Eat some high-test selenium foods — like seafood, poultry, mushrooms, sea vegetables, and wheat — and feel the effects for yourself.

**Carbohydrates.** If stress gets you down, a diet rich in carbohydrates might be just what the doctor ordered. Eating mostly carbohydrates during the day, suggests a recent European study, may make stressful situations more bearable for some people. The scientists fed people either a diet high in carbs and low in protein, or vice versa. Then the doctors put the subjects through a difficult mathematical task. The carbohydrate-rich diet worked to lower stress and depression in some of the subjects.

The carbohydrate diet appears to work by raising the level of tryptophan in your brain. Tryptophan is the amino acid your body needs to make serotonin, the "happy" neurotransmitter.

It's important to remember not all carbohydrates are equal. Nutritionally speaking, carbohydrates from fruits, vegetables, and whole grains and cereals are best. They'll save you from stress and boost your levels of vitamins, minerals, and fiber.

**Omega-3 fatty acids.** Don't be offended if someone calls you a fathead. You're in good company. Albert Einstein, Thomas Edison, Sir Isaac Newton, and Confucius can be called fatheads, too. That's because fat makes up about 60 percent of the human brain. But you do have a choice over what type of fathead you want to be. You can keep your brain running smoothly with the right kinds of fats or you can gum up the works with too much of the wrong kind. It all depends on what you eat.

Sound fishy? As a matter of fact, it is. The essential fats found in seafood, called omega-3 fatty acids, play a major role in brain function. They may even boost your mood. You need them but can't make them on your own. "Essential fatty acids only appear through your diet," says Dr. William Lands of the National Institutes of Health.

That means next time you're feeling blue, dip into the deep blue sea for your dinner. New medical evidence suggests the omega-3 fatty acids found in fish — called docosahexaenoic acid (DHA) and eicosapentaenoic acid (EPA) — can help drive away depression.

Dr. Andrew Stoll, a Harvard psychiatrist, found that fish oil capsules helped people with bipolar disorder, or manic depression, who go through periods of extreme highs and lows. He says, "The striking difference in relapse rates and response appeared to be highly clinically significant." Stoll suggests the omega-3 fatty acid in fish oil may slow down neurons in your brain, much like the drug Lithium, which is used to treat manic depression.

Another research group from England noticed depressed people had less omega-3 fatty acids in their red blood cells than healthy people. The more severe the depression, the less omega-3.

There is even evidence that EPA can help treat people with schizophrenia, a serious mental illness that can cause delusions, hallucinations, and disorganized behavior.

Some experts believe fish fights depression because neurotransmitters, the brain's Pony Express riders that carry messages from cell to cell, have an easier time wriggling through fat membranes made of fluid omega-3 than any other kind of fat. This means your brain's important messages get delivered.

Fish also has an effect on serotonin levels, one of your brain's good-news messengers. If you don't have enough serotonin, you're more likely to be depressed, violent, and suicidal. If you have low levels of DHA, you also have low levels of serotonin. More DHA means more serotonin.

Most antidepressants, including Prozac, raise brain levels of serotonin. You might be doing the same thing just by eating fish. In other words, gills may be as good as pills.

Whether you're depressed or not, work more omega-3 into your diet and perhaps cut down on omega-6, another type of essential fatty acid found in vegetable oils, meat, milk, and eggs.

Right now, the typical American eats at least 10 times more omega-6 than omega-3, or a ratio of 10-to-1. Some diets push that ratio to 25-to-1 or even higher. Eating fewer fruits, vegetables, and fish and more grain, farm-raised meat, and processed foods, puts the omega-6 to omega-3 ratio out of whack.

Not that omega-6 is bad, but too much leads to excess signaling in your brain. Fortunately, omega-3 can help stop the crazy antics of omega-6 and bring things back to normal.

So, to fix your balance of omega-6 and omega-3, the obvious first step is to eat more fish. Fatty fish, like salmon, herring, mackerel, and tuna, offer the most omega-3, but all seafood contains at least some. Aim for at least two fatty fish meals per week.

If you're an absolute landlubber who can't stand fish, get some omega-3's from flaxseed; walnuts; and collard, turnip, and mustard greens. Other good sources include dark green, leafy vegetables like spinach, arugula, kale, Swiss chard, and certain types of lettuce.

Remember though, the omega-3 in these foods is in the form of alpha-linolenic acid, which the brain can convert to DHA only in small amounts. To get the good stuff your brain prefers — the pre-formed DHA and EPA — you still need to eat fish.

You can take fish oil supplements, which are available in health food stores, pharmacies, and supermarkets. Just one caution — if you're taking blood thinners, check with your doctor before taking supplements since omega-3 also has blood-thinning effects.

Just as important to your fatty acid balance are the things not to eat, namely soybean and corn oils, both much too high in omega-6 and too low in omega-3. Eliminate all deep-fried foods and margarine and salad dressings that contain corn or soybean oil. Canola oil, which has a more favorable 2-to-1 ratio of omega-6 to omega-3, or olive oil, a monounsaturated oil with the least amount of omega-6, can do wonders for your essential fatty acid balance.

It all boils down to this — what type of fat you eat determines how your brain works. Moreover, your food determines your mood. Just by getting more omega-3 and less omega-6 into your diet, you can put your brain, and your spirits, in high gear. And that's no fish story.

# Diabetes

· · · · · · · · · · · · · · · · ·

| Eat | |
|---|---|
| High-fiber cereal | Oatmeal |
| Raisins | Figs |
| Vinegar | Beans |
| Peanut butter | Cornstarch |
| Oranges | Liver |
| | Tuna |
| | Grapefruit |
| **Avoid** | |
| High-glycemic foods, such as candy and refined grains | |

Diet has changed a [      ] 0 years. Instead of eating [      ] bles from old McDon [      ] more likely to drive through McDonald's for a high-fat, low-fiber meal with way too many calories. You have much more to choose from than your ancestors did, but many of those choices are unhealthy. Today's typical diet will make you overweight, but its lack of fiber-rich carbohydrates can make you feel hungry soon after eating. Worst of all, it can put you at risk for diabetes and heart disease.

Diabetes has become an epidemic in modern countries. About 16 million Americans have this blood sugar disorder that is divided into two categories — type 1 and type 2. Type 1, an autoimmune disease, usually attacks people under the age of 30 and has nothing to do with being overweight. But type 2, formerly called non-insulin-dependent, accounts for 90 to 95 percent of all cases. This form of diabetes stalks overweight, inactive people. Once a disease of the elderly, type 2 diabetes now appears even in overweight children.

If you have this type of diabetes, your body probably makes enough insulin but has "forgotten" how to use it. Your cells have become resistant to insulin so the glucose from the food you eat builds up in your blood instead of nourishing your cells. And high blood-sugar levels can start an avalanche of other medical problems including high cholesterol and high blood pressure. Type 2 diabetics risk blindness, amputations, heart disease, strokes, and nerve damage. And just because it's called "non-insulin-dependent" doesn't mean you'll never need insulin. Many people require insulin after several years with the disease.

If you want to avoid being diabetes' next victim, you'll have to rethink your diet. Healthy food choices can keep both your weight and blood sugar down. And regular exercise like brisk walking will go a long way toward keeping you fit. Even if you already have diabetes, a sensible diet can keep you from developing more health problems. Just make sure you check with your doctor before making any changes to your diet or exercise program.

## Nutritional blockbusters that fight diabetes

**High-fiber foods.** Fiber helps prevent diabetes because it slows down the process of converting carbohydrates into glucose, says Diana H. Noren, R.D., a certified diabetes counselor in Georgia. Also, if you eat a high-fiber carbohydrate, your body will respond with less insulin than it would if you eat a low-fiber food, she says. This is better for your overall health because high insulin levels could lead to weight gain and high blood pressure, among other problems.

In a study of nearly 36,000 older women in Iowa, the ones who ate several daily servings of high-fiber foods had a significantly lower risk of developing diabetes than women who ate little fiber.

Cereals are especially good at warding off diabetes. The women in the study who ate more than 7.5 grams of cereal fiber per day were 36 percent less likely to become diabetic than women who ate less than half that amount. And 7.5 grams is not a lot of fiber. A 1-ounce serving of bran flakes for breakfast will supply you with more than 8 grams of cereal fiber. Noren says you can actually eat a little more of a cereal that's high in fiber without harming your total carbohydrate count.

Fibrous foods that will help control your diabetes include:

◆ **Oats.** A good source of cereal fiber, oats contain a substance called beta glucan that breaks down slowly in your digestive tract. And longer digestion time means lower blood sugar for you. Start your day with a bowl of old-fashioned oatmeal flavored with a handful of raisins.

◆ **Legumes.** Use legumes in soups and casseroles, and cut back on meat. You'll lower your fat intake and increase your fiber at the same time. Legumes can fill you up and keep you satisfied.

◆ **Figs.** The American Diabetes Association recommends figs for a high-fiber treat that can satisfy your sweet tooth, too.

**Cornstarch.** More than just a thickener for gravy, cornstarch may help control blood-sugar levels and keep you from having an attack of hypoglycemia. This starch is digested and absorbed slowly so it's especially effective for type-1 diabetics prone to low blood-glucose levels overnight.

Researchers found that diabetics who drank a mixture of uncooked cornstarch dissolved in a non-sugary drink, such as milk or sugar-free soda, had fewer problems with low blood sugar when they woke up in the morning. If you have this problem, talk to your doctor about trying this natural solution.

You can also look for snack bars that contain sucrose, protein, and cornstarch. These ingredients release glucose at different speeds, giving you both immediate and long-term help for low blood sugar.

**Omega-3 fatty acids.** These essential fats all but disappeared when food became mass-produced. Most of the oils used today — corn, peanut, sesame, and safflower — are high in omega-6 fatty acids. These are also essential for good health, but if eaten without omega-3s, your immune system can start to break down. Researchers have shown that you need omega-3 fats to process insulin. Without them, you run the risk of not using your insulin properly. And insulin resistance is often the first stop on the road to diabetes.

You can find omega-3s in fatty fish like salmon and mackerel, along with walnuts and flaxseed. And inexpensive canola oil has a good blend of both omega-3 and omega-6 fats. Try eating fatty fish three times a week, and use canola oil for cooking. You can top salads with flaxseed oil, but you can't cook with it.

**Cod liver oil.** One oil that has high amounts of omega-3s is cod liver oil. Norwegians eat lots of it because they have so little sunlight, and they need the vitamin D found in the oil. A recent study in that country revealed that women who took cod liver oil during pregnancy reduced their child's risk of type 1 diabetes by more than 60 percent. Researchers think the

> ### When to ban peas and potatoes
>
> The long-held belief that sugary foods cause the biggest boost in blood sugar turns out to be untrue. Refined starches like finely milled breads are the biggest culprits. Even some innocent looking, natural foods like baked potatoes can make blood sugar jump. That's because they have a high glycemic index — a measure of how a food affects your blood sugar.
>
> But not everyone has the same response to every food so it's important to figure out your own glycemic index, says Dietician Diana Noren.
>
> "If I eat potatoes, and one-and-a-half hours later I test my blood sugar and it's in a fairly good range, then I know potatoes are OK for me," she says. "But if every time I eat peas my blood sugar goes way out of control, then I know I'm reacting to them and have a high index for that food."
>
> To keep your diabetes in line, fill up on typically low-glycemic foods such as coarsely ground whole-wheat breads; pastas made from durum wheat; long-grain and Basmati rice; lentils; and legumes.

omega-3 fats and vitamin D, either separately or combined, might be responsible for the lower risk.

**Vinegar.** Add red wine vinegar to your salads, and you can easily slow down the digestion of your meal. Because acidic foods are digested slowly, three teaspoons of vinegar can lower your blood sugar after a meal by as much as 30 percent. Lemon juice works well, too. Try squeezing a fresh lemon into water for a refreshing and healthful drink.

**Chromium.** Research shows that not getting enough chromium in your diet can make diabetes worse. That's because chromium helps your body process sugar. In the United States, people eat an average of 6 to 20 micrograms (mcg) of this essential element. But you should be eating 50 mcg per day. Good sources include liver, whole grains, cheeses, and nuts.

**Biotin.** This B-vitamin helps you digest fats and carbohydrates — important for diabetics. A deficiency can cause hair loss, a red rash, loss of appetite, depression, and a swollen tongue. But biotin is easy to get in a healthy diet. Good sources are peanut butter, liver, eggs, cereals, nuts, and legumes.

**Vitamin C**. Add an orange or grapefruit to your lunch. Research shows the antioxidants in vitamin C could keep you from developing problems with blood sugar. And if you already have diabetes, the acid in the fruit helps slow digestion, keeping your blood sugar more stable.

### A word of caution

Giving babies solid food or cow's milk before the age of four months can trigger type 1 diabetes. Researchers believe many children could avoid diabetes by drinking only mother's milk — or formula, if necessary — for at least four months.

# Diarrhea

• • • • • • • • • • • • • • •

| Eat | |
|---|---|
| Yogurt | Cinnamon |
| Broth | Rice |
| Bananas | Custard |
| Applesauce | Toast |
| Crackers | Water |

**Avoid**

Gas-producing foods
High-fiber foods
Milk products
Artificial sweetners

Everything you eat or drink seems to run through your system at breakneck speed when you have diarrhea.

The average adult has about four bouts of diarrhea every year. It usually lasts a couple of days, and then goes away on its own. If your diarrhea lasts longer, or if you have frequent bouts, it could be a sign of another problem.

Diarrhea can cause dehydration because your body loses body fluids very quickly. And because food passes through your intestines so fast, your bloodstream doesn't have time to absorb vitamins and minerals.

If your diarrhea lasts more than 48 hours, see a doctor to avoid complications from dehydration. For ordinary diarrhea, a few nutritional strategies will help you recover quickly and easily.

## Nutritional blockbusters that fight diarrhea

**Water.** Since dehydration is one of the greatest dangers of diarrhea, make sure you drink plenty of water. This means downing at least eight to 10 glasses of liquid each day. Water isn't the only fluid that helps. Broths and herbal teas are also good choices.

**Electrolytes.** While water is extremely important in battling dehydration, it doesn't contain electrolytes, which you also lose when you become dehydrated. Electrolytes are salts and minerals — such as potassium, sodium, calcium, and magnesium — normally found in your blood, tissue fluids, and cells. Loss of electrolytes can cause serious problems.

You can buy water with added electrolytes, or you can try an inexpensive method used in underdeveloped countries to battle diarrhea — drink the cooled water left in the pot after cooking rice. This liquid contains a lot of nutrients left from the boiled rice.

**Yogurt.** Bacteria are often the culprits that cause diarrhea, but you also have good bacteria in your digestive system. Acidophilus is a natural, "friendly" bacteria in your intestines. Sometimes, a poor diet or a course of antibiotics can affect how much acidophilus is active in your colon. If you have too little, you could suffer from digestive problems, including diarrhea. Eating yogurt containing active acidophilus cultures can help restore the balance of good and bad bacteria and ease your diarrhea.

**Cinnamon.** You may want to avoid spicy foods when you have diarrhea, but cinnamon could be an exception. Cinnamon can kill *E. coli* , a bacteria that causes severe diarrhea. In a recent study, cinnamon added to apple juice infected with *E. coli* destroyed more than 99 percent of the bacteria after three days at room temperature.

---

### A word of caution

Sorbitol, an artificial sweetener found in many sugar-free candies, chewing gums, and dietetic foods, might be causing your diarrhea. For some people, even small amounts of this sweetener can cause bloating and gas. Larger amounts can cause cramping and diarrhea.

If you are sensitive to Sorbitol, make sure you read labels before buying vitamin supplements and over-the-counter drugs. And ask your pharmacist if it's an ingredient in your prescription medications.

| Eat | |
|------|------|
| Whole grains | Brown rice |
| Oranges | Water |
| Collard greens | Lima beans |
| | Black beans |
| Kale | Blueberries |
| Apples | Broccoli |

| Avoid |
|-------|
| Red meat |
| White bread and pastries |
| Processed foods |

# Diverticular disease

· · · · · · · · · · · · · · ·

Diverticula are small pouches that can form in your intestinal wall. When you put too much pressure on your intestines, like when you're straining because of constipation, it weakens the wall and forms small, sac-like projections. It's a little like stretching part of a balloon before blowing it up. When you put air in it, the stretched part will form an extra pouch. Once this happens, you have what approximately one-third of the population over 45 in North America has — diverticulosis.

Like many people, you might have diverticulosis and not know it. The pouches are usually painless until bits of food get stuck in them. When this happens, little colonies of bacteria can form and lead to an infection. Called diverticulitis, this painful condition causes fever and severe pain, usually in your lower left abdomen. If you have these symptoms, see a doctor immediately. The infection could make a hole in your intestinal wall, requiring emergency surgery.

Some doctors and nutritionists think diverticulosis can be avoided by eating foods high in fiber, like fruits, vegetables, and whole grains. And even if you already have the little pouches, you can avoid infection by eating lots of fiber to keep your digestive system squeaky clean.

The late Dr. Denis Burkitt, a surgeon known for his research on fiber, called diverticular disease a "pressure disease." He blamed chronic constipation on diets high in refined foods and low in fiber.

"Diverticular disease," he once said, "is a disease of Western culture, almost unknown in the third world. Even in a relatively advanced city like New Delhi ... I found they had seen only eight cases of diverticular disease in 13 years. In Britain it is estimated that it is present in one in three adults over 60."

Why do so many people in industrialized countries get this disease while people in less developed countries don't? The answer is simple — diet. If you want to avoid diverticular disease, you'll have to forego white breads, pastries, and processed foods, and switch to a diet high in fiber.

## Nutritional blockbusters that fight diverticular disease

**Whole grains.** Trade in your white bread for whole grains, like whole wheat and rye and brown rice instead of white. It might take a while to get used to the heavier texture and nutty taste of these foods, but after a while, white bread and white rice will taste bland by comparison. Try replacing a hunk of red meat and a side of rice or potatoes with grains flavored with small amounts of meat. You can make brown rice casseroles, pilafs, and even whole-wheat pasta. Just be sure to add extra fiber gradually so your body can adjust to it. Otherwise, you might have uncomfortable gas and bloating.

**Fruits, vegetables, and legumes.** Whole fruits and vegetables give you a bonus that you don't get from juice — fiber. An orange will help your digestive tract a lot more than a glass of orange juice, even though both are nutritious. You can also use blueberries, raspberries and blackberries as a topping on cereal or yogurt for a morning or after-dinner treat.

Don't forget your greens. Green leafy vegetables and legumes are super sources of plant fiber. Try lima beans, black beans, spinach, romaine lettuce, escarole, collard greens, mustard greens, and kale. And lightly steamed or raw vegetables will do your colon more good than soggy, overcooked ones. So skip the mushy, canned vegetables whenever you can eat fresh produce. Your colon will thank you.

---

### A word of caution

Beef up your diet with chicken and fish and steer clear of red meats. Researchers think eating a lot of red meat might lead to diverticular disease because red meat creates unfriendly bacteria as it breaks down in your intestines. This can weaken the walls of your colon, making it easier for diverticula to form. In addition, the fat in red meat — unlike other kinds of fat — has been linked to diverticular disease.

---

**Water.** Many people are chronically dehydrated and don't even know it. If you always tend toward constipation, even when you eat a lot of fiber-rich foods, you might need more water. The old rule of drinking six to eight glasses of water daily still makes sense. Drinking lots of water should make your stools softer and decrease the chances that you'll develop diverticula. And if you already have the little pouches, extra water can help fiber flush out bits of food that could cause problems.

It's especially important to drink plenty of water if you add more fiber to your diet. If you don't, you could end up with a blockage in your intestines — something far worse than constipation.

### Benefits

Lowers cholesterol

Helps stop strokes

Controls blood pressure

Promotes weight loss

Battles diabetes

Combats cancer

# Figs

· · · · · · · ·

In the Garden of Eden, Adam and Eve used fig leaves for clothing. Fashions have changed a lot since then, but figs have never gone out of style.

These sweet fruits were mentioned in writings as far back as 3000 B.C. Cleopatra and the prophet Mohammed both enjoyed figs and the Roman writer Pliny the Elder praised them for their power to get rid of wrinkles. Today, you can find figs in a variety of forms, including the popular Fig Newton cookie — a healthy alternative to most desserts.

When you get down to it, figs mean fiber. Pound for pound, figs pack more of this precious stuff than any other fruit or vegetable. Five figs, fresh or dried, give you a whopping 9 grams of fiber, more than a third of the recommended dietary allowance. Besides fiber, figs are loaded with minerals and nutrients to help fend off heart disease, cancer, constipation, and even diabetes.

Plus, figs taste great. These chewy treats, sometimes called "inside-out strawberries," contain tiny, edible seeds. Bite into a deliciously healthy fig, and you'll feel just a little bit closer to paradise.

## 8 ways figs keep you healthy

**Cuts cholesterol.** "If you eat a lot of fiber, you will have a better cholesterol level," says Dr. Joe Vinson, chemistry professor at the University of Scranton in Pennsylvania and an expert on figs. The bottom line is lowering artery-clogging cholesterol lowers your risk of heart disease.

Figs also contain lots of polyphenols, plant compounds that act as antioxidants. Polyphenols stop low-density lipoprotein (LDL or "bad") cholesterol from oxidizing then building up in your arteries and they keep your blood from becoming sticky and clumping together.

**Saves you from strokes.** The triple punch of fiber, potassium, and magnesium in figs means extra protection from stroke, especially if you have high blood pressure. Even though fewer people are suffering from strokes these days — thanks to better treatments for hypertension — strokes still cause one out of every 15 deaths. Experts agree, more nutrient-rich fruits and vegetables should be your first line of defense.

**Halts high blood pressure.** Because they provide potassium and calcium, experts recommend figs for people with high blood pressure. Both minerals, in combination with eating less sodium, keep your blood pressure under control.

**Manages weight.** Remember fiber can help you lose weight, which will not only shrink your waistline but your risk of heart disease and other health problems, too. "Figs are very filling," Vinson explains, "so you'd decrease your consumption of other things if you ate more figs They're not super-high in calories or fat, either." You'll get just 48 calories and almost no fat in every dried fig.

**Deals with diabetes.** If you're worried about high blood sugar but still want a tasty treat, look no further than the fig.

"Figs are not a high-carbohydrate food," says Vinson, "so they would be typically a good thing for someone who has diabetes to consume. And fiber will lower your glucose." Keep in mind, fiber slows the amount of glucose your body absorbs from your small intestines.

The evidence backs Vinson up, too. A recent study found that a high-fiber diet — 50 grams per day — helped keep blood sugar, insulin, and cholesterol under control in people with diabetes.

Eating chewy, delicious figs is a terrifically tasty way to get more fiber. In fact, the American Diabetes Association suggests recipes that include figs.

**Guards against cancer.** When you make figs part of your diet, you also welcome a host of polyphenols, those naturally occurring plant chemicals that act as antioxidants. These crusaders go after the free radicals that can damage your body and cause cancer. That's one reason nearly every major health organization encourages you to eat more fruits and vegetables.

"If you get more antioxidants into your body, you'll be better off," Vinson says. "As you age, there's more and more damage to the cells and organs of your body as a result of constant bombardment from these free radicals."

Of course, figs' large helping of fiber also protects you from cancer, especially colon cancer. In a 25-year study, adding 10 grams of fiber — roughly six figs — to a daily diet slashed the risk of dying from colon cancer by 33 percent.

Other possible anti-cancer agents found in figs include substances called coumarins, studied for treating skin and prostate cancers, and benzaldehyde, which might have anti-tumor powers.

**Combats kidney stones.** If you have kidney stones, you probably know oxalate is an enemy. This substance, found in foods like spinach, tomatoes, cranberries, rhubarb, peanuts, coffee, tea, and chocolate, may cause this painful condition.

But another nutrient, calcium, is really on your side. When you eat high-calcium foods with high-oxalate foods, the calcium keeps your body from absorbing the oxalate. This makes you less likely to form oxalate-based kidney stones. However, don't load up on calcium supplements — you might actually increase your risk of calcium-based kidney stones. Your best bet is to get calcium through whole foods. Eating 10 dried figs gives you 33 percent of the recommended dietary allowance (RDA) of calcium.

Stave off kidney stones as well with the plentiful potassium in dried figs. Low potassium means a higher risk of forming stones. Ten dried figs provides more than half your daily needs.

**Foils constipation.** The main advantage of eating figs is still their astonishingly high fiber content.

"That seems to be what's unusual about them relative to other foods," says Vinson. "That's good because fiber can improve the digestive tract. It has a laxative effect on people and speeds up the movement through the digestive tract."

So say hello to figs and goodbye to irregularity.

## A word of caution

If you have rosacea, a condition that makes your nose and cheeks red and bumpy, you might want to avoid figs. They contain histamine which causes flushing and can further irritate your skin. If you just can't say no to these sweet little treats, try taking an antihistamine about two hours before you eat any figs.

Figs can also cause high blood pressure, headaches, and neck pain if you're taking a certain type of antidepressant called a monoamine oxidase (MAO) inhibitor. Certain liver enzymes usually destroy a substance in figs called tyramine. However, MAO inhibitors reduce these enzymes allowing tyramine to build up to dangerous levels in your body. See your doctor if you experience any of these symptoms.

## Pantry pointers

Figs are usually sold dried, but you can also find them fresh from June to October. Refrigerate fresh figs and try to eat them within two to three days because they go bad quickly. Figs can be round or oval and come in a range of colors from dark purple to nearly white.

Besides fresh or dried, you can find candied or canned figs. In health food stores, you can even buy fig concentrate, a seedless purée used to flavor desserts or as an ice cream topping. Eat figs as a snack, add them to dishes, or bake with them.

### Benefits

Combats cancer

Protects your heart

Supports immune system

Boosts memory

Eases arthritis

# Fish

· · · · · · · ·

Mothers everywhere used to dose their families with cod liver oil for good health. That oil might have left a bad taste in your mouth, but, as usual, your mother was right. Fish oil really can keep you healthy.

Fish is an excellent source of omega-3 fatty acids — something your body needs but can't make by itself. You can only get these fats in food, along with equally important omega-6 fatty acids. Nutritionists now know that a balance of these two fatty acids can protect you from heart disease, arthritis, mental illness, and a host of other medical problems.

How can you balance your diet? You won't have any problem finding omega-6. There's plenty of it in crackers, cookies, baked goods, salad dressing, and fried foods. You name it — if it's got oil in it, it's probably omega-6. The problem, though, is getting enough omega-3. These fats are found mostly in fish and green leafy vegetables — foods that you probably don't eat quite as heartily as the omega-6 foods. And food companies usually don't use omega-3 fats in their products because they tend to spoil fast.

But there's no need to flounder on the shores of poor health when you can dive into the sea for nutritious meals.

## 5 ways fish keeps you healthy

**Keeps cancer at bay.** The antioxidant powers of fatty fish come from a substance called astaxanthin. This antioxidant hunts down and destroys free radicals that might damage cells in your body. When animals with lymphoma, a type of cancer, were given fish oil and the amino acid arginine, they lived longer and had longer periods without the disease than animals who were not treated. In addition, researchers have found that omega-3 can slow the growth of cancers — the exact opposite of what they found for omega-6, which can help cancers grow.

But astaxanthin does even more. Studies show it can protect you from skin cancer, too. The pinkish color of a salmon and the reddish hue of a lobster come from astaxanthin — a natural protector against the sun's harmful ultraviolet rays. Since skin cancer has been linked to sunburns, it makes sense to protect yourself as much as possible. When mice were fed astaxanthin in their diets, then exposed to ultraviolet radiation — similar to the rays of the sun — their skin was less damaged than mice that weren't fed the antioxidant.

An added bonus of eating lots of fatty fish is healthier looking skin. If your skin is dry and rough, it could be a sign that you need more oil. Eating foods with omega-3 fats should give your skin a healthy sheen.

More research needs to be done, but all signs indicate fish is a winner in the fight against cancer.

**Helps your heart.** Studies show that fish oil keeps your blood from sticking together, keeps your veins open, and helps your heart to beat regularly. Keeping veins open and blood flowing easily is important in preventing heart attacks and strokes. In a 20-year study of more than 2,000 men from seven European countries, researchers found that regularly eating fatty fish like salmon and mackerel can protect you from heart disease. Eating lean fish such as flounder or haddock won't give you the same protection.

In a recent long-term study involving more than 20,000 doctors, those who ate at least one fish meal a week were half as likely to die suddenly of a heart attack as those who ate less than one serving of fish per month. And when a group of post-menopausal women were given eight fish-oil capsules a day for a month, they had much lower cholesterol levels. This is good news for women since heart disease is the leading cause of death in post-menopausal women.

**Tames your immune system.** If you have arthritis, multiple sclerosis, or asthma, you may have an immune system that's turned on you. Instead of going after germs like it should, it's busy attacking your body as though it were the enemy. But fish could help you get your immune system back on your side.

Dr. Artemis P. Simopoulos, author of *The Omega Diet,* thinks omega-3 fats are directly related to autoimmune disorders. "We now know omega-3 fatty acids can apply the brakes to an immune system that has gotten out of control," she says.

Research shows fish oil may do this by blocking an enzyme in your body that causes inflammation. This may be why arthritis sufferers who took fish oil supplements found their joints were less stiff in the morning. Fish oil also helped a group of people with the autoimmune disorder multiple sclerosis. They had fewer and less severe attacks when they added it to their diets along with omega-6 fats.

Asthma, which affects more and more children every year, is another autoimmune condition. Some researchers think the high amounts of omega-6 fats children eat are partially to blame. But researchers noticed that children who eat fish a couple times a week are less likely to have asthma. It's not clear, however, whether fish can help adults with asthma.

**Slows kidney disease.** Fish oil may be a tonic to your kidneys. When 55 people with a serious kidney disease called IgA nephropathy took fish oil over a two-year period, their kidney disease slowed down. In a follow-up study, researchers also gave fish oil to the group previously taking a placebo, and after six years found their disease had stabilized as much as those in the long-term fish oil group.

**Blankets your brain.** If you've heard that fish is brain food, you heard right. Researchers have found that breast-fed babies have higher intelligence than bottle-fed babies, probably because of the omega-3 found in mother's milk. And it doesn't help just babies. A study showed that older men who ate fish regularly had better working brains than men who didn't eat fish.

Fish oil even helped migraine sufferers have fewer and less severe headaches. And there is strong evidence that omega-3 fats can help with a host of mental illnesses including depression, mood disorders, and even schizophrenia. (See the *Depression* chapter.) Some doctors even think the epidemic amounts of mental illness in modern societies can be traced back to the omega imbalance in the food supply.

## A word of caution

Be sure to eat a variety of foods with vitamins A, C, and E if you eat lots of fatty fish. Some studies suggest that eating fish reduces the amount of these antioxidants available to you. This isn't bad, though, since it means the fish oils are working to protect your cells — they just need help doing it.

There is some evidence that eating lots of fatty fish without a well-balanced diet could be worse than no fish at all because you'll deplete your reserves of vitamins, which can lead to disease.

## Pantry pointers

Salmon, mackerel, tuna, pacific herring, anchovy, and bluefish are all good sources of omega-3. The flesh of the fish should be firm and not smell too strong. Fresh fish kept in the refrigerator should be used within a few days.

You can grill most of these fish with a light marinade of olive oil, salt, pepper, and garlic. Fish cooks quickly, so grill no more than 15 minutes for each inch of thickness. When done, fish should flake apart easily with a fork.

### Benefits

Aids digestion

Eases arthritis pain

Protects your heart

Battles diabetes

Improves mental health

Boosts your immune system

# Flax

People used to eat foods with about a 50/50 balance of both fatty acids your body needs — omega-3 and omega-6. But that was before food became mass produced. Since omega-3 fats go bad quickly, food manufacturers replaced them with longer lasting omega-6 fats and hydrogenated oils — oils with hydrogen added to make them more stable. Now food companies don't have to worry about their products spoiling too soon. But you have to worry about not getting enough omega-3 and possibly getting too much omega-6.

Where can you find the omega-3 fats you need? Fatty fish is a good source. But if you're like most people, you can only eat so much fish before you start feeling like Flipper. Luckily, you have another option.

Flax is an herb that is high in omega-3, which is unusual for a plant. You might know it by the name linseed, because it's the plant linen is made from. For thousands of years, certain types of the flax plant have been grown for the edible seeds and the oil that can be pressed from them. But don't confuse this edible oil with linseed oil for wood, which is made from a different variety of the plant.

Some doctors think the epidemic of heart disease, high blood pressure, inflammatory disorders, mental illnesses, and even cancer in modern societies can be traced back to imbalances in essential fatty acids. (See the *Depression* chapter.) Artemis P. Simopoulos, M.D., has spent decades studying how nutrition affects health. In her book *The Omega Diet,* Simopoulos explains why you should add omega-3 fats back to your diet.

"One of the most important findings to come out of the research program," she says, "is that our bodies function most efficiently when we eat fats that contain a balanced ratio of the two families of essential fatty acids — omega-6 and omega-3 fatty acids. The ratio in the typical American diet has been estimated to be as high as 20 to 1."

But you can fight back. You can cut down on omega-6 fats by avoiding fried foods and foods made with corn, cottonseed, and tropical oils. And you can boost your omega-3 intake by eating lots of fatty fish and using flaxseed oil on vegetables, salads, and in baking.

## 5 ways flax keeps you healthy

**Soothes your gastrointestinal tract.** As a rule, Eskimos don't get inflammatory bowel disease because of all the omega-3 they get from eating fish. Fish oil can help if you have trouble with an irritated bowel. But you might not like the fishy aftertaste, burping, and bad breath that comes with it. In many studies, people who were given fish oil capsules stopped taking them because of these side effects.

But flaxseed oil, with its mild flavor, can give you the same benefits of fish oil. So if you can't bring yourself to eat one more serving of fish, why not add this oil to a salad of dark green, leafy vegetables? You'll boost your omega-3 intake and soothe your intestines at the same time.

**Chases away arthritis pain.** If you were born in Japan, chances are you would never get arthritis. What protects this population? The same substance that keeps Eskimos healthy — omega-3. Having the right balance of fatty acids in your body can protect your immune system from breaking down and causing diseases like arthritis.

Dr. Donald Rudin, a Harvard-trained physician and medical researcher, believes immune disorders can often be traced to out-of-balance omegas in your body. He explains the effect of fatty acids on the immune system in his book *Omega-3 Oils: A Practical Guide.*

"Normally, the immune system is kept under control by the body's essential fatty acid-based regulatory system," he says. "But dietary distortions, especially a shortage of the omega-3 fatty acids, are now known to contribute to — or even prompt — the breakdown of the immune system."

Rudin recommends one tablespoon of flaxseed oil per day for a 100-pound person who is deficient in omega-3. He also suggests you take a multivitamin. If you have food allergies, though, you should start with less oil and gradually add more. But don't overdo it. Taking more than six tablespoons daily might actually make your symptoms worse.

**Shields your heart.** Omega-3 fats contain alpha linolenic acid (ALA), an ingredient that should be near and dear to your heart. Eating ALA-rich foods like flax can make your blood less sticky, which keeps it from clotting too fast and causing a blockage. It also helps keep your blood pressure down and your heart beating regularly.

The people who live on the island of Kohama, Japan have the longest life expectancy in the world and the lowest rate of heart disease. They also have very high levels of ALA in their blood. Coincidence? Scientists think not.

Experts suggest you eat about four fatty fish meals a week and use a vegetable oil high in ALA like canola or flaxseed oil.

**Dethrones diabetes.** If diabetes runs in your family, and you eat a typical modern-day diet, your chances of getting this blood sugar disorder are high.

But who says you have to? Researchers are finding that diet is as closely linked to diabetes as family history. It seems the more omega-6 fats you eat, the more likely you are to be overweight. You're also more likely to become resistant to insulin — a double whammy that sets you up for diabetes.

Omega-3 fats don't treat you so cruelly. In fact, they help you. When laboratory animals were fed a high omega-6 diet, no one was surprised when they got fat. But animals fed the same amount and calories of omega-3 fats weighed an amazing 33 percent less. That's the difference between a 150 and 225 pound person. Maybe you don't need to eat all that tasteless low-fat food to stay slim. Maybe you're just eating the wrong kind of fat.

Besides keeping you thin, this friendly oil also helps your blood sugar. When a group of people with insulin resistance were switched to omega-3 fats instead of omega-6, they got better. They had lower blood pressure, lower blood sugar, and less harmful fat floating in their blood.

**Calms a troubled mind.** Until about 100 years ago, many poor people got a disease called pellagra, which is Italian for "rough skin." Besides dry, rough skin, they had ringing in their ears, exhaustion, and mental problems. It took a long time for doctors to figure out that these people were missing vitamin B in their diets. When the vitamin was finally added to staple foods like rice, the disease became history. Or did it?

Pellagra may have returned in — of all places — wealthy countries where people eat highly processed foods. Sure, there's plenty of vitamin B in foods now, but your body also needs a certain amount of omega-3 acids to use vitamin B. So you could be well fed but malnourished. Some doctors think the high rates of mental illness wherever you find modern diets is proof of the connection.

> ### Scramble a healthier egg
>
> Here's an egg-ceptional way to get more omega-3 in your diet — crack an egg. Some chicken farmers are feeding their hens a special diet containing flaxseed. According to the Flax Council of Canada, these hens are laying eggs that look and taste the same, but contain eight to 10 times more omega-3 fatty acids than regular eggs. Look for "modified fat" eggs or ones labeled "omega-3 enriched."

When Rudin put several patients with mental illness on one to six tablespoons of flaxseed oil daily, most of them got noticeably better. His patients included people with manic depression, fear of open spaces, and even schizophrenia — a severe thought disorder. Some patients reported feeling calm for the first time in years.

## Pantry pointers

You can buy flax as seeds in most health food stores and in some grocery stores. Sprinkle them on baked goods, or add them to granola. For the most nutrition, grind the seeds with a coffee grinder and use them immediately. Flax meal is now also available in many health food stores. Store it in the refrigerator to keep it fresh.

You'll find flaxseed oil sold in brown, pint-size bottles in most health food stores. Check the expiration date to be sure it's fresh. Store it in the refrigerator and use it within two months. If it smells overly fishy, it's probably gone bad and you shouldn't use it. Flax oil will keep in the freezer without freezing for up to one year. You can use the oil on salads and on vegetables instead of butter.

Don't try to fry anything in flaxseed oil since it breaks down in very high heat and could even be harmful.

# Gallstones

· · · · · · · · · · · · · · · · · · · · ·

| Eat | |
| --- | --- |
| High-fiber cereal | Oranges |
| Cantaloupe | Sweet red peppers |
| Whole-wheat bread | Coffee |
| | Barley |
| **Avoid** | |
| Foods high in saturated fat, such as red meat | |
| Foods high in refined sugars, such as pastries | |

Horses never have gallstones because, like many animals, they don't have gallbladders. The gallbladder is an organ you can live without, too.

Your gallbladder stores bile, a digestive fluid made by the liver. Sometimes substances in your bile — usually cholesterol — crystallize into gallstones. Some stones don't cause any symptoms. They are called "silent" stones and don't require treatment.

When gallstones grow large or block any of the ducts that carry bile from the liver to the small intestine, they can set off intense pain in your right side or upper abdomen. The pain may also radiate to your right shoulder or between your shoulder blades. These symptoms, which frequently occur after eating or at night, are often mistaken for those of a heart attack, appendicitis, ulcers, or irritable bowel syndrome.

If any of the ducts remain blocked for a significant period of time, severe damage can occur to the gallbladder, liver, and the pancreas. Warning signs of a serious problem are constant pain, fever, and jaundice (a yellow tint of your skin or eyes). Treatment sometimes involves surgically removing the gallstones or the gallbladder. If the gallbladder is removed, bile flows out of the liver and goes directly into the small intestine.

Many health experts say you can avoid painful gallstones by changing your diet and lifestyle. A recent study at the University of Buffalo found that a typical Western lifestyle — too much saturated fat and refined sugar and too little exercise and fiber — increases your risk for gallstones. Lead author Maurizio Trevisan says, "This study confirms that gallbladder disease is one of the diseases of Western civilization. It is one more message that a diet high in fat and refined sugar and a pattern of low physical activity can get you into all kinds of trouble." And anyone who has experienced the pain of gallstones can tell you it is definitely trouble.

## Nutritional blockbusters that fight gallstones

**Fiber.** Fill up on fiber instead of fat, and you may protect yourself from gallbladder disease. Vegetarians are less likely to get gallstones, possibly because they eat less saturated fat and more fiber. Fiber increases movement of food through your colon, which could reduce the amount of bile acids in your gallbladder.

A high-fiber diet could also help reduce your risk of gallstones by helping to control your weight. Being overweight is a well-known risk factor for gallbladder disease.

**Caffeine.** If you can't get moving until you've had your second cup of coffee in the morning, you may be protecting yourself from the pain of gallstones. A recent study found that men who drank two to three cups of coffee every day were 40 percent less likely to develop painful stones than those who didn't drink coffee.

Results of a later study found that coffee did not protect against gallstones, yet it did reduce symptoms in women who already had them. Researchers think the caffeine in coffee might prevent symptoms of gallstones, but not the gallstones themselves.

**Vitamin C.** Women are the unlucky recipients of more than two-thirds of all gallstones. You may be able to change your luck if you eat foods high in vitamin C, like citrus fruits, sweet red peppers, green peppers, strawberries, and cantaloupe.

In a large study, researchers found that a high blood level of vitamin C was associated with a lower rate of gallbladder disease in women, but not in men.

Scientists think women may be more likely to develop gallstones because estrogen increases the amount of cholesterol in the bile. Since most gallstones are made of excess cholesterol, vitamin C may protect women because it helps convert cholesterol into bile acids.

---

### A word of caution

Sack the sugar and you might avoid gallstones. People who eat a lot of sugar are more likely to develop gallbladder disease. Researchers think it could be because sugar increases insulin production, which in turn increases cholesterol. And since most gallstones are made of cholesterol, anything that causes more cholesterol in your bile could increase your risk of developing stones.

One of the best ways to lower your cholesterol is to cut your intake of saturated fats. Foods high in saturated fats include meat, egg yolks, whole milk, butter, cheese, as well as a few vegetable fats like coconut oil, palm oil, and hydrogenated vegetable shortenings. Eating less saturated fat is good for your gallbladder and your heart.

Lowers cholesterol

Controls blood
 pressure

Combats cancer

Kills bacteria

Fights fungus

# Garlic

• • • • • • • • • •

Vampires must not be very healthy. Or very smart. Otherwise, they would gobble up garlic instead of fleeing from it.

Garlic has been appreciated for thousands of years for its healing powers as well as its flavor. The ancient Egyptian and Chinese cultures used the fragrant bulb as medicine. Slaves building the pyramids ate garlic to keep up their strength. Aristotle praised its medicinal powers. Roman warriors ate it to give them courage in battle. Even the Bible mentions garlic. During their long trek through the desert after leaving Egypt, the Israelites said garlic was one of the foods they missed.

Not only is garlic just as popular today, but scientific research proves eating garlic does indeed provide health benefits. In fact, garlic may protect you from just about everything from the common cold to heart disease and cancer. It might even help you live longer.

So what is it about garlic that makes it so special? Crush garlic and it produces a powerful, penicillin-like compound called allicin. Allicin, in turn, breaks down to create several sulfur compounds plus a substance called ajoene. These compounds, which give garlic its distinctive smell, fight the bulk of the battle against heart disease. In addition, garlic is chock-full of antioxidants that protect you from damaging free radicals and is a good source of selenium, an important trace element.

For its positive effects on the heart, experts recommend eating 4 grams of garlic, or about one clove, per day. But why stop at one clove? Pep up your food with garlic, and you're not just adding flavor, you're also unleashing a potent weapon in the crusade to stay healthy.

# 9 ways garlic keeps you healthy

**Attacks atherosclerosis.** Imagine trying to walk through thick, gooey mud. Now imagine that same mud oozing through a straw, and you get an idea of how cholesterol can damage your arteries.

As cholesterol builds up in your arteries, your heart has to work harder to pump blood through them. This leads to high blood pressure. High cholesterol and high blood pressure help trigger atherosclerosis, or thickening and hardening of the arteries — the leading cause of death in the Western world. In fact, heart attacks happen when one or more of the coronary arteries get too clogged or completely blocked.

By lowering cholesterol and your blood pressure, garlic protects your arteries from potential disaster. Garlic also slows the stiffening of arteries that happens with age. One study of healthy adults ages 50 to 80 found garlic helped keep the aorta, the body's main artery, elastic.

**Clobbers cholesterol.** Like a nutritional superhero, garlic goes after your bad LDL cholesterol without harming your good HDL cholesterol. The result is less fat built up in your arteries, lower triglyceride levels, and generally healthier circulation. Just a half to one clove of garlic a day (or an equal amount in supplements) may be all you need to decrease your cholesterol levels.

**Brings down blood pressure.** With less cholesterol causing traffic jams in your arteries, your blood can zip through your body more easily. That means less stress on your heart and lower blood pressure. Some studies show garlic can actually bring down your blood pressure by several points.

**Crushes clots.** Ajoene, along with garlic's other compounds, stops your blood from clumping and clotting. This keeps your blood flowing more smoothly and reduces your risk for a heart attack or stroke.

**Cripples cancer.** In China, researchers discovered people who ate a lot of garlic had fewer cases of cancer in the stomach and esophagus than those who didn't. It's probably not a coincidence.

Garlic's hard-working antioxidants, including its sulfur compounds, vitamin C, and flavonoids, capture free radicals and keep them from damaging your body and causing cancer. Allicin and its many sulfur compounds also order more of your body's mighty immune cells into battle. These tiny soldiers kill tumors and cancer cells.

Experts keep finding more evidence of garlic's cancer-fighting powers. A Penn State study demonstrated that garlic and selenium prevented breast cancer in animals exposed to a strong cancer-causing substance. Other studies have linked eating garlic with lower risks of colon, prostate, skin, bladder, and lung cancers.

**Banishes bacteria, viruses, and more.** When penicillin was scarce during World War II, Russian soldiers used garlic to fight off infection. War-time studies also showed that soldiers who ate garlic had fewer cases of dysentery than those who didn't.

That's because of allicin, a potent antibiotic that kills a variety of bacteria, viruses, fungi, molds, yeasts, and parasites. Some of garlic's victims include *H. pylori, Salmonella, staph, E. coli ,* and *Candida.* Allicin is so powerful that it appears to conquer some infections that normally stand up to antibiotics.

This is helpful to remember when cooking hamburgers or other ground beef dishes. If *E. coli* is present in undercooked meat, it can cause severe illness and even death. Researchers at Kansas State University recently discovered that adding 3 to 5 teaspoons of garlic powder to 2 pounds of ground beef helps protect you against *E. coli* poisoning.

**Intensifies your immune system.** Tired of blowing your nose? Reach for garlic instead of a box of tissues. Garlic boosts your immune system, so you're less likely to get sick with colds or flu. Once again, the sulfur compounds in garlic do the work by prodding your immune cells into action. Garlic also makes you sweat, which is one of your body's ways to get rid of waste.

**Stamps out blood sugar.** Worried about diabetes? Garlic also lowers your blood sugar. High blood sugar is a key symptom of diabetes. In fact, because garlic also lowers cholesterol and blood pressure, adding some to your diet might help if you're diabetic or at risk of developing diabetes.

**Rubs out rheumatoid arthritis.** If your body has low levels of antioxidants and selenium, you could be at greater risk for rheumatoid arthritis. Because garlic contains plenty of both, it can help stop this form of arthritis before it starts.

## Pantry pointers

When shopping for garlic, choose firm bulbs with white, papery skin. Avoid brown cloves. Do not store garlic in plastic bags, sealed containers or direct sunlight. If you keep garlic in a cool, dry place without too much humidity, it can last four to six months.

One odd but effective way to store garlic is the pantyhose method. Take a pair of pantyhose and cut off the legs. Drop a bulb of garlic into the toe and tie a knot above the bulb. Then drop in

### A note of caution

While garlic's ability to prevent your blood from clotting may help reduce the risk of a heart attack or stroke, it could be dangerous if you are taking warfarin or other blood-thinning medication. Check with your doctor before adding garlic to your diet.

Garlic has a few other unpleasant side effects. Too much garlic might give you heartburn, indigestion, or gas. After eating garlic, you'll also have "garlic breath," which might prevent you from getting too close to that special someone (or anyone, for that matter). Try chewing a sprig of parsley after a garlicky meal to mask the smell.

a second bulb and tie another knot. Keep doing this until you run out of room, then hang the leg in a dark, cool place. Every time you need a new bulb, just snip off a section of the pantyhose.

Garlic should be minced or crushed to make the most of its healing powers. There's some evidence that waiting 10 minutes between chopping and cooking preserves its powers better than if you cook it right away. Also, do not overcook it or you'll lessen its healing potential.

---

### Benefits

Neutralizes nausea

Combats cancer

Aids digestion

Tames arthritis pain

Enhances blood flow

Soothes heartburn

---

# Ginger

● ● ● ● ● ● ● ● ● ● ● ●

You probably think of ginger as just one more spice in the rack — only appearing for Chinese stir fries and Indian curries. But if you knew what else ginger was good for, you might use it a lot more.

Ginger makes your body healthier while it makes your food tastier. For thousands of years, it's been an herbal superstar. People from all over the world have relied on it to aid digestion, improve circulation, calm nausea, and soothe headaches and other pain. It works so well that one pound of it was once worth the price of a sheep.

Ginger is much cheaper nowadays, but it still works wonders on everyday ailments. Incredibly, ginger might also be a powerful weapon against more serious problems, like cancer and heart disease.

Now you know about them, take advantage of ginger's spicy powers more often. Toss some chopped ginger into a rice dish, or steep some in a pot of tea. Eat candied or pickled ginger by the handful, or take ginger supplements. Any way you slice it, ginger's just too good — and good for you — to pass up.

# 6 ways ginger keeps you healthy

**Calms your queasiness.** Researchers now know what Chinese sailors figured out thousands of years ago; ginger fights motion sickness without annoying side effects. It takes care of dizziness, nausea, and vomiting when you're in just about anything that bumps and shakes — a boat, plane, or car. By relaxing the nerves and muscles in your digestive tract, ginger promises one quiet ride.

In one of the latest studies on motion sickness, scientists followed almost 2,000 people on a whale safari. Out of the seven different sea sickness medicines used on the trip, ginger stood out like a champ. It worked as well as any of the heavy-duty drugs, but unlike them, ginger didn't make anyone drowsy.

Even though some doctors are big fans of ginger, others are not convinced. Just know that ginger might not work for everyone. To see if it helps you, pick up ginger supplements at any natural food store and take two 500-milligram (mg) pills about an hour before travel. If you still feel sick, take one or two more every four hours. You can also use candied or crystalized ginger. A piece 1 inch square and one-quarter inch thick is equal to a 500-mg pill. You can find candied ginger at most grocery stores or in Asian markets.

**Soothes other nausea, too.** Ginger doesn't stop with motion sickness, either. It may also prevent nausea from surgery, chemotherapy, and morning sickness. Just be sure and talk to your doctor before taking ginger and don't take unusually large doses.

**Closes the door on cancer.** Ginger is chock full of nutrients called phytochemicals that give all fruits and vegetables their color, flavor, smell, and texture. More importantly, many of them are antioxidants that may ward off diseases like cancer. Experts discovered ginger contains at least 12 different phytochemicals, making it one of the most potent food sources of antioxidants. Out of the dozen, curcumin stands out as a potential tumor fighter. Like all antioxidants, it helps your body capture and flush out cancer-causing free radicals.

**Cleans up blood clots.** Two other phytochemicals in ginger, gingerol and shogaol, could protect your heart by preventing blood clots. Recent studies using varying amounts of fresh and dried ginger seemed to show this connection. Just don't put all of your hopes for a healthy heart on ginger since this link is still controversial. Simply make ginger one part of a wholesome diet full of other fruits and vegetables.

**Treats tummy troubles.** For thousands of years, herbalists have prescribed ginger for bloating and heartburn, and today's experts see little reason to go against this practice. The German government's Commission E, similar to America's FDA, even recommends ginger on a daily basis to improve digestion. They suggest eating 2 to 4 grams a day, which is equal to about a 1-inch chunk of fresh ginger or 500 to 1,000 mg of ginger supplements.

**Provides pain relief.** Many pain medicines — even aspirin — hurt as much as they help. Even when you take them for just a short while, you have to be careful of their side effects.

> ### A ginger for all seasons
>
> When you shop for ginger, you might have to look for it under another name — ginger root. The plant looks like something you'd pull out of the ground, but it's not a root — it's a rhizome, a thick underground stem.
>
> To see for yourself how ginger grows, plant your own — it's one of the easiest herbs to grow. Just slice off 2 inches from a piece of fresh ginger. Make sure it has a bud, or eye, on it like you would find on a potato. Then plant it, cut side down, in a 4-inch pot — about 1 inch under the soil — and place in a sunny window. Keep it moist and in about a month, your baby ginger plant should appear.

Ginger, on the other hand, might ease your discomforts without this problem. Researchers in Denmark suggest ginger could relieve everyday muscle pain, migraines, and take the ache and inflammation out of arthritis — without any aftereffects. It's no wonder, then, that the Arthritis Foundation lists ginger as an herbal remedy for pain.

Even though the research looks promising, arthritis is a serious condition. Talk with your doctor before you trade in your medication for ginger.

# Pantry pointers

Ginger's not the prettiest vegetable in the produce department. But don't judge the book by its cover — ginger is a healthy, delicious addition to your shopping cart. Your best choice is a piece with thick branches and tight skin. If it's shriveled or cracked, pass it by.

When you bring your fresh ginger home, store it like a potato — at room temperature. If you're worried about pests, keep it in the fridge. Just make sure to wrap it in paper towels to keep away mold.

To use your ginger, first remove the skin and slice, grate, or chop as much as you need. Then toss it in your stir-fry, marinade, stew, sauce, or salad. Or boil some in water for 10 minutes to make tea. Whatever you do, try a little at first — it can have a strong, sometimes spicy flavor — and don't substitute dried or powdered ginger in a recipe calling for fresh. You'll be disappointed in the results.

### A word of caution

Although most people can enjoy fresh or powdered ginger without any side effects, check with your doctor before taking supplements if you regularly take nonsteroidal anti-inflammatory drugs (NSAIDs) or blood thinning medication, like warfarin. Because ginger can keep blood from clotting, it may cause you bruising and bleeding problems.

If you're scheduled for surgery, stop any herbal supplements well in advance. In addition to bleeding problems, you might experience an interaction with anesthesia.

Talk to your doctor about ginger if you have gallstones. And before you recommend ginger to your pregnant friends, please note that it may not be safe for unborn babies.

# Gout

• • • • • • • • • •

**Eat**

Cherries    Ginger
Turmeric    Water
Yogurt    Milk
Grapefruit    Curry

**Avoid**

Purine-rich foods, such as turkey, anchovies, bacon, dried peas and beans, cauliflower and seafood

High-fat foods

"The gout," Charles Dickens once wrote, "is a complaint as arises from too much ease and comfort." Since ancient times, people believed gout only troubled kings, barons, and other rich folk who splurged on food and alcohol. That's why they called it "the disease of kings."

Experts now know gout is a form of arthritis that tends to run in families. If you suffer from gout, your body has problems dealing with uric acid, a natural byproduct of metabolism. Either your body produces too much, or your kidneys can't flush it out. This causes uric acid to build up in your blood, leading to sudden and repeated attacks of gout.

In fact, you may fall asleep one night feeling fine, only to wake up with a red, aching, swollen big toe. That's how gout strikes. Crystals of uric acid are deposited in your joints — especially joints farthest from your chest, like your big toe — triggering the fiery inflammation. A painful attack can keep you bedridden for days or weeks.

Older people should be wary of taking aspirin frequently. As little as 75 milligrams (a little less than one children's aspirin) a day can affect the way your kidneys release uric acid.

If you have symptoms of gout, see your doctor. He can get at the root of the problem and prescribe medication to prevent future outbreaks. Failure to treat gout could cause permanently disfigured joints and kidney stones.

Being overweight and having high blood pressure are two major causes of gout. So play it safe — cut down on fatty foods;

punch up your daily intake of fruits, vegetables, and whole grains; and exercise regularly. Alcohol can also bring on an attack, making moderation a sensible practice if you drink at all.

## Nutritional blockbusters that fight gout

**Cherries.** According to research from Michigan State University, if gout attacks, chew on some cherries. Dr. Muralee Nair, lead author of the study, suggests eating about 20 or so cherries a day to reduce the swelling and ache of a sudden gout attack. "Daily consumption of cherries," Nair says, "has the potential to reduce pain related to inflammation, arthritis, and gout."

Some researchers think cherries might work as well as drugs, without the side effects. Nair's test-tube studies show that cherry compounds are very effective when compared with aspirin, ibuprofen, and other nonsteroidal anti-inflammatory drugs (NSAIDs).

These amazing cherry compounds are the same ones that give the fruit its red color. Called anthocyanins, they stop your body from producing prostaglandins, chemicals that cause inflammation.

If eating a whole bowl of cherries sounds like a task fit for Hercules, dried cherries can provide a more concentrated dose.

**Ginger and turmeric.** According to the Arthritis Foundation, ginger and turmeric might be two more natural weapons against gout. Both spices contain curcumin, a phytochemical renown for its antioxidant and anti-inflammatory powers. It may even work as well as ibuprofen and other NSAIDs, according to recent research.

To try curcumin's healing powers, add fresh ginger to your next stir-fry or brew some ginger tea. And getting turmeric is as easy as ordering curry at your local Indian restaurant.

If you have gallbladder trouble or take NSAIDs or blood thinning medication, like warfarin, talk with your doctor before treating your gout with these spices.

---

### A word of caution

If you have gout, don't eat foods high in purines. They can make your gout worse.

Purines cause your body to produce too much uric acid. This can trigger uric acid crystals to form in your joints, leading to inflammation and pain.

High purine foods include dried peas and beans, turkey, salmon, bacon, anchovies, liver, and cauliflower. Check with your doctor about following a low-purine diet.

---

**Water.** Your body needs at least eight 6-ounce glasses of water every day. Water not only helps prevent dehydration, it flushes out uric acid.

Try to stick with plain old water. Sugary drinks — even the fashionable sports beverages that promise quick hydration — are loaded with empty calories.

**Dairy.** If you don't want another gout attack, soothe your system with dairy foods. According to a recent study from Canada, eating at least 30 grams of dairy protein a day can help keep the amount of uric acid circulating in your blood under control. Considering that one serving of yogurt has 12 grams of protein and a cup of milk has 8 grams, getting enough protein from dairy foods is easy to do.

### Benefits

Protects against heart attacks

Promotes weight loss

Helps stop strokes

Combats lung, breast and prostate cancer

Lowers cholesterol

# Grapefruit

Grapefruit is a relative newcomer to the world of fruits and vegetables, having been around only about 200 years. Compared to the apple, which scientists believe was eaten in prehistoric times, grapefruit is just an infant — but what a healthy baby, brimming with nutrition.

This luscious fruit contains potassium as well as the B vitamin inositol and is an excellent source of vitamin C — just a half grapefruit will give you a full day's supply. By eating the red- and pink-fleshed varieties, you'll benefit from lycopene, which appears to protect against several health problems, including cancer. And best of all, it's low calorie and fat-free.

You can thank the Jamaicans for giving us this healthy and tasty fruit. Grapefruit was first grown on the shores of this small Caribbean country and got its name from the way it grows in clusters, like grapes. Grapefruit trees were introduced to Florida in the 1820s, and today, half the world's supply of grapefruit is grown in that state.

## 4 ways grapefruit keeps you healthy

**Provides triple protection against heart disease.** Grapefruit, like all plant foods, is cholesterol free. It also protects your heart from the damaging effects of cholesterol with a trio of nutrients.

◆ **Pectin** — Grapefruit contains pectin, a kind of soluble fiber that lowers cholesterol. In one study, grapefruit pectin decreased unhealthy LDL cholesterol by more than 10 percent. A study of pigs with high cholesterol found that grapefruit pectin did not lower cholesterol levels, but it reduced narrowing of the coronary arteries by about 50 percent. This means pectin might have a beneficial effect on your arteries even if it doesn't lower your cholesterol.

◆ **Vitamin C** — Vitamin C helps keep LDL cholesterol from oxidizing, which could protect against heart disease. Numerous studies have found that high levels of vitamin C are associated with lower levels of LDL cholesterol and higher levels of good HDL cholesterol.

◆ **Lycopene** — Red and pink grapefruit contain lycopene, a carotenoid that gives the fruit its color. One study found that the risk of heart attack was 60 percent lower in people with the highest concentration of lycopene in their bodies compared to people with the least amount of lycopene.

**Helps take the weight off.** Some form of the "grapefruit diet" has been around since the 1930s when the Hollywood Diet, which consisted of a few select foods, became popular. Grapefruit was included several times a day because it supposedly contained a fat-burning enzyme. Other versions of the same diet have popped up over the years.

Registered dietitian Kim Gaddy warns that basing any diet around a single food long-term is probably a bad idea. "The main reason I don't encourage this type of eating plan is that major nutrients are left out. For example, if following an all-grapefruit diet, missing nutrients are protein, calcium, and many more. Any time you restrict food groups, you place yourself at risk of nutrient deficiencies."

Although you shouldn't rely on grapefruit alone to help you lose weight, it is still a healthy, low-calorie food, and can be an important part of a weight-loss plan. For a balanced diet plan that includes grapefruit, visit the Florida Citrus Web site on the Internet at <www.floridajuice.com/floridacitrus/diet.html>, or write to the Florida Department of Citrus, P.O. Box 148, 1115 East Memorial Boulevard, Lakeland, FL 33802-0148. This particular diet was studied at Johns Hopkins University and is endorsed by fitness expert Denise Austin.

**Cuts your cancer risk.** Include grapefruit in your morning breakfast, and you may give yourself some natural cancer protection. White grapefruit contains a flavonoid called naringin that may be responsible for its cancer protective effect. A study at the University of Hawaii found the people who ate the most white grapefruit were 50 percent less likely to develop lung cancer than the ones who ate the least. And animal studies find that naringin may help prevent breast cancer.

If pink grapefruit is your favorite, you may be doing your prostate a big favor. Studies have found that eating foods containing lycopene can lower your risk of prostate cancer. And that goes for men who already have prostate disease as well.

**Stops stroke in its tracks.** Eating grapefruit can really pay off in stroke protection. A study of more than 100,000 people found those who ate the most fruits and vegetables had a 30 percent lower risk of stroke. And each serving of fruits or veggies you add to your daily diet gives you a 6 percent lower risk of stroke — up to six servings. More than that apparently doesn't help, the study found.

Citrus fruit and juice were among the most beneficial of the foods studied. Researchers think the potassium in grapefruit may make it especially protective against stroke. One large study found that men who ate the most potassium had a 38 percent lower risk of stroke.

### A word of caution

If you love grapefruit juice, you have two things to watch out for — drug interactions and kidney stones.

Grapefruit juice can affect the way your body handles certain drugs. Sometimes it blocks absorption, and other times it makes your body absorb the drug faster. Always check with your doctor or pharmacist before taking any medication with grapefruit juice.

If you're prone to kidney stones, research shows you can lower your risk by drinking more fluids. But don't choose grapefruit juice. In a recent study, an 8-ounce serving of wine lowered the risk of kidney stones by 59 percent, while coffee and tea reduced risk by 8 to 10 percent. But grapefruit juice *increased* risk by 44 percent.

## Pantry pointers

Grapefruit isn't picked until it's ripe, so you don't have to worry about getting a "green" one. Choose one that feels heavy for its size, and you'll get a fruit that's juicy and tasty. You can store grapefruit at room temperature for a week or in the refrigerator for six to eight weeks. For a juicier treat, let it sit at room temperature for a while before eating.

| Benefits |
| --- |
| Protects your heart |
| Combats cancer |
| Saves your eyesight |
| Conquers kidney stones |
| Enhances blood flow |

# Grapes

• • • • • • • • • • • • • •

Ring in the New Year in Spain and you'll get quite a mouthful, that is if you follow Spanish tradition. Legend has it if you can eat 12 grapes — one for each month — during the final 12 seconds before midnight, you'll have good luck the whole year through. And as long as you don't choke on the grapes, you might have good health, too.

Grapes practically overflow with polyphenols, plant compounds that act as antioxidants and protect you from heart disease and cancer. They also have fiber, small amounts of vitamins, and important minerals like potassium, calcium, manganese, and iron. No wonder grapes were a popular food as far back as 3000 B.C. Today, grapes grow on vines and shrubs in warm areas around the world.

It's not hard to make these delicious fruits part of your diet. Try grape jam or red wine, and don't forget chewy raisins. But the best way might be the most simple — just grab a handful of grapes for a snack.

And remember, unless it's New Year's Eve, there's no hurry.

# 4 ways grapes keep you healthy

**Calls a halt to heart disease.** Perhaps you've heard of the "French Paradox." It's the combination of an apparently unhealthy lifestyle — eating high fat foods, smoking, getting little exercise, and drinking wine — and a low rate of heart disease. Many experts say the red wine is the key. Several European studies suggest drinking red wine in moderation — anywhere from one to two glasses a day — reduces your risk of dying from heart disease by about 40 percent.

The secret is in the skin. Grape skins contain resveratrol, a type of plant estrogen, also called a phytoestrogen. In your body resveratrol fights inflammation and prevents blood clots.

Grape skins also contain the powerful flavonoid quercetin. It works as an antioxidant to prevent the low-density lipoprotein (LDL or "bad") cholesterol from building up in your artery walls and blocking blood flow to your heart and brain. It also stops your blood from turning sticky and clumping together. Blood moves through your arteries more easily, taking some of the pressure off your heart and reducing your risk of stroke.

And that's why red wine, which uses the grape skin, helps your heart while white wine does not. If you indulge in a bit of champagne, you're getting more flavonoids than from most white wines. That's because those healthy grape skins are left in the juice during part of the champagne fermenting process.

But just because red wine may ward off heart disease doesn't mean you should start drinking. If alcohol isn't your choice, you can get similar benefits from non-alcoholic wine or grape juice, which has about half the flavonoids of red wine. Or you can eat more grapes. If you do drink, remember moderation is the secret to good health.

**Combats cancer.** When it comes to battling cancer, resveratrol is something of a superhero. Researchers at the University of Illinois found this plant estrogen foils cancer at every turn by acting as an antioxidant and fighting inflammation, cell mutation, and tumors.

Throw in the powerful antioxidant action of quercetin and other flavonoids — including the anthocyanins that give grapes their red color — and you've got an even stronger defense against dangerous free radicals that damage your cells and cause cancer.

You'll be glad to know research bears this out. In studies, moderate wine drinking lowered cancer deaths by 22 percent. Just remember, heavy drinking — more than a couple of glasses of wine per day — greatly increases your risk of cancer.

And again, you don't need to drink wine to get these anti-cancer benefits. Grapes and grape juice also guard against this disease. In fact, experts link eating more grapes to a lower risk of oral cancer.

**Avoids eye problems.** If you're worried about your eyesight, you might want to start seeing red — red grapes, that is. Red seedless grapes are a good source of the carotenoids lutein and zeaxanthin. These carotenoids may protect against age-related macular degeneration, the leading cause of vision loss in people over 50.

**Crushes kidney stones.** The pain of kidney stones is enough to drive anyone to drink. Oddly enough, that may be one good solution. Drinking more fluids helps flush stone-causing toxins out of your body, but wine is even more beneficial than your average fluid. Harvard studies indicate every 8-ounce daily glass of wine reduces the risk of stone formation by 39 percent for men and a whopping 59 percent for women.

## Pantry pointers

Grapes, like wine, can be classified as red or white. Their skin color ranges from pale green to purplish black. Some grapes have seeds, while others are seedless. Some varieties are used for wine, others for food products like grape juice, jams, and jellies. Still others are table grapes — the sweet, juicy kind you can just pop in your mouth.

When shopping for table grapes, choose plump fruit still attached to the stem. You can store them in a plastic bag in the refrigerator for about a week. Before eating, make sure you rinse them well in case they were sprayed with insecticide.

# Green tea

· · · · · · · · · · · · · · · · · ·

| Benefits |
| --- |
| Combats cancer |
| Protects your heart |
| Helps stop strokes |
| Promotes weight loss |
| Strengthens bones |
| Kills bacteria |

It's hard to believe something as soothing as a warm cup of tea could protect you from disease, but it's true. And for thousands of years the Oriental world has known the health secrets of this simple beverage.

According to legend, the Chinese Emperor Shen-Nung discovered this tasty drink by accident in 2737 BC. As the story goes, the emperor was boiling a kettle of water on a terrace when some leaves from a nearby bush happened to drift by and fall into the water. The emperor tasted the brew and found it delicious. It wasn't long before people were adding the leaves to kettles all over China and the Far East and enjoying the protective benefits of this plant.

Dutch traders brought tea to the Western world around 1600, and the British soon began a similar trade route, preferring the taste of black tea. To this day, the Western world drinks mostly black tea, while the Chinese and Japanese typically drink green.

Both black and green teas are made from the same bush, native to China and India, *Camellia sinensis*. Green tea is different only in how it is prepared. Unlike black tea, which is fermented, green tea leaves are steamed soon after being picked. This steaming process helps preserve the plant's antioxidants, called tannins or polyphenols.

Scientists believe green tea antioxidants are more powerful than those found in most vegetables. Green tea also contains B vitamins and vitamin C and is lower in caffeine than black tea. Because of the powerful ability of one of its antioxidants to fight cell-damaging free radicals, this natural drink is gaining a reputation as a warrior against aging and disease.

Many clinical studies recommend drinking certain amounts of tea every day. Just remember not all teacups are created equal. Traditional Japanese cups are quite small and hold only a few ounces, while most coffee mugs are huge in comparison. Your best bet is to choose a cup somewhere in between.

## 8 ways green tea keeps you healthy

**Says sayonara to sickness.** Thousands of women who practice the ancient Japanese tea ceremony called Chanoyu cut their risk of dying from several fatal diseases in half — and it's what they're pouring in their cups that counts.

It's common knowledge green tea extract fights many bacteria that cause diarrhea and sickness, even some strains of *E. coli.* It can also keep the germs that cause plaque build-up and cavities from growing in your mouth. But researchers think the custom of drinking green tea in small amounts throughout the day might be the secret to keeping antioxidants circulating in your body. You don't need a ceremony to get these same benefits — just keep filling up that cup.

**Cancels out cancer.** If cancer is a frequent visitor to your family tree, green tea might be your new best friend. Studies show it fights cancers of the breast, stomach, colon, prostate, and skin. But it doesn't stop there. Green tea can even help chemotherapy patients get the most out of their treatment. Often during chemotherapy, cancer cells stop responding to the drugs. But a study in Germany showed green tea could make the resistant cancer cells start responding again.

**Drowns your risk of mouth cancer.** If slowing down isn't your cup of tea, consider this — slowly drinking and holding green tea in your mouth for a few seconds at a time keeps high levels of antioxidants in your mouth and throat. Scientists believe this could be why green tea drinkers get fewer oral and esophageal cancers than other people. What a great reason to relax over a cup.

Another good protection against cancers of the mouth and throat might be as simple as a meal spiced with turmeric and washed down with lots of green tea. Researchers at Memorial Sloan-Kettering Cancer Center in New York discovered that green tea combined with curcumin, from the spice turmeric, creates a cancer-fighting superhero that drastically slows the growth of cancer cells from a human mouth.

**Battles breast cancer.** There's good news for women who regularly drink green tea. Five or more cups a day could mean you have a better chance of surviving breast cancer. In addition, if your doctor discovers the cancer in an early stage, it's less likely to spread to lymph nodes. More than eight cups a day, for postmenopausal women, might mean even extra protection. Overall, green tea drinkers are more likely to have types of cancer that respond to medical treatment, and are less likely to get cancer again than other women.

**Heads off heart disease and stroke.** While you are lingering over another cup, green tea is getting down to work lowering your blood pressure and cholesterol. That means less risk of suffering a heart attack or stroke. A long-term study of older men in the Netherlands showed a relationship between heart disease and stroke risk and how much fruit, vegetables, and tea the men consumed. Those with the highest intake of these antioxidant-rich foods and drink were the least likely to die from heart disease or stroke.

If you're a heavy coffee drinker, you might want to switch at least some of your hot drinks to this wonder liquid. A Harvard Medical School study found that tea drinkers had a lower risk of heart attack than java lovers. Scientists believe an amino acid in green tea, called theanine, is responsible for keeping blood less sticky so it can move smoothly through your arteries. Preventing plaque build-up this way can reduce your risk of heart disease, stroke, and other health problems.

> ### The Japanese tea ceremony
>
> The Japanese, who've been perfecting the art of drinking tea for centuries, have developed a tea ceremony that can be a social, artistic, and sometimes religious event.
>
> Although tea can be a casual get-together for friends, the very formal tea, called a chaji, can last anywhere from three to five hours. This special event can require a meal of several courses and an intermission in a garden. Each server's movement is considered important to the overall experience, and serious tea servers will even practice the positions of their fingers. Some will go so far as to sculpt the ashes for the fire used to heat the water.

**Loves your liver.** A weekly cup of green tea may be able to keep toxins from damaging your liver cells. But drinking more than 10 cups per day can be good protection against liver disease. Since tea has caffeine in it, you might want to choose decaffeinated if you drink this much.

**Beats brittle bone disease.** Did you know your teacup can be a powerful weapon against osteoporosis? More than 1,000 tea-drinking women in England had their bone density measured. Surprisingly, they had stronger bones than the women who avoided tea. And even though these British women were drinking black tea, the benefit came from antioxidants found in both green and black teas. In addition, it didn't seem to matter if the women smoked, used hormone replacement therapy, drank coffee, or added milk to their tea — the results were the same.

According to the U.S. Department of Health and Human Services, one-fourth of women over 65 and half the women over 85 will suffer from osteoporosis. This means tea could become an important part of every woman's diet.

**Lets you drink up and slim down.** As if green tea weren't busy enough saving the world from diseases, it can also help you lose weight. In several tests, researchers gave a group of people green tea extracts — equal to between three and five cups of tea — at each meal. Their metabolism increased even more than the group taking caffeine pills. This is great news for dieters since a higher metabolism means you burn calories faster. What's more, green tea can help you lose excess water weight — the kind that makes you feel bloated. Just think, sipping tea for good health might also help you fit back into your skinny clothes.

## Pantry pointers

You can buy green tea in most grocery and health food stores, either loose or in tea bags. Store it in a dark, airtight container, and keep the container in a cool, dry place. It's best to use green tea within a month or two to get the best health benefits.

Because boiling water destroys some of the antioxidants in tea, you should steep green tea in water that is hot, but not boiling, for about three minutes. Drink it before it gets too cool and the tea turns to a darker brown — a sign that the antioxidants are no longer active. Try it without any additional sweeteners, but if you just can't deny your sweet tooth, add a half teaspoon of honey per cup. Topping it with a bit of skim milk will sneak some extra calcium into your diet but won't change the health benefits of the tea.

### A word of caution

Although green tea has less caffeine than black tea and about one-third as much as coffee, too much of this good thing might keep you awake at night or feeling jangled during the day. Also, some people experience stomach irritation the more they drink. If this is true for you, switch to a decaffeinated tea, either green or black, that will still give you super antioxidant protection without these side effects

| Benefits |
| --- |
| Controls blood pressure |
| Lowers cholesterol |
| Battles diabetes |
| Combats cancer |
| Protects prostate |

# Guava

• • • • • • • • • • •

Guava gets a "C" on the nutritional grading scale — "C" for champion, that is. If you thought oranges and other citrus fruits were the kings of vitamin C, you need to meet the guava. One guava has 165 milligrams (mg) of vitamin C, while one orange has a mere 69 mg. This delicious fruit is also a good source of beta carotene, lycopene, potassium, and soluble fiber.

Guava is thought to have originated in Central America over 2,000 years ago. It's difficult to grow in some areas, but in tropical regions like the Caribbean where conditions are right, guava can spread rapidly and is considered a nuisance. It also grows in Hawaii, California, and Florida.

Although Tampa, Fla., isn't a major producer of guava, it's called the "Big Guava," a take-off of New York's "Big Apple" nickname. Every year at Halloween, Tampa hosts the annual Latin-style "Guavaween Festival" in the Ybor City area — complete with a "Guava Love It" cooking contest.

Why not broaden your fruit horizons and try some guava — or have guava jelly on your toast instead of the usual grape or apple jelly.

## 3 ways guava keeps you healthy

**Helps your heart.** Guava can improve your heart health by helping to control your blood pressure and cholesterol.

In one study, researchers gave guava to people with high blood pressure before meals for 12 weeks. By the end of the study, average systolic (top number) blood pressure dropped by 8 points and diastolic (bottom number) fell by 9 points.

Guava's ability to lower blood pressure could be the result of potassium. This mineral is an electrolyte that's essential to electrical reactions in your body, including your heart. It also keeps your heartbeat steady, and it assists your kidneys in removing waste from your body.

In addition, the study participants' total cholesterol dropped almost 10 percent. Experts think guava's cholesterol lowering effect may be due to its soluble fiber content. Soluble fiber softens and forms a gel that binds cholesterol and carries it out of your body.

> **Unusual way to treat diarrhea**
>
> The fruit of the guava plant may be tasty and nutritious, but the leaves have been used as medicine for centuries. Natives of the areas where guavas grow use the leaves for digestive problems, particularly diarrhea. They also put the crushed leaves on wounds and chew the leaves to relieve toothaches. Although most of these folk remedies have little scientific evidence to back them up, one study did find that there might be some truth to the anti-diarrheal effect of guava leaves.

The vitamin C found in guava might be a particularly effective antioxidant against heart disease. Studies show it raises good HDL cholesterol, and it helps prevent bad LDL cholesterol from becoming oxidized and turning into artery-clogging plaques. Vitamin C can also help keep your small blood vessels springy and healthy.

**Curtails cancer.** Guava is a good source of lycopene. This carotenoid, which gives many plant foods their red or pink coloring, may help prevent cancer, as well as boost heart health.

The evidence for lycopene's cancer-protective effect is strongest for prostate cancer, lung cancer, and stomach cancer.

Tomatoes and tomato-based products are a major source of lycopene for most people. That's why much of the research on cancer and lycopene has focused on tomato products.

The vitamin C in guava may also protect you against cancer. Studies find that a high intake of vitamin C may lower your risk of developing colon, stomach, breast, and lung cancers.

**Treats diabetes.** According to folklore, guava has been used in Chinese medicine to treat diabetes for a very long time. And now, a recent study proves that it could lower blood sugar. The effect wasn't as potent as chlorpropamide and metformin, drugs commonly used to lower blood sugar. Nevertheless, it may be a natural way to help treat or prevent diabetes.

## Pantry pointers

Ever seen a guava? This exotic fruit has a thin, light yellow or slightly greenish skin. When buying guava, look for ones that "give" to gentle pressure. But keep in mind that ripe guava bruises easily, so handle with care.

Once they're ripe, eat them quickly because they're only at their peak for about two days. You can refrigerate them for a short period, but they get tough after a couple of days.

Guavas ripen practically year-round, but fresh guava is most likely to be available in your supermarket, or Hispanic markets, from late spring to early fall. Canned guava, guava paste, and guava juice are good alternatives to fresh guava. Guava also makes excellent jam and jelly.

# Headaches and migraines

· · · · · · · · · · · · · · · · ·

| Eat | |
|---|---|
| Tuna | Salmon |
| Ginger | Brown rice |
| Popcorn | Oatmeal |
| Broccoli | Green peas |
| Acorn | Potatoes |
| squash | Shrimp |
| Clams | Skim milk |

**Avoid**

Specific foods that may
trigger your headache

Thank goodness headache remedies aren't what they used to be. In ancient times, people believed evil spirits caused this some-times-unbearable pain. They would drill holes in the sufferer's head to let these evil spirits out. The headache must have felt downright pleasant compared to the cure. Fortunately, today, many experts believe you can find relief from headache pain just by watching what you eat.

About 90 percent of all headaches are tension headaches. These feel like you've got a tight band around your head causing pain in your forehead and temples or in the back of your head and neck. Less common are cluster headaches, with their typical sharp, sudden pain behind one eye. Men get these much more often than women do. Women, however, have nearly three times as many migraine headaches as men. With a migraine, you feel a strong pain, usually on one side of your head. Light and sound bother your eyes and ears, and you might feel dizzy and sick to your stomach.

Whatever you call it, many things can cause a headache — stress, fatigue, loud noise, bright lights, and changes in a woman's estrogen levels, such as during her period. Even skipping meals or eating the wrong foods — especially those containing substances that affect blood flow to your brain — can spell trouble. Some of the most common migraine triggers include red wine, cheese, and chocolate. Hot dogs, bacon, the Chinese food additive MSG, nuts, and citrus fruits may also lead to head pain.

The good news is you don't have to eliminate all of these foods from your diet. Different foods affect people differently. To find out which, if any, foods give you trouble, try keeping a headache and food diary. If you see a pattern — for example, your headaches always come after you've snacked on a chocolate bar — you might think twice before eating that food.

Just as some foods can trigger headaches, some foods can help prevent them. To stop the pain before it starts, choose a menu with plenty of these nutrients.

## Nutritional blockbusters that fight headaches and migraines

**Magnesium.** People who suffer from migraines — an estimated 28 million in the United States alone — have lower levels of this mineral in their red blood cells and brain than other people. Because of this, researchers think a magnesium deficiency might cause migraines.

German researchers tested this idea and found magnesium supplements helped reduce the number and severity of migraines. You would have to eat nearly 11 cups of oatmeal or 26 sweet potatoes to get as much natural magnesium as they used in this study, but don't despair. Simply making healthy, magnesium-rich foods like brown rice, popcorn, broccoli, green peas, potatoes, shrimp, clams, and skim milk part of your daily menu could be enough to soothe your aching head.

**Riboflavin.** This B vitamin can be just as effective as aspirin in easing the pain of migraines. In one study, people with migraines who took daily supplements of riboflavin experienced as much improvement as those who took riboflavin plus aspirin.

Like magnesium, this vitamin was studied in large doses. But that doesn't mean you can't boost your levels of riboflavin through diet. Milk, eggs, meat, poultry, fish, and green, leafy vegetables give you hefty amounts of this key vitamin.

**Calcium and vitamin D.** If you're a woman who gets migraines around the time of your period, extra calcium and vitamin D could mean fewer headaches and fewer PMS symptoms, too. This combination helped postmenopausal women with migraines as well. To get this therapy in one gulp, drink more vitamin D-fortified milk.

**Omega-3 fatty acids.** Battles take place every day between omega-3 and omega-6 fatty acids — with your body as the battlefield. You need both of these essential fatty acids, and you must get them through your diet because your body can't make them on its own. But you need them in the right amounts. When one type of fatty acid drastically outnumbers the other, things can go haywire.

> ### Caffeine: friend or foe?
>
> In Operation Headache, caffeine acts as a double agent. On one hand, drinking too much caffeine or withdrawing from caffeine can trigger headaches. On the other, small amounts of caffeine can help relieve the pain of a headache once it starts.
>
> Caffeine constricts, or narrows, your blood vessels. This helps that pain in your cranium because your blood vessels often swell before a headache. Caffeine also helps other headache medications work better, so you need less of them.
>
> Just remember, caffeine is a drug — one you can grow to depend on. The National Headache Foundation recommends limiting yourself to two caffeinated beverages a day. If you drink a lot more coffee than that, cut back gradually. Giving it up all at once could trigger what's called a "rebound" headache.

Experts say most people get more than enough omega-6 from a diet loaded with common vegetable oils. Too much of this omega-6 leads to too much signaling in your brain. This chaos triggers inflammation, which can give you all sorts of problems, including headaches.

"It's the fast-moving omega-6's that, when they're excessive, are the headache — literally and figuratively," says Dr. William Lands of the National Institutes of Health. "Billions of dollars are being spent to develop things that will slow down excessive omega-6 signaling."

A cheaper strategy, however — and one you can control — is to get more of the omega-3 fatty acids that calm down the hyperactive omega-6. The best source of omega-3 is fish, especially fatty fish like salmon, mackerel, or tuna. But you'll also find it in walnuts, wheat germ, and some green, leafy vegetables.

**Ginger.** This spice has long been hailed for its powers to ward off nausea. Because an unsettled stomach often accompanies migraines, eating ginger may help lessen the agony of a migraine attack.

A woman in Denmark took between 500 and 600 milligrams of powdered ginger at the first sign of a migraine. Within half an hour, she felt better. What's more, she made raw ginger a part of her daily diet and had fewer and less severe migraines.

Although there's no scientific proof concerning ginger and migraines, try drinking up to 2 grams of powdered ginger in water throughout the day or slicing fresh ginger into your favorite recipes.

| Eat | |
|---|---|
| High-fiber cereal | Olive oil |
| Bananas | Wheat germ |
| Broccoli | Spinach |
| Tuna | Oranges |
| Tomatoes | Salmon |
| | Brown rice |

**Avoid**

Foods high in saturated fat, such as red meat and whole-milk dairy products

# Heart disease

• • • • • • • • • • • • •

Japan has a longer healthy life expectancy than any other country in the world, according to statistics from the World Health Organization.

Why did Japan come out on the top end of the life expectancy figures? Largely because the traditional low-fat Japanese diet helps keep hearts healthy.

Heart disease is the leading cause of death in the United States and other developed countries, but it's rapidly becoming more of a problem worldwide. The good news is heart disease is one disease you can do something about — no matter where you live.

Because heart disease is such a serious problem, the American Heart Association (AHA) issues dietary guidelines to help people battle this killer disease. The AHA recommendations include eating at least five servings of various fruits and vegetables daily; six or more servings of grains daily; two or more servings of fish weekly; and limiting your intake of saturated fat, cholesterol, salt, and alcohol.

## Nutritional blockbusters that fight heart disease

**Fiber.** Do you want an easy way to follow the American Heart Association's recommendations for a heart-healthy diet? Just add two bowls of high-fiber cereal to your diet every day.

In a recent study, men who ate two servings of high-fiber cereal each day — one for breakfast and one later in the day as a snack — changed their diets enough to meet the AHA's recommendations for fat and cholesterol. Eating cereal for breakfast meant they ate fewer fatty breakfast foods, like omelets, pastries, and breakfast sandwiches. And some of the men ate cereal as an after-dinner snack, instead of their usual bowl of ice cream.

Researchers didn't tell them to make any changes except adding the cereal to their regular diets, but the men found that they automatically ate fewer fatty foods because the fiber was so filling.

Because fiber helps lower cholesterol, the AHA recommends eating soluble fiber, found in foods such as oatmeal, oat bran, rice bran, beans, barley, citrus fruits, strawberries, and apples, as well as insoluble fiber found in whole-wheat breads and cereals, brown rice and many fruits and vegetables.

**Folate.** Homocysteine, an amino acid your body produces as a by-product of protein metabolism, could be as damaging to your heart and blood vessels as cholesterol. Scientists have found that people with heart disease, strokes, or clogged arteries in their legs are much more likely to have high levels of homocysteine in their blood.

Luckily, it's easy to fight homocysteine with the right foods. Folate and other B-vitamins break down homocysteine in your body. That's why people with high levels of folate usually have low levels of homocysteine.

To boost your folate level, eat lots of green leafy vegetables, beans, citrus fruits, and fortified cereals and breads.

**Omega-3.** If you want to keep your heart healthy, eat fish more often. A large study on male doctors found that those who ate at least one fish meal a week were 52 percent less likely to die from a sudden heart attack than those who ate fish less than once a month.

Omega-3 fatty acids are the heart heroes in fish. Research indicates that omega-3 can lower your blood pressure, reduce the stickiness of your blood, and help regulate your heartbeat. Fatty fish, such as tuna and salmon, contain lots of omega-3. If you're not a big fan of fish, you can also get omega-3 in flaxseed oil and some green leafy vegetables, like spinach and kale.

**Antioxidants.** The AHA recommends you eat at least five servings of fruits and vegetables every day. Fresh fruits and vegetables are loaded with antioxidants, which may prevent LDL cholesterol from becoming oxidized. Dr. Lori J. Mosca, director of preventive cardiology research and education at the University of Michigan, says, "When a fat such as LDL undergoes oxidation, it is more prone to collect in blood vessels to form plaque. Over time, the plaque narrows the blood vessels, or unleashes a blood clot, which can result in a heart attack or stroke. When LDL is not oxidized, it does not seem to cause problems."

These powerful antioxidants can help keep your heart healthy.

◆ **Vitamin E.** Because vitamin E is a fat-soluble vitamin, it is stored in fat cells in your body. That puts it right where the action is, preventing LDL cholesterol from becoming oxidized. One study found that women who ate lots of vitamin E-rich foods were less likely to have oxidized LDL in their blood. An earlier study found that women who ate foods high in vitamin E were 62 percent less likely to die from a heart attack as women with low vitamin E intakes. Foods high in vitamin E include nuts, vegetable oils, whole grains, and wheat germ.

◆ **Vitamin C.** Besides protecting cells from oxidation, vitamin C also helps keep blood vessels open wide, and it works well with vitamin E for an extra antioxidant punch. Citrus fruits, strawberries, cantaloupe, tomatoes, brussels sprouts, and broccoli provide beneficial amounts of vitamin C.

◆ **Flavonoids.** If you shoot for the AHA's recommendation of five or more servings of fruits and vegetables every day, you'll easily get a healthy dose of heart friendly flavonoids. Flavonoids work like antioxidants and protect your heart by preventing the build up of plaque in your arteries. One study found that broccoli was particularly protective. Tea, onions, and apples came out the heart-protective winners in another study.

**Unsaturated fats.** If you often shout, "Cheeseburger, fries, and a chocolate shake, please," into a speaker from your car, you're a perfect example of why heart disease is the leading cause of death in most developed countries. People eat too much fat.

Yet, not all fats are created equal when it comes to keeping your heart healthy. Fats born on sunny Mediterranean shores may actually do your heart good. People who eat a typical Mediterranean diet, rich in olive oil, are less likely to have heart disease.

To protect your heart from harmful fats, eat less saturated fat, found in meat, dairy products, and some vegetable oils, like coconut oil and palm oil.

### A word of caution

Eating the right foods can help keep your heart healthy, but eating too much at one time may be a fatal mistake.

A recent study found that you could be four times more likely to have a heart attack within two hours after eating a heavy meal.

Overeating could trigger a heart attack in much the same way as outbursts of anger and extreme physical exertion, especially in people who have heart disease.

Eating smaller, more frequent meals could stop a heart attack before it starts.

**Vegetarian diet.** Studies find that vegetarians are less likely to develop heart disease than meat eaters. Dr. Dean Ornish's well-known program for reversing heart disease includes following a very low-fat vegetarian diet. The program also includes getting regular exercise, managing stress, and stopping smoking. If you decide to follow Dr. Ornish's program, try it at least three or four weeks. It takes that long to break bad habits and establish a new, healthy lifestyle.

| Eat | |
|---|---|
| Yogurt | Brown rice |
| Water | Whole-wheat |
| Watercress | bread |
| Ginger | Chamomile |
| Artichokes | tea |
| Oat bran | Barley |

**Avoid**

Foods high in acid, such as tomatoes, oranges, and grapefruit

# Heartburn and indigestion

More than 60 million Americans suffer from heartburn and indigestion. If you burp a lot — sometimes with a burning taste in your mouth — and feel bloated and uncomfortable after meals, you're probably one of them. These symptoms often get worse during times of stress. Maybe you have resigned yourself to the discomfort, figuring nothing will help the burning feeling in your gut. But you shouldn't ignore it completely. Even though heartburn is not a disease, it could be a symptom of something more serious.

That burning in your throat after eating is probably acid reflux, a condition you get when stomach acid washes back up your throat. This can lead to nausea and vomiting. Acid reflux, also called GERD (gastroesophageal reflux disease) is serious because it can damage your esophagus and lead to severe bleeding. It also increases your risk of esophageal cancer. If your indigestion makes you vomit blood or comes with a severe, burning pain in your stomach, see your doctor immediately. You might have gastritis — an inflammation of the stomach that needs treatment.

The cause of many heartburn cases is simply poor eating habits. What you eat and the medicines you take directly affect your digestive system. For instance, eating too much fat and red meat and not enough fruits and vegetables can easily cause acid reflux. Taking antibiotics may wipe out both good and bad bacteria, leading to indigestion and other problems. And constantly popping antacids for heartburn can backfire by prompting your body to make more acid.

Why not get to the root of your heartburn — what you are or aren't eating. If your doctor has ruled out disease, try healing your heartburn and indigestion with nutrition.

## Nutritional blockbusters that fight heartburn and indigestion

**Water.** Drink plenty of water during the day. Six to eight 8-ounce glasses should help with your indigestion. Water washes acid out of your throat and dilutes the acids in your stomach. But don't drink liquids with meals since you need stomach acid to digest your food. An hour before or after is best.

Dr. Fereydoon Batmanghelidj, author of *Your Body's Many Cries For Water,* says your body needs lots of water for proper digestion. And if you fill up with coffee and colas, you actually lose water since the caffeine in these drinks signals your kidneys to pump water out of your body. Dr. B., as his patients call him, has had much success treating indigestion with plain, old water.

"Dyspeptic pain," he explains, "is the most important signal for the human body. It denotes dehydration. It is a thirst signal of the body. It can occur in the very young as well as in older people."

The next time your stomach cries for help, give it a couple glasses of water to quench the fire.

**Yogurt.** Yogurt is a "probiotic" food, which means it helps good bacteria grow. Even if most milk products cause your indigestion to kick in, you can probably eat yogurt since the friendly bacteria in yogurt have predigested the milk sugar for you. Yogurt is especially good if you've recently taken antibiotics. To be sure you get these helpful bacteria, and not just milk and sugar, check the label to see if the yogurt has active cultures. Buy plain yogurt and flavor it with some fresh blueberries or peaches.

**Low-fat, low-acid foods.** Replace high-fat meats and fried foods that promote stomach acid with low-acid fruits, vegetables,

---

### Do's and don'ts for gastritis

If you suffer from the pain of gastritis, Registered Dietitian Yun Blair of the Vanderbilt University Medical Center has this advice:

#### Do

- Eat small, frequent meals that don't stretch your stomach.
- Drink liquids between meals and not with meals.
- Eat plenty of fiber-rich foods like fruits, vegetables, and oat bran. Also, a fiber supplement like Metamucil might help.
- Engage in some form of regular physical activity like walking or swimming three times per week.

#### Don't

- Eat less than four hours before bedtime.
- Eat fried foods or other foods high in fat.
- Drink caffeine.
- Use any spices that irritate your stomach.
- Eat high-acid foods like citrus fruits, sodas, and orange juice.

and whole grains like whole-wheat bread and brown rice. These natural foods should keep you feeling satisfied but not stuffed. And the grains should help soak up excess acid. Stay away from acidic foods like tomatoes, oranges, grapefruits, radishes, alcohol, coffee, tea, and cola.

**Bitters.** Dogs may be smarter than people when it comes to soothing an upset stomach. When a dog's stomach hurts, it finds some bitter grass to eat. That's pretty smart since bitter herbs help get your digestive juices flowing.

Some people have too much stomach acid, and some have too little — especially older people. If you don't have enough acid, your food may sit undigested in your stomach too long, causing pain. To fight this kind of indigestion, eat bitter plants like watercress, endive, dandelion, artichokes, and grated orange peel (but not the fruit). Ginger, a bitter spice, has been used for centuries to treat indigestion. Steep a teaspoon of grated ginger in hot water for 10 minutes, and drink throughout the day as needed.

**Chamomile tea.** Another ancient remedy, chamomile tea settles the stomach and helps digestion. Drink a cup between meals three or four times per day. You can buy chamomile flower heads at a natural-food store. Steep a heaping tablespoon 10 to 15 minutes before drinking. Be careful, however, if you are allergic to ragweed. You might also be allergic to chamomile.

---

### A word of caution

Sometimes eating too much, too fast can cause acid indigestion. Gulping your meal makes you swallow air with your food, resulting in gas and a bloated feeling. And if you haven't chewed your food properly, your stomach gets large pieces of food that are harder to digest than small ones. So slow down, chew carefully, and eat small portions of low-fat, healthy foods.

To avoid nighttime indigestion, eat several hours before you go to bed. If you still get reflux, try putting blocks under the legs of your headboard to keep your head higher than your stomach.

**Eat**

Bananas      Prunes
Whole-wheat  Broccoli
 bread       Mackerel
Garlic       Oranges
Flaxseed     Canola oil

**Avoid**

Foods high in saturated
fat, such as red meat

Salt and alcohol in large
amounts

# High blood pressure

• • • • • • • • • • • • • • •

How hard does your heart work? For many people, the answer is "too hard," and they don't even know it.

High blood pressure, also called hypertension, sneaks up on you — no symptoms, no signs, no warnings. This silent killer, if left untreated, can lead to heart disease, kidney disease, and stroke. If you don't get your blood pressure checked regularly, you might never know it's too high until it's too late.

Here's how to tell if you're at risk. Blood pressure readings have two numbers. The top number, called systolic blood pressure, measures the force of your blood against your artery walls as your heart beats. The bottom number, called diastolic blood pressure, measures the force between beats. A blood pressure of 130/85 or lower is normal, and anything above 140/90 is high. That means your heart is working too hard to pump blood through your arteries.

As you get older, your risk of high blood pressure skyrockets. Half of all people over 60 have high blood pressure. If you're black, you might be at even greater risk. Some risk factors, such as age and race, can't be controlled. But you can lose weight and watch what you eat — key ways to manage this dangerous condition.

The National Heart, Lung, and Blood Institute's Dietary Approaches to Stop Hypertension (DASH) recommends cutting down on salt, alcohol, saturated and total fat, and cholesterol. It also encourages you to eat more fruits, vegetables, whole grains, and low-fat dairy products.

Add the following items to your diet and give your hard-working heart a rest.

## Nutritional blockbusters that fight high blood pressure

**Minerals.** Like the Three Musketeers, potassium, calcium, and magnesium join forces to duel with high blood pressure. The DASH diet includes two to three times more of these minerals than the average American diet.

◆ **Potassium.** This vital mineral leads the charge against high blood pressure. It neutralizes sodium, often the enemy when it comes to controlling your blood pressure, by flushing it out in your urine. Potassium also relaxes your blood vessels, which improves blood flow. Eat more peas, beans, apricots, peaches, bananas, prunes, oranges, spinach, stewed tomatoes, sweet potatoes, avocados, and figs if you want more potassium in your diet.

◆ **Magnesium.** This mineral also helps lower blood pressure by relaxing your blood vessels. And it balances the amount of sodium and potassium in your blood cells — less sodium, more potassium. Magnesium-rich foods include whole-wheat breads and cereals, broccoli, chard, spinach, okra, oysters, scallops, sea bass, mackerel, beans, nuts, and seeds.

◆ **Calcium.** People who get very little calcium in their diet often have high blood pressure. Like potassium, calcium works by helping your body get rid of sodium through your urine. Cheese, milk, yogurt, broccoli, spinach, turnip greens, mackerel, perch, and salmon are good sources of calcium.

**Vitamin C.** High C means low blood pressure. Several studies show that people with higher levels of vitamin C in their blood have lower blood pressure — and those with low levels of vitamin C have higher blood pressure.

This antioxidant vitamin may reduce high blood pressure by strengthening the connective tissue, or collagen, that supports your blood vessel walls. That makes your blood vessels more capable of handling the pressure of the pumping blood.

Researchers from the Boston University School of Medicine reported that a daily dose of 500 milligrams (mg) of vitamin C lowered systolic blood pressure an average of 13 points after one month. That would be like eating seven oranges or drinking five glasses of orange juice a day.

Other good sources of vitamin C include sweet red peppers, green peppers, strawberries, cantaloupe, black currants, brussels sprouts, broccoli, tomato juice, collard greens, and cabbage.

**Omega-3 fatty acids.** Watch out for fats, but remember — some fats are good for you. Omega-3 fatty acids, the polyunsaturated type found in fish, offer help for your high blood pressure.

Most people eat much more omega-6, a polyunsaturated fat found in vegetable oils, than omega-3. Your body converts omega-6 into a substance that constricts your arteries. That makes your heart work harder to pump blood throughout your body, which increases your blood pressure. Several studies show that eating fish or taking fish oil supplements lowers blood pressure. That's because your body converts omega-3 into a gentler substance that doesn't tighten your arteries as much. Switching from omega-6 to omega-3 can be an easy way to lower your blood pressure.

You get omega-3 mainly from fatty fish, such as salmon, mackerel, and tuna. Other foods with omega-3 include flaxseed, canola oil, walnuts, wheat germ, and some green leafy vegetables, like collard and turnip greens.

**Monounsaturated fat.** Further evidence that not all fats are bad comes from olive oil. This staple of the Mediterranean diet contains mostly monounsaturated fat. In a recent study comparing diets rich in olive oil and sunflower oil, a polyunsaturated fat, the olive oil diet drastically lowered blood pressure while the sunflower oil diet only lowered it slightly. The olive oil diet made such a difference that many people on the diet cut in half the amount of blood pressure medication they were taking, under the guidance of their doctors.

**Fiber.** You already know you should eat fiber for protection against heart disease, stroke, and cancer. Well, here's one more reason. A four-year follow-up study found that women who ate more than 25 grams of fiber a day were about 25 percent less likely to develop high blood pressure as women who ate less than 10 grams of fiber every day.

Fruits, vegetables, and whole-grain breads and cereals are good sources of fiber. For example, one potato with skin has 5 grams of fiber, an orange has 3 grams, and a cup of raisin bran has 8 grams.

Fiber works best over the long term. Don't get discouraged if your blood pressure doesn't drop right away.

> ### Eating vegetarian
>
> Going green might bring your blood pressure out of the red zone, but make sure you plan before switching to a vegetarian diet.
>
> Fruits and vegetables have plenty of fiber, vitamins, and minerals, like potassium, magnesium, and calcium. You also get very little fat and sodium, and they are cholesterol free. All that adds up to a great strategy to fight high blood pressure.
>
> Nevertheless, vegetarians often lack protein and iron. And if you don't eat fish and cook with only soybean or corn oil, your ratio of omega-6 to omega-3 fatty acids might be way out of whack as well.
>
> To make sure you're getting all the nutrients you need, add these foods to your eating plan — beans and legumes for protein, oatmeal and whole wheat for iron, and walnuts and canola oil for omega-3.

**Garlic.** This fragrant herb does more than add flavor to meals. It also lowers cholesterol and protects your arteries from clogging. That way, your blood can zip through with less "oomph" from your heart. Some studies show garlic lowers your systolic blood pressure by nearly 7 percent and your diastolic blood pressure by almost 8 percent.

DASH recommends using both garlic and its cousin, the onion, as tasty cooking alternatives to salt.

**Eat**

| | |
|---|---|
| Oat bran | Apples |
| Barley | Avocados |
| Walnuts | Garlic |
| Onions | Wheat germ |
| Cranberries | Kale |
| Spinach | Beans |

**Avoid**

Foods high in saturated fat, such as red meat and whole-milk dairy products

# High cholesterol

•••••••••••••••••

It's almost impossible not to hear about cholesterol. Advertisements tout foods with no or low cholesterol, while others claim to lower your cholesterol. As if that's not enough, health advice always includes watching your cholesterol.

What exactly is cholesterol? Believe it or not, it's a fat your body needs to help form certain hormones, cell membranes, and bile. Unfortunately, too much of this soft, waxy substance means trouble.

Because cholesterol can't dissolve in your blood, like some nutrients, carrier molecules called lipoproteins must transport it. The two main types of lipoproteins are low-density lipoprotein (LDL) and high-density lipoprotein (HDL).

Often, LDL cholesterol goes by the name "bad" cholesterol because it can build up on the walls of your arteries and form a hard deposit called plaque. Plaque can make your arteries so narrow your heart has trouble pumping blood through them. A blood clot can also form near the site of the plaque. If it blocks the flow of blood to your heart, it can cause a heart attack. When a clot blocks the flow of blood to your brain, it can cause a stroke.

On the other hand, HDL cholesterol whisks cholesterol away from your arteries to your liver and, eventually, out of your body. This "good" cholesterol actually protects you from heart disease and stroke.

Like high blood pressure, high cholesterol comes with no symptoms. You'll never know you have high cholesterol unless you get a blood test and talk with your doctor about the results.

These numbers should be a warning to you — total cholesterol over 240, LDL cholesterol over 160, and HDL cholesterol below 35. They could indicate an increased risk of heart disease. To lower your risk, your total cholesterol should be below 200 and your LDL below 130. HDL cholesterol should be between 35 and 90.

If you're worried about high cholesterol, eat more fruits, vegetables, and whole grains and less meat, cheese, eggs, whole milk, processed foods, and baked goods.

You'll also be glad to know that foods high in the following nutrients have the power to lower high cholesterol, and help reduce cholesterol build-up in your arteries.

## Nutritional blockbusters that fight high cholesterol

**Fiber.** Oat bran became a big sensation when scientists discovered it could lower cholesterol. A type of soluble fiber called beta-glucan gives oat bran its power.

According to Dr. Barbara Schneeman, a researcher with the U.S. Department of Agriculture, this fiber sparks a process called "reverse cholesterol transport." Here's how it works. These gummy beta-glucans slow down your food as it travels through your stomach and small intestine. That way, HDL cholesterol has more time to pick up cholesterol and take it out of the bloodstream — and LDL cholesterol has less opportunity to carry cholesterol to your artery walls.

Most health organizations recommend getting between 25 and 35 grams of fiber into your daily diet. You certainly don't have to get it all from oat bran. Other good sources of soluble fiber include barley, beans, oatmeal, apples, and other fruits and vegetables.

**Unsaturated fats.** Trimming fat from your diet helps trim your cholesterol levels — but don't go overboard. Like some kinds of cholesterol, certain fats actually help you. Some even lower LDL cholesterol.

Monounsaturated fat wipes out bad LDL cholesterol without harming good HDL cholesterol. An Australian study of avocados, which contain 30 grams of mostly monounsaturated fat, showed that as little as half an avocado a day could shrink your total cholesterol by more than 8 percent without lowering good HDL cholesterol. According to a Mexican study, avocados might even boost your levels of HDL by 11 percent. You can also get monounsaturated fat from olive oil and nuts.

Walnuts, in addition to some monounsaturated fat, also have a polyunsaturated fat called alpha-linolenic acid. This fat, part of the omega-3 family, gives walnuts their proven cholesterol-lowering ability. Omega-3 mostly comes from fatty fish, like tuna, mackerel, or salmon, but you can also find it in flaxseed, wheat germ, and green, leafy vegetables, like kale and spinach.

Substituting either monounsaturated or omega-3 fats for saturated fats may be a more effective cholesterol-fighting strategy than switching to a very low-fat, low-cholesterol diet. Very low-fat diets will lower your cholesterol — but they'll get rid of your protective HDL cholesterol, too.

**Antioxidants.** Put a muzzle on a vicious dog, and it can't bite you. Antioxidants use the same approach when it comes to LDL cholesterol. These roving do-gooders muzzle free radicals, keeping them from oxidizing LDL. Once oxidized, LDL travels much more quickly to your artery walls, where it can build up and cause damage.

Dr. Lori J. Mosca of the University of Michigan found that vitamin E in foods — but not in supplements — prevented LDL oxidation. You can find vitamin E in wheat germ, nuts, seeds, and vegetable oils. Other antioxidant vitamins include vitamin C and beta carotene, both found in a variety of fruits and vegetables.

Fruits and vegetables also contain more antioxidant substances called flavonoids that fight high cholesterol. For example, Dr. Ted Wilson of the University of Wisconsin-La Crosse found that the flavonoids in cranberries prevented LDL oxidation. Other hardworking flavonoids include quercetin, found in onions, apples, and tea, and lycopene in tomatoes.

**Garlic.** Making garlic a staple of your kitchen can make a big difference in your battle against high cholesterol. This flavorful herb has a surplus of sulfur compounds that hunt down LDL cholesterol without harming the HDL variety. As little as one-third of a clove of garlic can reduce total cholesterol by about 12 percent and LDL cholesterol by 14 percent.

## Understanding the Cholestin controversy

Cholestin is made from rice fermented in red yeast. The Chinese have used it for centuries to add a brilliant red color to certain dishes, like Peking duck and spareribs. Today, it's also used as a natural and effective way to lower cholesterol. But Cholestin has come under heavy scrutiny in the United States.

Although the scientific evidence that Cholestin works is convincing, the controversy centers on just what kind of product it is. If it's a drug, the Food and Drug Administration (FDA) must regulate it. If it's a dietary supplement, Cholestin can be produced and sold without government supervision. The problem is Cholestin contains lovastatin, the same ingredient that's in Mevacor, a prescription cholesterol-lowering drug.

"Many people may assume that a naturally occurring substance, such as the red yeast rice, would be a more desirable choice for lowering their cholesterol, in comparison to prescription medications," says Thomas A. Pearson, M.D., Ph.D., chairman of the American Heart Association's population science committee.

"However, people need to take into consideration that comprehensive studies have been done only on the prescription statins, and we don't know if the naturally occurring statins behave in exactly the same way."

Pearson says the red yeast fermented on rice used in Chinese cooking is in much smaller quantities than the food supplement sold in the United States. He warns that people may be venturing into the unknown by using the substance in much higher amounts than was used in Chinese cooking. For instance, there has been at least one case of a dangerous allergic reaction to red yeast rice powder.

The FDA and the company marketing Cholestin are battling the issue in government courts. Whatever the final decision, don't risk possible side effects by mixing Cholestin with your current cholesterol-lowering prescription drugs. Make sure you talk to your doctor before switching from a tested and effective prescription statin to any over-the-counter remedies for high cholesterol.

---

### Benefits

Heals wounds

Aids digestion

Guards against ulcers

Fights allergies

Increases energy

Smoothes skin

# Honey

●●●●●●●●●●●●

For thousands of years, honey has been a symbol of prosperity. In ancient times it was so valuable merchants and landowners accepted it as a form of money. Even the Bible refers to the Holy Land as "the land of milk and honey." But don't consider this sweet syrup just a treat. Experts say it's a valuable medicine, too — one that can destroy dangerous infections, quiet a painful stomach ulcer, clean dirty wounds, revive dry skin, and soothe an upset tummy. Honey even pours on antioxidants that defeat cancer-causing free radicals.

In recent years honey has taken a back seat to man-made antibiotics and to processed sweeteners. But modern science shows honey kills bacteria that even the most powerful antibiotics can't handle. And since it contains traces of vitamins, minerals, proteins, and other nutrients — which sugar doesn't have — it is the sweetener of choice again for many people.

So be sure to keep a honey bear in your pantry — and maybe in your medicine cabinet and your first-aid kit, too.

## 7 ways honey keeps you healthy

**Heals with a touch.** The next time you get a scald or scrape, reach for your honey pot — just a dab will perform several healing tasks at once.

Honey forms a protective barrier over your wound while cleaning it of debris; it allows, even encourages, your skin to re-grow; it reduces swelling; and prevents scarring. It doesn't irritate your tissues and is virtually painless to apply and remove. Most importantly, it spells doom for bacteria by slowly releasing antiseptic hydrogen peroxide over several hours.

In fact, hospitals around the world are using honey as a healing salve in hundreds of cases and on all kinds of wounds — abrasions, burns, amputations, diabetic ulcers, bed sores, surgical wounds, and others. The success rate is extraordinary.

Dr. Peter Molan, a leading expert on honey's healing powers for 20 years, reports, "Excellent results are being obtained with cases that have gone unhealed for long periods of time with the best modern conventional treatment."

Molan recommends using honey for minor wounds and for emergency first aid. Stir or warm the honey very slightly, then for a 4-inch square wound, spread about an ounce on a bandage. For more serious injuries he cautions, "It is important to get a doctor's opinion as a new wound may need stitches, and a persistently non-healing wound may be malignant or have a failure in the blood circulation system beneath it."

While all honeys are antibacterial to some extent, some are more potent healers than others. In particular, honey made from specific flowers in New Zealand have amazing antibacterial qualities. You may be able to find this manuka honey at a health store, but it's more likely you'll have to order it directly from the bee-keepers in New Zealand or one of their distributors near you. Your best bet is to get hold of a computer and search the Internet to compare prices. Simply search under the term "active manuka honey," and you should come up with several ordering options.

Just remember if your honey has been heat-processed, important antibacterial enzymes are destroyed. In addition, look in specialty health food stores for brands of honey with an antibacterial — or UMF — rating of at least 10.

**Coats an upset stomach.** Like that famous pink, over-the-counter remedy, honey spreads soothing relief throughout your belly. Against diarrhea caused by bacteria, for instance, research shows it could ease that bloated and cramped feeling. Next time you're laid low by a stomach bug, mix three teaspoons of honey into every 10 ounces of clear, non-caffeinated beverage you drink.

**Overcomes an ulcer.** Bacteria called *Helicobacter pylori* — not stress or spicy foods — cause up to 90 percent of all ulcers. Honey's antibacterial properties can be just as effective against this kind of pesky bug as against those that infect cuts and scrapes. Researchers say eat the honey one hour before meals, with no fluids, and again at bedtime. Spread a tablespoon on a piece of bread. This keeps the honey in your stomach longer.

Making honey your everyday sweetener may also shield your stomach from other irritants that can cause ulcers — like non-steroidal anti-inflammatory drugs (NSAIDs) and alcohol.

**Sweeps away allergies.** "Pollen is not really bad for you," Dr. T.V. Rajan of the University of Connecticut Health Center states. "It's your body's overreaction to pollen that brings on the runny eyes, sneezing, and wheezing."

To stop this allergic reaction without drugs and uncomfortable side effects, Rajan is feeding people honey. Not just any kind of honey, but honey from local flowers full of local pollen.

"Your immune system is trained not to attack anything ingested by mouth," Rajan explains. Eat the pollen-laced honey, he believes, and you tell your immune system this pollen is not bad for you. Then when you breathe in the same type of pollen later, your immune system recognizes and accepts it.

Though Rajan stresses his findings are not definite, he recommends you test his theory out for yourself. Buy locally collected honey at your nearby farmer's market or health food store, and take one tablespoon each day. However, Rajan warns, if you have diabetes, heart disease, or other serious illness talk to your doctor first.

**Adds on antioxidants.** Buy the darkest honey you can find and you'll be getting the most antioxidant bang for your buck. Dr. Nicki Engeseth, professor of food science at the University of Illinois, has tested the antioxidant properties of honey. She's found many varieties are full of phenols and flavonoids — known cancer fighters even more powerful than vitamin E.

> ### 8 foods to smooth, younger-looking skin
>
> Before you spend hundreds on anti-wrinkle creams and moisturizers, try an easy, home-made tonic first. Foods in your kitchen cupboard are some of the main ingredients in those expensive store-bought creams.
>
> For instance, banish crow's feet with a few dabs of olive oil before bed. Or blend 2 tablespoons of honey with 2 teaspoons of milk. Smooth this moisturizing mask over your face and throat and leave it on for 10 minutes. Rinse and you'll have a soft glow Cleopatra would envy.
>
> Also try experimenting with yogurt, lemon or lime juice, papaya, cucumber, and even mayonnaise.

**Fends off free radicals.** According to Engeseth, "Honey is extremely effective in reducing oxidation in meat." Normally, oxygen in the air starts a chain reaction in meat, creating a horde of free radicals. Not only are they unhealthy, but these free radicals steal your food's flavor. To stop them in their tracks, lightly coat cold cuts, leftovers, or ground meats with honey. "The best time to add antioxidants," Engeseth says, "is when the meat is fresh."

**Energizes your workout.** If you are exercising to stay healthy, you need extra energy to stick with your workout routine. Carbohydrates are a great source. They also help your muscles get stronger, repair any tissue damage, and help maintain a strong immune system.

Dr. Richard Kreider of the University of Memphis Exercise and Sports Nutrition Laboratory says, "Honey can serve as a good carbohydrate source for people who are even moderately active. Adding it to a drink is a good way to get some natural carbohydrates." Kreider found that the sweet treat works just like expensive power gels athletes use, but at a fraction of the cost. You can take honey before a walk or aerobics class, but it's more important after exercise, when your body needs the carbohydrates to replace the ones you burned.

## Pantry pointers

Every type of honey, whether it's blueberry, clover, or eucalyptus, comes from a different flower and thus has a different taste. Just remember that darker honeys tend to be stronger.

Store your honey bear or jar in your pantry or on your kitchen counter at room temperature and away from sunlight. Colder temperatures, like in your refrigerator, make honey crystallize. Even worse, direct sunlight saps its healing powers.

### A word of caution

Honey is healthy and safe for most children and adults, but babies less than 12 months old don't have resistance to certain bacteria in it. To be safe, save the honey until children can ask for it by name.

# Insomnia

· · · · · · · · · · · · ·

**Eat**

| | |
|---|---|
| Oats | Ginger |
| Barley | Bananas |
| Cottage | Turkey |
| cheese | Beef |
| Corn | Potatoes |
| Avocados | Peanut |
| Skim milk | butter |

**Avoid**

Foods and beverages containing caffeine

After a good night's sleep, your body — and your brain — feel refreshed and energetic. That's because while you were hitting the hay, your internal systems were hard at work replenishing blood cells and repairing muscles, bones, skin, and other organs. Sleeping eight hours every night is about enough for most people. If you need a little more or a little less, that's all right, too. Just as long as you feel rested and alert during the day, you're probably getting enough.

But what if you spend every night restless and get up tired every morning? In some cases an illness or a medication may be causing your unsettled nights. Talk to your doctor about this. Or perhaps you have certain habits — too much caffeine close to bedtime, an irregular sleep schedule, too little exercise, or exercising just before bedtime — that keep you awake.

Or it could be you don't have enough melatonin, a hormone that regulates your sleep cycle. As you age, your melatonin production slows down. But, according to research scientist Russel J. Reiter, author of *Melatonin: Your Body's Natural Wonder Drug,* older people can still sleep well. You just need to help your body make more of that magic melatonin.

## Nutritional blockbusters that fight insomnia

**Melatonin.** "If you want to raise your melatonin levels naturally," says Reiter, "start by eating a bedtime snack of foods high in melatonin. This simple practice may help you sleep better, strengthen your immune system, heighten your antioxidant protection, and partially offset the age-related decline of melatonin production."

To follow his advice, choose oats, sweet corn, and rice — foods with the highest levels of melatonin. Reiter recommends you experiment with these and other melatonin-rich foods to see which ones help you sleep best. A banana and milk smoothie, for example, may send you snoozing. Or maybe a bowl of tomato soup is your ticket to dreamland.

Whatever you choose, eat it an hour or so before bed. According to Reiter, this gives your body enough time to absorb the melatonin and send you gently off to sleep.

**Tryptophan plus carbohydrates.** You get up from the Thanksgiving table and head straight for the couch. You're not being lazy, your body is just reacting to a certain amino acid in the turkey called tryptophan. After a pasta supper with friends, you can barely keep your eyes open. It's not the company, it's the carbohydrates. Experts have found you can use tryptophan and carbohydrates together to tell your body it's time to go to sleep.

"The tryptophan in foods such as milk and tuna fish do promote sleep," says Lenore Greenstein, a dietitian and nutrition columnist for the Naples Daily News in Florida. "Add a carb snack and you'll promote the release of melatonin which causes relaxation as well." The carbohydrates help the tryptophan that's in the blood stream get to the brain. There your pineal gland converts this essential amino acid to serotonin, then to melatonin.

You'll find tryptophan mostly in animal and fish protein, but you can also get it in soy nuts, cottage cheese, pumpkin seeds, tofu, and almonds. Grains, dairy products, and vegetables like corn, potatoes, and beans are good sources of carbohydrates.

So next time you find yourself counting sheep, try tuna on whole wheat or cereal with milk. Combinations like these will deliver a double dose of exactly what it takes to make you sleepy.

**Calcium and magnesium.** You'll never get any shut-eye unless your muscles are relaxed and your brain is calm. For that, you need melatonin. And according to Greenstein, you need calcium and magnesium to produce the melatonin that quiets and soothes your body.

It's easy to make these nutrients a part of your regular diet. Spread peanut butter on whole grain crackers for magnesium and pour a glass of milk for calcium. Yogurt and sardines are other calcium-rich foods and you can get plenty of magnesium from nuts and green leafy vegetables. If you're on a high protein diet, you're probably eating lots of meat, fish, and dairy products — all foods low in magnesium. To avoid becoming deficient, talk to your doctor about taking supplements.

According to Reiter, nutritionists aren't sure what amounts of these nutrients will help combat insomnia. He suggests you start by taking 500 milligrams of magnesium and 1000 milligrams of calcium just before bedtime. "But first," he says, "ask your physician if there is any reason you should not be taking these supplements in these amounts."

**B vitamins.** Just two little B vitamins could mean the end of nights spent tossing and turning. B3 or niacin and B6 or pyridoxine both play important roles in your body's production of sleep-inducing melatonin.

Your body can make niacin out of tryptophan, but remember, you need tryptophan to make serotonin then melatonin. So, Reiter suggests you get extra B3 from your diet. This way you won't have to use up your own supply of tryptophan. Dried apricots, peanuts, barley, chicken, and turkey are good sources.

Vitamin B6 also helps convert tryptophan to serotonin. You may not have enough B6 if you smoke, drink alcohol, take birth control pills or estrogen, have carpal tunnel syndrome, suffer from depression, or eat a lot of refined foods. Seniors, also, seem to be at risk. To increase your B6, eat avocados, bananas, carrots, rice, and shrimp. If you want to kill two birds with one stone, eat brewer's

---

### A word of caution

Avoid sleep thieves. While some foods make you drowsy, others can have the opposite effect. You probably know caffeine — in coffee, tea, chocolate, and colas — is a stimulant that can keep you awake. But don't think a nightcap is a better choice to end the day. While alcohol may help you fall asleep faster, it's likely to make you wide-eyed and restless later in the night.

Instead, make your last meal of the day a light one. Leave off spicy, sugary, or fatty foods, which can interfere with sound slumber. Think about your eating and sleeping habits, together. "Many times," says Greenstein, "when people overeat they are really compensating for lack of sleep."

---

yeast, salmon, sunflower seeds, tuna, and wheat bran — you'll be getting a dose of both B3 and B6.

If your doctor approves, Reiter suggests taking a supplement of 100 milligrams of B3 just before going to bed and 50 milligrams of B6 early in the day. The B6 could make you feel more alert rather than sleepy if you wait until bedtime to take it.

### Eat

| | |
|---|---|
| Whole-wheat bread | Brown rice |
| | Flaxseed |
| High-fiber cereal | Skim milk |
| | Cantaloupe |
| Oatmeal | Figs |
| Apricots | Prunes |
| Water | Peaches |

### Avoid

Gas-producing foods, such as beans and cabbage

# Irritable bowel syndrome

You avoid social situations where food will be served or outdoor events where you may not find a bathroom. Getting to work on time and keeping appointments is sometimes a problem because of your unpredictable bowel habits. If this sounds like you, you may be suffering from irritable bowel syndrome (IBS), also known as spastic colon. It's a condition that causes abdominal pain, bloating, constipation, and diarrhea, and can wreak havoc with your social life.

Although there is nothing physically wrong with your gastrointestinal tract, you may have a sensitive colon that reacts to things that wouldn't bother other people. IBS symptoms usually start after eating and are more common when you're under stress. It's possible that stress triggers hormonal changes that can cause too much stomach acid or changes in digestion.

If your symptoms only occur when you drink milk, it's more likely you have lactose intolerance. That means you can't digest the natural sugar in milk. You need to add lactase enzyme (sold in drugstores) to milk products, or in extreme cases, avoid all foods containing milk.

Some doctors and nutritionists blame packaged foods for the increase in IBS. Instead of eating mostly plant-based and natural foods, people now eat refined foods with added chemicals. Maybe you're one of those whose stomach is protesting. But the good news is, you can take control of this irritating condition. Many IBS sufferers have found that a carefully chosen, nutritious diet helps their symptoms.

Dr. Steven R. Peikin, author of *Gastrointestinal Health*, agrees. "By far the best approach for the long-term management of IBS symptoms is diet," he says. "A high-fiber diet significantly affects the colon, or large intestine, throughout its entire course."

> ### Find your trigger foods
>
> People with IBS find that many ordinary foods cause their bowels to act up. Try keeping a diary for a week or so, and make notes of how you react to certain foods. You may find that every time you eat lunchmeats, you are in pain within the hour. Or maybe high-sugar foods cause gas and bloating. By keeping track, you can eliminate the offending foods from your diet. But don't forget about nutrition. For example, if you stop drinking milk, you'll need to take calcium supplements and eat lots of green leafy vegetables to keep your bones strong.

## Nutritional blockbusters that fight IBS

**Fiber.** If most of the bread, rice, and pasta you eat is made with white flour, your stomach ends up full of something like the flour-and-water paste you made in kindergarten. And that's a recipe for a stomachache. On the other hand, fiber-rich grains like whole-wheat bread and brown rice can help keep your bowels humming along.

Peikin explains that fiber is like a sponge, soaking up moisture to lessen diarrhea and creating bulk to help with constipation. Try using brown rice in your casseroles and as a side dish, and switch to whole-grain breads for sandwiches. But be careful not to eat too much bran, which can bother people with IBS. Instead, try cooked vegetables and fresh, non-citrus fruits, which are good sources of fiber.

### Get natural relief from psyllium

Psyllium comes from the husks of plant seeds and forms a gel in liquid. It is often recommended for IBS because the gel helps slow diarrhea but also fights constipation by keeping stools soft. It's sold commercially as Metamucil, but you'll also find it in breakfast cereals such as Kellogg's Bran Buds. Check your favorite cereals to see if they have been fortified with this helpful fiber.

Add these foods to your diet gradually. Most people have to build up a tolerance for fiber and will experience some gas and bloating at first. You might want to avoid cruciferous vegetables like cabbage and cauliflower, though, since these are harder to digest.

**Low-fat foods.** For IBS, low fat is where it's at. Cut way down on foods rich in cream and butter. Also, avoid nuts and seeds since they are high in fat and can cause gas. If you drink milk, be sure it's skim, and drink it with some food for better digestion. Peikin recommends you eat small, frequent meals to avoid overloading your stomach, which can lead to cramping and diarrhea. According to Peikin, a single serving of high-fat food can trigger an attack on your gastrointestinal tract.

**Flaxseed.** This seed of the flax plant is rich in omega-3 oils when crushed. If you use it whole, it works as fiber, bulking up in your stool for an easy ride through your system. It also absorbs extra fluid that might lead to diarrhea. You can sprinkle flaxseed on hot cereals or salads or bake them into breads and muffins.

Add flaxseed oil to your diet to replace some unhealthy foods like store-bought cookies, crackers, and other processed foods. Try using flaxseed oil on salads and vegetables instead of butter. It has a nutty, slightly fishy flavor and might take some getting used to. Available in health food stores, flaxseed oil must be stored in the refrigerator and never used for frying. Be sure to check the expiration date since it's only good for a few months.

# Kale

• • • • • • •

**Benefits**

Saves your eyesight

Strengthens bones

Combats cancer

Promotes weight loss

Banishes bruises

Boosts your immune system

There's more to kale than just a pretty plate. With its scalloped edges and variety of colors, this member of the cabbage family is a chef's favorite garnish. And it's also one of the few vegetables grown for ornamental purposes.

But kale and its country cousin, collard greens, are healthy additions to your menu, too. Low in calories and fat, kale is high in vitamin C, contains moderate amounts of calcium and other minerals, and is rich in antioxidants, especially the carotenoid beta carotene.

In fact, kale has the highest Oxygen Radical Absorbance Capacity (ORAC) score — a measure of the total amount of antioxidants in a food — of any vegetable. (Prunes came out a winner with the highest score overall.)

So next season plant a crop of kale and it will beautify your yard, your dinner table, and your body.

## 3 ways kale keeps you healthy

**Keeps eyes eagle-sharp.** As you grow older, you're more likely to develop sight-stealing conditions, such as cataracts and age-related macular degeneration (AMD). To save your vision, experts say eat more foods containing the plant chemicals called carotenoids. These act like antioxidants in your body and, according to research, are linked to a lower rate of AMD.

Lutein is the carotenoid researchers think is responsible for the sight-protective effect, and fresh kale has more lutein than any other food classified by the USDA. Even though cooking any food reduces the amount of lutein available, a recent study found you will absorb more of that protective substance if you add a little bit of fat when cooking. However, if you also want to protect your heart, use olive oil instead of animal fats.

**Builds better bones.** Do you need or want "cowless" calcium? If you don't eat dairy products, either because you're lactose intolerant or because you follow a vegetarian diet, plant sources of calcium can be important. Although some vegetables contain calcium, your body may have difficulty absorbing it. The calcium in kale, on the other hand, is very easily absorbed. That makes it a smart, bone-strengthening food.

But it's not just the calcium in kale that helps your bones, it's also the vitamin K. Women with low levels of K seem to have low bone mineral density and experience more bone fractures. According to research, senior women who get more than the recommended dietary allowance of vitamin K — 65 micrograms (mcg) per day — may cut their risk of hip fracture by up to 30 percent. You can get almost four times the RDA in just one ounce of raw kale.

**Stands firm against cancer.** Eating lots of vegetables and other plant foods can reduce your risk of developing cancer. And the *brassica* family of vegetables — including kale, cabbage, brussels sprouts, broccoli, and turnips — may be especially protective. Researchers think these vegetables are beneficial because they contain naturally occurring chemicals called glucosinolates which block the cancer-forming process.

> ### To cook or not to cook
>
> Although fresh is usually best, raw isn't always better when it comes to eating vegetables. You may absorb as much as three times more beta carotene from some cooked and puréed vegetables than from raw ones. To get the most nutrition from your diet, eat plenty of both.

The protective effect seems to be strongest for lung, stomach, colon, and rectal cancer. What's more, eating the recommended five or more daily servings of fruits and vegetables — with the specific nutrients found in kale such as vitamin A, vitamin C, and lutein — may provide some protection against breast cancer in women.

## Pantry pointers

When buying kale or collards, look for a fresh green color and crispy leaves. Avoid greens that are turning brown or yellow, or ones with wilted leaves or tiny holes — usually from insects.

Store your greens in the refrigerator and use them within a day or two. You may want to remove the tough center stalks before cooking. Wash the leaves well, since they tend to have dirt and sand clinging in the crevices.

If you want Southern-style kale or collards without the traditional bacon or fatback, try this healthier version. Sauté onions and garlic in olive oil. Then add a little liquid smoke and your greens and cover with water or vegetable broth. Boil for about an hour or until the leaves are tender.

**Eat**

| | |
|---|---|
| Skim milk | Sardines |
| Figs | Water |
| Avocados | Bananas |
| Potatoes | Broccoli |
| Lemonade | Beans |
| Limeade | Prunes |

**Avoid**

Foods high in oxalates, such as spinach and beets

# Kidney stones

• • • • • • • • • • • • •

Having a kidney stone can be one of the most painful experiences of your life, one you won't want to repeat. Unfortunately, once you've had one kidney stone, you're more likely to have another. Preventing kidney stones is important, not only to avoid pain, but because large stones can damage your kidneys.

Your kidneys perform an essential job — filtering waste from your blood and removing it from your body as urine. They contain almost 40 miles of tubes that process about 100 gallons of blood daily. To do their job properly, they need the right balance of liquids and dissolved solids. When this balance is out of whack, a kidney stone can form.

These hard, crystal lumps develop from dissolved solids in your urine. They can be tinier than a grain of sand or as big as a golf ball.

Kidney stones are made of different substances. Calcium oxalate or calcium phosphate accounts for 70 to 80 percent of them. Other types of kidney stones include struvite stones, caused by urinary infections, and uric acid stones, caused by too much uric acid in the urine.

If you think you have a kidney stone, get medical attention right away. Symptoms include:

◆ Extreme pain in your back or side that will not go away.

◆ Blood in your urine.

◆ Fever and chills.

◆ Vomiting.

◆ Urine that smells bad or looks cloudy.

◆ A burning feeling when you urinate.

## Nutritional blockbusters that fight kidney stones

**Water.** People who live in the "stone belt," a region of the southeastern United States, are more likely to develop kidney stones. Researchers think it's because the hot weather causes increased perspiration and reduced urine output. Drinking lots of water can help because it dilutes your urine and washes potential stone-causing particles out of your body.

If you've had a kidney stone, research shows drinking extra water could cut in half your risk of having a second stone. Try to drink three to four quarts of water a day. Drink even more during hot weather or when exercising.

**Calcium.** Because most kidney stones contain calcium, doctors once recommended eating fewer dairy products and other sources of calcium. Recent studies found that the people with the highest intake of dietary calcium are actually less likely to develop kidney stones, although calcium supplements may increase risk. Researchers think calcium from food sources may help prevent kidney stones by binding to oxalate in your digestive system.

Eating foods high in calcium also keeps your bones strong and protects them from osteoporosis. Good sources include dairy products, sardines, and peanuts.

**Vitamin B6.** Calcium oxalate stones are by far the most common type. Getting enough vitamin B6 in your diet may help you avoid these stones, because it works to convert oxalate into other substances in your body. Research indicates that a deficiency of B6 causes an increased risk of kidney stones. Foods high in B6 include avocados, beans, bananas, potatoes, and prunes.

> ### A word of caution
>
> According to recent research, eating fewer foods high in oxalate might help prevent calcium oxalate stones. Although most plant foods contain some oxalate, a recent study found that only eight foods caused an increase in urinary oxalate — spinach, rhubarb, beets, nuts, chocolate, tea, wheat bran, and strawberries.
>
> Limiting the amount of sugar and salt in your diet may also reduce your risk of kidney stones.

**Potassium.** This mineral reduces the amount of calcium in your urine, which lowers your risk of kidney stones. Dietary sources of potassium include bananas, avocados, figs, beans, and potatoes.

**Magnesium.** Add some magnesium to your potassium, and you could cut your risk of kidney stones dramatically. Magnesium may help your body convert oxalates into other substances, just like vitamin B6. Foods high in magnesium include seeds, nuts, beans, avocados, and broccoli. Add any of these to your next salad for a healthy treat.

**Plant protein.** Kidney stones are more common in developed countries, and a high intake of animal protein may be to blame. High levels of dietary protein can increase urinary calcium and decrease urinary citrate, which raises your risk of kidney stones. Animal protein is also a major source of purines, which can increase the risk of uric acid stones.

Severely limiting your protein intake can cause other health problems. Here's a better solution — get your protein from plant sources. Good sources include barley, beans, nuts, and broccoli.

**Citric acid.** If you're drinking glass after glass of water to help avoid kidney stones, fill one up with refreshing lemonade for a change. A high level of urinary citrate may lower your risk of kidney stones, and lemonade may increase your citrate level. One small study found that drinking lemonade every day — made with

4 ounces of lemon juice, 2 quarts of water, and very little sweetener — increased urinary citrate levels in 11 of 12 volunteers.

Not just any citrus juice will do. Lemon juice has about five times more citric acid than orange juice. And studies have found that drinking grapefruit juice may actually increase your risk of kidney stones.

# Lemons and limes

. . . . . . . . . . . . . . . . .

| **Benefits** |
| --- |
| Combats cancer |
| Protects your heart |
| Controls blood pressure |
| Smoothes skin |
| Stops scurvy |

No matter how many times you squeeze lemons and limes into your diet, it's probably not enough — and here's why. These fragrant citrus fruits offer a quick boost of disease-fighting nutrients. Just one tablespoon of lemon juice gives you more than 10 percent of the RDA for vitamin C.

Just ask the sailors of the British navy. They learned the hard way just how healthy limes can be. For centuries, sailors suffered from scurvy, a vitamin C deficiency, during their long sea voyages. Scottish naval surgeon James Lind discovered in the 1700s that citrus fruits could cure the disease. After that, British sailors always carried limes onboard with them.

Today, lemons and limes grow in California, Florida, and Arizona by the millions. These citrus fruits abound with antioxidants and other phytochemicals, which team up to fight heart disease, cancer, and infection.

It's easy to eat more lemons and limes. Just be creative — grate the peel, or zest, on grilled salmon; squeeze the juice on vegetables and salads; or whip up a refreshing pitcher of ice-cold lemonade.

---

### A tasty way to fight cancer

It's no secret that marinades make grilled meats tastier, but you might not know they make them healthier, too. "Scientists have found that marinades may be the single most effective way of reducing the formation of cancer-causing substances created during grilling," says Melanie Polk, the Director of Nutrition Education at the American Institute for Cancer Research. They may be as much as 99 percent effective.

The exact ingredients of your marinade are up to you. Just make sure to include a food from these three groups of ingredients — a flavoring (like garlic or onion), a base (honey or oil), and, most importantly, an acidic liquid, like lemon juice.

---

# 3 ways lemons and limes keep you healthy

**Protects your skin from cancer.** "Just by adding a slice of lemon to your beverages, or zest to your baking, or even squeezing fresh lemon juice on your food before eating," says Dr. Iman Hakim of the Arizona Cancer Center, "will make a difference in the long run." This big difference, according to Dr. Hakim's study of almost 500 people, may mean not getting squamous cell skin cancer.

The key to lemons' anti-cancer power, Dr. Hakim suggests, is d-limonene, a chemical that gives citrus fruits their smell. It's mostly in the zest, so you'll need to shave off this outermost, colored section of the peel to get the cancer fighter. But as Dr. Hakim recommends, "Incorporating citrus peel into your food is easy and tasty and can afford extra protection against chronic diseases." Just use the smaller teeth of a hand grater or a sharp knife. You can even buy a tool called a citrus zester that's perfect for the job.

**Puts the squeeze on heart disease.** Vitamin C is a powerful antioxidant. Studies show it raises good HDL cholesterol and helps prevent bad LDL cholesterol from becoming oxidized and forming plaques, which can clog your arteries. Vitamin C also helps lower blood pressure and strengthens your capillaries.

**Gives tea more punch.** A little lemon juice can go a long way. According to a recent study from India, just a squirt or two in a cup of tea unleashes that drink's full power to stop free radicals. Tea contains potent antioxidants, but your body can't take full advantage of them until you add lemon. The lemon juice breaks down the antioxidants in the tea, making them easier for your stomach to absorb.

## Pantry pointers

Buying a lemon or lime is like looking for a kitchen decoration. Only the prettiest will do — and the most fragrant. They should fill the room with their flowery smell and shiny, unblemished color. So when you bring lemons home, leave them out to brighten your kitchen, only putting them in the refrigerator after slicing them.

Like a paperweight, fresh lemons should also feel heavy for their size. That means they're loaded with juice. To get the most juice from a lemon, roll it against your kitchen countertop using the palm of your hand. This softens it up for better squeezing.

You'll get more juice from a lemon that's at room temperature. If your lemon is cold, try zapping it in the microwave for about 15 seconds.

> ### The secret to younger-looking skin
>
> Lemons contain an antioxidant that may protect your skin from the ravages of time. According to scientists from Italy, this chemical — called Lem1 — stopped the free radicals that cause the signs of aging even better than vitamin E.
>
> Lemon juice can irritate your skin, so don't use it by itself. Instead, mix it with other healing ingredients. For instance, to fade sunspots try adding the juice of a lime and a lemon to 2 tablespoons of honey and 2 ounces of yogurt. Rub the mixture into the spot at least once a week.

Here's another healthy tip. Anytime you cook vegetables, their vitamin C literally disappears, and the nutrient's benefits vanish with it. If you want to replenish the vitamin C in cooked foods, squirt some lime or lemon juice on your food right before you eat it.

### Eat

| | |
|---|---|
| Collard greens | Spinach |
| Carrots | Corn |
| Whole grains | Egg yolk |
| Poultry | Crab meat |
| Yogurt | Soybeans |
| | Apricots |

### Avoid

Foods high in saturated fat, such as red meat and whole-milk dairy products

# Macular degeneration, age-related (AMD)

As you stroll through your neighborhood, you may notice the vibrant colors of nature — red, orange, gold, and green. Look for these same colors on your plate at mealtime, and you'll increase your chances of keeping the sights around you in sharp focus.

Eating lots of brightly colored fruits and vegetables can reduce your risk of age-related macular degeneration (AMD), the number one cause of blindness in older people. AMD occurs when the macula, the central part of your retina, begins to break down. Nobody knows for sure why this happens, but free radical damage from light exposure is probably one contributing factor.

You won't feel any pain with macular degeneration. It just becomes harder to make out fine details as your central vision blurs or distorts. You're considered at risk of AMD if you're far-sighted, smoke, have light-colored eyes, have been exposed throughout your life to the sun, and have a family history of AMD or heart disease.

There are two kinds of AMD, wet and dry — both irreversible. Most people have the dry kind which progresses slowly and generally causes less serious vision loss. About 10 percent, however, have the wet kind that can cause permanent vision loss within weeks or even days. Although there are some new medications and surgeries for AMD, so far they've had only limited success. The experts say prevention is still the best medicine and a good place to start is with your diet.

Since high blood pressure and heart disease are risk factors, if you cut fat, especially saturated fat, from your diet, you'll be ahead of the game. Then eat lots of dark green leafy vegetables. One research study found those who ate the most collard greens and spinach had a far lower rate of AMD. Read on to find out more about the nutrients you need to keep your vision sharp.

## Nutritional blockbusters that fight AMD

**Vitamins and minerals.** You know how important teamwork can be in a family or when playing a sport. Vitamins and minerals work together in the same way to help prevent macular degeneration. Healthy eyes have a high concentration of the antioxidant vitamins C and E. They help each other do their job and end up protecting your retinas from free radical damage. Another team player is selenium, a trace mineral that combines with vitamin E to protect your eyes from the dangers of oxidation.

You can get these important team players from the food you eat. Meat, shellfish, fresh vegetables, and unprocessed grains provide plenty of selenium. And you'll absorb lots of vitamins C and E from brightly colored vegetables and fruits, like apricots, carrots, and red and green peppers. Supplements don't seem to give the same protection, and they certainly don't offer the delicious flavors or the fun crunchiness of these foods.

**Carotenoids.** Fruits and vegetables get their bright colors from a group of chemicals called carotenoids. And the antioxidant power of these nutrients can really brighten up your eyesight as well. Two in particular — lutein and zeaxanthin — accumulate in the macula of your eye where they help filter out damaging light rays.

To get lots of lutein, dish up an extra helping of corn and a big serving of those green leafy vegetables. One of the best ways to get zeaxanthin is to add some chopped orange peppers to your green salad. You'll find plenty of both of these carotenoids in zucchini, yellow squash, orange juice, and kiwi fruit. A good non-vegetable source is egg yolk.

**Zinc.** You don't need much zinc, but it's amazing what your body does with just a little. This mineral shows up in every organ, helping with many body processes that keep you healthy. It's especially concentrated in your retinas where it fights free radicals and helps in other ways to protect your eyes from AMD. Researchers have found a relationship between low levels of zinc and a higher risk of AMD.

You probably get plenty of zinc from your diet, but young children, pregnant women, and seniors can sometimes be deficient. Foods that contain zinc include oysters, crab meat, beefsteak, poultry, soybeans, enriched cereal, and yogurt. Your body absorbs zinc best from meat, but vegetarians who eat whole-grain breads leavened with yeast shouldn't have a problem.

Some doctors treat macular degeneration with zinc supplements. If you have AMD and think these might help you, be sure to discuss it with your doctor first. There is a real danger of getting too much zinc from supplements.

**Fatty fish.** To reduce your risk of AMD even more, make fatty fish, like salmon or tuna, a regular part of your weekly menu. The omega-3 fatty acids found in these kinds of fish may protect and restore the cell membranes in your retina. But eating fish more often isn't necessarily better. Too much omega-3 fatty acids can interfere with your body's ability to use the vitamin E your eyes need.

**Wine.** Getting important flavonoids from an occasional glass of wine can mean less chance of developing AMD. Pour a glass just once a month and you'll receive the benefits. On the other hand, research shows those who drink beer increase their risk of AMD.

# Mangoes

• • • • • • • • • • • • • •

| Benefits |
|---|
| Combats cancer |
| Boosts memory |
| Regulates thyroid |
| Shields against Alzheimer's |
| Aids digestion |

Eaten a mango lately? Apparently, a lot of people have. More fresh mangoes are eaten worldwide than any other fruit. This "apple of the tropics" may be considered exotic in some neighborhoods, but to much of the world's population, it's a common part of the diet.

The first mango tree probably grew in India, and that country is by far the world's leading producer of mangoes. In addition to being an important food source, the mango tree is also seen as a symbol of love in India, because according to legend, Buddha was given a grove of mango trees in which to rest.

Mangoes provide healthy amounts of beta carotene, vitamin C, vitamin B6, vitamin E, and potassium. Interestingly, while the fruit of the mango tree is beneficial, the leaves are toxic and can kill cattle or other grazing animals.

## 3 ways mangoes keep you healthy

**Cuts down cancer.** Add a juicy mango to your diet occasionally, and you may help ward off cancer. Mangoes are high in antioxidants, those nutritional powerhouses that help fight off disease. The

National Cancer Society recommends five fruits and vegetables a day, and just half a mango counts as one serving.

In addition, a substance in mangoes called mangiferin has shown an anti-tumor effect in test tube and animal studies. One study on mice found that mangiferin slowed tumor growth and helped the mice live almost two weeks longer than the non-mangiferin-treated mice.

**Heads off hypothyroidism.** Your thyroid is a small gland that causes big problems when it doesn't work as well as it should. It produces hormones that affect almost every part of your body. When the gland doesn't make enough of these hormones, you suffer from hypothyroidism.

The mango may be the perfect food to help regulate your thyroid. This gland needs vitamin A, and your body makes it from beta carotene, which the mango has in abundance. Mangoes also contain vitamin B6, vitamin C, and vitamin E, all important vitamins in making thyroid hormones.

**Keeps your memory sharp.** If you want to keep your brain fit and help stave off Alzheimer's, make mangoes a regular part of your diet. Scientists have found that the antioxidant vitamins E, C, and beta carotene may help save your memories, and mangoes are a great source of all three. If you're a woman, you'll get 100 percent of your daily requirement for vitamin A (beta carotene), 95 percent

---

### Tender, tasty, and healthy grilling

The next time you grill out, add a mango to your marinade. Besides making your meat more tender and tasty, it may help you avoid stomach problems and perhaps even cancer.

Mangoes make a super meat tenderizer because they contain an enzyme that breaks down protein. This enzyme may also help with digestion, which is probably why mangoes have been used for centuries as a stomach soother.

The American Institute for Cancer Research recommends marinating meat before grilling to reduce cancer risk. Just combine the mango with an acidic ingredient such as lemon, lime, or orange juice, and throw in a few herbs and spices. Your food will have a sweet and extra healthy punch.

of your vitamin C, and almost a third of your vitamin E from eating just one mango.

## Pantry pointers

Spring and summer bring fresh mangoes to the market, although you can buy the canned fruit year-round. When picking out a mango, give it a gentle squeeze. A fresh one will yield slightly to the pressure.

Although different varieties have different colors, one that is totally green or greenish-gray is probably not ripe. Like bananas, mangoes tend to get black speckles on the skin as they ripen, so too much black probably means it's overripe. Mangoes will ripen at room temperature, but if you want to speed up the process, toss them in a paper bag with another mango (or a banana).

Peeling and eating a fresh mango may be a challenging experience because the juicy fruit can be quite messy, but once you bite into the sweet flesh, it's all worth it.

# Memory loss

· · · · · · · · · · · · · · · · · · · · · · · ·

| Eat | |
|---|---|
| Blueberries | Strawberries |
| Kale | Spinach |
| Beets | Olive oil |
| Avocados | Liver |
| Asparagus | Oatmeal |
| Barley | Tuna |

**Avoid**

Foods high in saturated fat, such as red meat and whole-milk dairy products

Age doesn't have to take a toll on your mind. If you're experiencing memory loss, maybe all you need is a new, healthier diet.

Eat fresh foods rich in fiber, nutrients, and antioxidants, and eat plenty of them. You'll be helping your body combat serious illnesses that can affect your memory, like heart disease, and you'll be stimulating your appetite at the same time. Sometimes, medications, denture problems, or loneliness can steal your desire for food. Poor nutrition will put you at greater risk for memory problems.

If, despite a healthy menu, you or someone you know experiences a serious memory loss, see a doctor. It may be a sign of a bigger problem, like Alzheimer's disease. With professional help, you can chart a course of treatment.

## Nutritional blockbusters that fight memory loss

**Antioxidants.** Free radicals, remember, are unstable molecules your body makes as it processes oxygen. They zip around damaging your cells and making you more likely to fall prey to health problems — like memory loss. Luckily, antioxidants, substances in certain foods, get rid of free radicals.

According to scientists at the USDA-ARS Human Nutrition Research Center on Aging, your brain needs antioxidants to keep sharp. Otherwise, its cells wear down after years of free radical bombardment. Your memory becomes a little fuzzier, just like the picture in an old television.

Your best sources of antioxidants are vitamin E, vitamin C, beta carotene, and flavonoids. All together, the USDA experts believe these antioxidants can fix free radical damage done in the past, as well as prevent damage in the future. Fruits and vegetables pack an arsenal of antioxidants. So, eat strawberries, blueberries, prunes, brussels sprouts, and kale. They're like television repairmen for your head.

**Carbohydrates.** Eat a potato for breakfast and you might think better all day. At least that's what an exciting new study from Canada says. Subjects started their day with mashed potatoes, cooked barley, or a sugary drink. All three meals boosted memory and IQ test scores. The secret behind this morning miracle — energy. Your brain needs it and carbohydrates provide it.

All carbohydrates, though, aren't equal. Those from fruits, vegetables, and whole grains are better all-round sources of energy. Plus, whole grains and fruits tend to have a low glycemic index, which improves brainpower the most. (See the *Diabetes* chapter for an explanation of the glycemic index.)

Eat hearty carbohydrates — like oatmeal, bran, bananas, barley, and whole-wheat toast — for breakfast and throughout the day. Your brain will thank you by being alert, clear, and able to remember where you left your wallet.

**B vitamins.** Folate, thiamine, B6, and B12 — these B vitamins may be important ingredients in many of your brain chemicals. And that could be why people with B deficiencies scored lower on memory and problem solving tests, while people receiving a boost of B vitamins performed better. Chronic B vitamin deficiencies may also be one cause of serious mental conditions like Alzheimer's disease.

Make sure to eat spinach, beets, avocados, asparagus, and other vegetables for folate; low-fat cheeses, fish, and poultry for B12; and potatoes, beans, and watermelon for B6 and thiamin.

**Olive oil.** Pour on the olive oil, says a recent study from Italy, and you'll pour on the recall. Out of nearly 300 seniors, those who ate at least 5 tablespoons of olive oil a day tested best on memory and problem solving skills.

Give monounsaturated fatty acids (MUFAs) the credit. These "good" fat molecules appear to buffer brains against memory loss for one simple reason — your brain is made up of fat. And as you age, your brain needs more and more fatty acids to patch itself up.

You'll find MUFAs in almost any oil, but olive was the oil of choice because it contains vitamin E and other powerful antioxidants, as well as no cholesterol and no "bad" saturated fats.

**Iron.** You might need to iron out a problem in your diet if your brain feels sluggish. An iron deficiency could mean a muddled mind. Besides memory problems, other symptoms include pale skin, tiredness, and depression. Watch out for these signs if you regularly take nonsteroidal anti-inflammatory drugs (NSAIDs), if you are a menstruating woman, or if you are a vegetarian. All these put you at risk for iron deficiency and even anemia.

Meats are the prime source of this mineral, but legumes and green leafy vegetables work, too. Make sure to top these foods with a rich source of vitamin C like lemon juice, which helps your body absorb the iron from plant sources.

If you take NSAIDs and suspect you're low on iron, notify your doctor. The medication might be causing internal bleeding.

## Soy linked to higher rates of senility

If you've started eating tofu burgers instead of hamburgers because you think soy is healthier — you may be in for a surprise. New research suggests eating tofu may make your brain age faster, leading to serious problems with memory and learning in later years.

Even if you never eat tofu — a custard-like food made from puréed soybeans — you're still not in the clear. Soy or soybean oil is in everything from salad dressings, mayonnaise, and margarine to breakfast cereals and energy bars, making it the most widely used oil. About 60 percent of all processed foods contain soy protein. And since it is added to cattle and other livestock feed, you may consume it indirectly just by eating your usual steak or hamburger.

Researchers in Hawaii concluded that soy might contribute to brain aging after examining the diets of more than 8,000 Japanese-American men for over 30 years. They found those who ate two or more servings of tofu a week were much more likely to become senile or forgetful as they grew older compared with men who ate little or no tofu.

The more tofu the subjects ate, the more learning and memory problems they suffered in later life. Loss of mental function occurred in 4 percent of the men who ate the least amount of tofu compared with 19 percent of the men who ate the greatest amount of tofu.

These are shocking results for a food touted for its health benefits and recently given FDA approval to make health claims on package labels.

Dr. Lon White, lead researcher of the Hawaiian study, suggests the study's findings should make people think twice about the amount of soy they eat. "What we have here is a scary idea that may turn out to be dead wrong," he says. "Or it could turn out to be the first uncovering of an important health-negative effect of a food that we believe may have a lot of good going for it."

White's study included subjects ranging from 46 to 65 years old. The men were asked whether they ate certain foods associated with a traditional Japanese diet or an American diet. They were interviewed about their dietary habits again in the early 1970s and were tested for cognitive function — including attention, concentration, memory, language skills, and judgment — in the early 1990s when they were 71 to 93 years old. They were also given a brain scan at that time.

The results were disturbing. Out of 26 foods studied, only tofu was significantly related to brain function. Men who had a high intake of tofu not only scored lower on tests of mental ability, but their brains were more likely to show signs of advanced age and shrinkage. Their test scores were typical of a person four years older.

Although the study was done on men, researchers also interviewed and tested 502 wives of the men in the study — and came up with similar findings.

The study has created a stir because it contradicts previous research that found soy to be beneficial. Earlier studies have shown soy may fight cancer and heart disease, prevent osteoporosis, and relieve menopause symptoms. Researchers credit estrogen-like molecules called isoflavones for soy's apparent disease-fighting properties. But those same substances could have negative effects on the body as well, White notes. He says people need to understand that isoflavones are complex chemicals that act like drugs and change the body's chemistry.

"The great things they [consumers] have been hearing about soy foods in recent years have little to do with nutrients — carbohydrates, proteins, fats, minerals, vitamins," he says. "All that hype is related to the idea that soy contains other kinds of molecules that act like medicines ... they alter the way our body chemistry works."

The isoflavones in soy are a type of phytoestrogen or plant estrogen, which mimics the estrogen produced naturally in your body. Brain cells have receptors that link up with estrogen to help maintain brain function, and White believes phytoestrogens may compete with the body's natural estrogens for these receptors.

Many think soy's isoflavones interfere with enzymes and amino acids in the brain. One of soy's main isoflavones, genistein, limits the enzyme tyrosine kinase in the hippocampus — the brain's memory center. By interfering with the activity of this enzyme, genistein blocks a process called "long-term potentiation" that is central to learning and memory.

Dr. Larrian Gillespie, author of *The Menopause Diet,* says eating too much soy could result in other problems as well. She has found that consuming 40 milligrams (mg) of isoflavones a day can slow down thyroid function, resulting in hypothyroidism. Most isoflavone supplements come in a 40-mg dose, and just 6 ounces of tofu or 2 cups of soy milk would supply the same amount.

Also, because isoflavones act like estrogen, some studies suggest that postmenopausal women who eat a lot of soy may increase their risk of breast cancer. And scientists have questioned the potential effects of soy on infants as well. One study found infants who drank soy formula received six to 11 times as many phytoestrogens as the amount known to have hormonal effects in adults.

Some think this could lead to early puberty, which is associated with a greater risk for breast cancer and ovarian cysts.

This leads to the question of whether soy's good aspects outweigh the negative ones.

"Whatever good effects come with the gift [soy], will also come at some cost," White says. "We do not know yet just what those costs are, just as we really don't know yet the full and honest extent of their health benefits. We're flying blind ... and my data ... are very, very disturbing."

The Hawaiian study was a long-term, well-designed, controlled study, but it was just one study. The results are strong enough to make you sit up and take notice, but only more research can confirm them. If you eat soy, you may want to err on the side of caution. Be sure you know the amount of soy isoflavones you consume each day, and avoid soy supplements and soy-enriched foods (like some nutritional bars) until more research is done.

The following chart will help you determine the isoflavone content of some common soy products.

| How many soy isoflavones do you consume each day? | | |
|---|---|---|
| Food | Milligrams of isoflavones* | Serving size (approximate) |
| Bacon, meatless | 1.9 | 2 strips (1/2 ounce) |
| Granola bar (hard, plain) | .1 | 3.5 ounces |
| Harvest Burger, (all vegetable protein patty) | 8.2 | 1 patty |
| Infant formula, Prosobee® and Isomil® with iron, ready-to-feed | 8 | 1 cup |

| How many soy isoflavones do you consume each day? | | |
|---|---|---|
| Food | Milligrams of isoflavones* | Serving size (approximate) |
| Miso | 43.0 | 1/2 cup |
| Peanuts, raw | .3 | 1/2 cup |
| Soy breakfast links (45 g) | 1.7 | 2 links |
| Soy cheese, cheddar | 7 | 3.5 ounces |
| Soy flour (textured) | 148 | 1/2 cup |
| Soy hot dog (51 g) | 3 | 2 hot dogs |
| Soy milk | 20 | 1 cup |
| Soy powder (vanilla shake) | 14 – 42 ** | 1 scoop |
| Soy protein nutritional bar | 14 – 42 ** | 1 bar |
| Soy sauce, made from hydrolyzed vegetable protein | .1 | 1/2 cup |
| Soy sauce, made from soy and wheat | 1.6 | 1/2 cup |
| Soybean chips | 54 | 1/2 cup |
| Soybeans (roasted) | 128 | 1/2 cup |
| Tempeh | 44 | 1/2 cup |
| Tofu (silken, firm) | 28 | 1/2 cup |
| Tofu, yogurt | 16 | 1/2 cup |
| USDA Commodity, beef patties with Vegetable Protein Product (VPP), frozen, cooked ◆ | 1.9 | 3.5 ounces |

\*　Data from USDA – Iowa State University Database on the *Isoflavone Content of Food – 1999.*

\*\*　Data derived from Protein Technologies International.

◆　VPP is often used in school lunch programs.

# Menopause

· · · · · · · · · · · · · · · · · ·

| Eat | |
|---|---|
| Oats | Wheat |
| Corn | Apples |
| Skim milk | Wheat germ |
| Chinese | Almonds |
| cabbage | Peanuts |

**Avoid**

Foods high in saturated fat, such as red meat

Salt and alcohol in large amounts

For half of all women, menopause, which means the end of menstruation, takes place by age 50. You might experience this "change of life" several years earlier — especially if you smoke — or later depending on your genes.

Menopause occurs when your ovaries stop producing eggs each month. It can happen all at once, as it does when ovaries are surgically removed, or more gradually, over several years. Some women hardly notice a difference during this time, while others report vaginal dryness, indigestion, loss of sleep, hot flashes, mood swings, and depression.

You can trace most of these unpleasant side effects to plummeting hormone levels, especially estrogen. What's more, once your estrogen production tapers off, you're at greater risk of heart disease and osteoporosis.

◆ Estrogen dramatically lowers your "bad" LDL cholesterol levels and increases your "good" HDL cholesterol. It also keeps your fibrinogen levels low. Fibrinogen is the sticky substance that helps your blood clot. Having too much of it is a major factor in heart disease. Because of falling levels of estrogen, heart disease is a threat to women after menopause.

◆ Estrogen also helps your body absorb calcium better and actually kills off some of the cells in your skeleton whose job it is to break down your bones. That means without enough estrogen, osteoporosis, the crippling, bone-thinning disease that affects many older women, could be just around the corner.

While each woman experiences menopause in a unique way, all women need a healthy diet during this transition. In fact, there is evidence that good nutrition can keep you feeling well and happy during this important time of change.

According to the American Academy of Family Physicians, lifestyle changes may ease the symptoms of menopause. They advise a high-fiber, low-fat diet rich in antioxidants and including soy products. They feel this can decrease coronary heart disease risk, improve your cholesterol level and decrease hot flashes and other menopausal symptoms.

## Nutritional blockbusters that fight symptoms of menopause

**Phytoestrogens.** You don't have to despair when your personal supply of estrogen runs low because of menopause. People aren't the only ones who make estrogen — plants do too, called phytoestrogens. Eating plant foods with phytoestrogens can give you some of the protective benefits of estrogen. Sources are oats, wheat, corn, apples, almonds, cashews, and peanuts.

Isoflavones, a specific kind of phytoestrogen, are found mostly in soy-based foods like soybeans, tofu, miso, and soy nuts. Asian women eat about one type of soy food every day and report very few hot flashes and mood swings during menopause. This could mean they're getting some estrogen from their diet. (New research claims that soy may accelerate brain aging. For more information, see the *Memory loss* chapter.)

**Calcium.** More than ever, your body needs calcium during menopause to keep your bones strong and to avoid osteoporosis. In fact, experts recommend menopausal women get 1,200 milligrams of calcium every day. In addition to building strong bones, some nutritionists believe calcium might also help with hot flashes. If you have trouble digesting milk, as many adults do, try a product like Lactaid, which has the intestinal enzyme you are missing.

Other good sources of calcium are yogurt, which is easier to digest than milk, Chinese cabbage, spinach, molasses, legumes, seeds, and almonds. And if you haven't already, switch to juices fortified with calcium. The juice doesn't taste any different and cup for cup you'll get at least as much calcium as from milk — if not more.

**Vitamin E.** You can counterattack the threat of postmenopausal heart disease with vitamin E, a natural aid to your heart. As an antioxidant, it fights potential cancer-causing substances and keeps blood cholesterol from damaging your arteries. Researchers found evidence that eating foods high in vitamin E lowers the risk of death from coronary heart disease for postmenopausal women. The vitamin E, however, must come from food, not supplements.

To lessen those bothersome hot flashes and keep your skin feeling soft and looking younger, eat more E. Good sources are nuts, seeds, creamy salad dressings, mayonnaise, and avocados. Look for products made with canola oil to get the added benefits of omega-3 fatty acids. Just remember these are all high fat foods. If you add more vitamin E-rich foods to your diet without cutting down on other fats, you'll gain weight.

Although many women choose replacement hormones during menopause, talk to your doctor about what's best for you.

---

### A word of caution

Drop the saltshaker and no one gets hurt. Too much salt in your diet will make you feel bloated, and might make hot flashes worse. In addition, excess salt is bad for your heart and can contribute to bone loss by chasing away calcium.

If you crave salt, try using different herbs and spices on your food instead and drink lots of water. Water will help flush extra salt out of your body while keeping your skin and internal organs in good shape.

**Benefits**

Controls blood
  pressure

Lowers cholesterol

Kills bacteria

Combats cancer

Strengthens bones

# Mushrooms

• • • • • • • • • • • • • • • • • • • • • •

It would be nice if mushrooms could do what the ancient Egyptians believed — make you live forever. And what if they could grant you super strength or help you find lost objects? Throughout history and around the world, people from Mexico to Russia have given mushrooms magical powers. In reality, there's nothing miraculous about these fungi at all, but they can make you healthier.

Although mushrooms are largely made up of water, they are also high in protein, carbohydrates, and fiber. They are a potent source of vitamin D, riboflavin, and niacin, plus minerals like potassium, selenium, and copper. They are low in fat, salt, and calories. If that's not enough, mushrooms are literally made of disease-fighting ingredients called polysaccharides — giant chains of small sugar particles that link together to fight cancer, heart disease, and infection.

Next time you're at the grocery store, keep an eye out for all the varieties of mushrooms, particularly those with exotic names like shiitake (she-tah-key), maitake (my-tah-key), and chanterelle (shan-ta-rel). These specialty mushrooms are the most nutritious of the bunch.

## 5 ways mushrooms keep you healthy

**Controls cholesterol.** It's no secret — high cholesterol leads to trouble with your ticker. But mushrooms may be one way to lower your blood cholesterol by as much as 12 percent. Research from Japan shows that shiitake mushrooms may do just that. Although people in the study ate five or more mushrooms every day to get these results, add a few to your menu and look forward to some benefits.

**Levels off blood pressure.** Just half a cup of dried shiitake mushrooms has more potassium than a banana. That's important if you have high blood pressure, since getting enough potassium may be as necessary as cutting back on salt for getting your pressure on an even keel. You'll find many other mushrooms are rich in this mineral, as well.

**Zaps bacteria and viruses.** When cold and flu season next rolls around, many experts say reach for a blanket and some mushrooms. Certain chemicals in shiitake mushrooms help fight the flu virus as well as the top man-made drugs. And they seem to increase your resistance to fungi, parasites, and other viruses, too. Extracts from shiitake and maitake mushrooms may also jump start your immune system into making more natural killer cells. While the connection between eating whole mushrooms and these benefits is still controversial, adding a few of these delicacies to your daily menu can't hurt when it's cold and blustery outside.

**Cans cancer.** Consider mushrooms, too, when it comes to cancer prevention. Eating certain kinds — shiitake, maitake, oyster, and other exotic types — may cut your risk. However, experts agree they need to do a lot more research. Most of the focus so far has been on extracts of mushroom polysaccharides, not the whole mushrooms. These chemicals, studied for twenty-five years, seem to increase cancer survival by boosting resistance to tumors and reducing harsh side effects of chemotherapy.

### No open season on mushrooms

"There are old mushroom hunters, and bold mushroom hunters," the old saying goes, "but there are no old, bold mushroom hunters." Out of the thousands of mushrooms in the world, only a few hundred are edible. That means many more are poisonous. So unless you are a mycologist (a mushroom expert), only hunt for mushrooms in the grocery store. Eating mushrooms you uncover in the woods or in your backyard could be a fatal mistake.

In addition to providing a healthy dose of polysaccharides, whole mushrooms give you selenium. According to Dr. Peter E. Newberger, a professor working with the American Institute for Cancer Research, "Selenium is a potent antioxidant which can block cell DNA damage that may lead to cancer." Several studies show that it may prevent lung, colon, breast, throat, and prostate cancer. Eight dried shiitake mushrooms have almost all your recommended daily amount of selenium.

**Builds up your bones.** Mushrooms are the only non-animal food that can give you vitamin D — an important fact if you're a vegetarian. Mushrooms and their vitamin D may also be important to postmenopausal women fighting osteoporosis and people who are lactose intolerant and don't get vitamin D through fortified dairy products. Look for the chanterelle and shiitake varieties for big vitamin D boosts.

## Pantry pointers

Shopping for mushrooms may seem tricky at first, since there are so many kinds to choose from. But with a little know-how, you can have fun hunting for the one that gets your taste buds talking. Start with this list — experiment with dried or jarred varieties, too — and see for yourself.

◆ **Button.** This is probably the most common type of mushroom, but see the warning information later in this chapter.

◆ **Portobello (Roma).** You might think this giant mushroom is exotic, but it's actually just an overgrown button mushroom that's great for grilling.

◆ **Cepe (Bolete or Porcini).** Consider eating this dark, thick-stemmed mushroom instead of the regular buttons. It might cost a little more, but the flavor is worth it.

◆ **Enoki.** This native Japanese mushroom is small with a long stem. You'll get the best flavor from this delicate fungus if you eat it raw or just lightly cooked.

◆ **Shiitake ("Chinese black mushroom").** Although it's been popular in Asia for thousands of years, it is only now popping up in restaurants and markets throughout the rest of the world. Shiitake mushrooms have a strong, earthy taste and large, umbrella-like caps.

◆ **Maitake.** This mushroom is another delicacy in Asia, but it also grows wild in North America. Maitakes are sometimes called "hen-of-the-woods" because some claim they taste like chicken.

◆ **Chanterelle (Girolle).** Shaped like a bugle, this specialty fungus comes in a rainbow of colors — from golden yellow to black. The flavor varies, too, from light and fruity to peppery and robust.

◆ **Morel.** You'll probably only find morels grown wild, but they are especially popular because of their hearty flavor.

◆ **Oyster.** You have your pick of colors with oyster mushrooms — including pink and yellow. They taste mild, but their chewiness mixes well with crunchy vegetables.

---

### A word of caution

It may be time to turn in your everyday button mushrooms for a fancier type. Along with portobellos and false morels, buttons contain hydrazines — chemicals that some experts believe cause cancer. While the evidence is still limited, be on the lookout for more information.

If button mushrooms are your favorite and you don't want to give them up, then at least avoid eating them raw. Cooking them, especially for extended periods of time, seems to destroy some of the hydrazines.

◆ **Truffle.** This is the fanciest of the fancy mushrooms, and the most expensive at $400 a pound. If you plan on harvesting your own, you'll need to take a specially trained dog or pig to certain areas of France or Italy.

When buying any of these mushrooms fresh, choose ones that are firm and dry. Store them in a loosely closed paper bag. Too much moisture will make mushrooms rot so use very little water to clean them and don't store them in your refrigerator's crisper.

## Benefits

Lowers cholesterol

Combats cancer

Battles diabetes

Prevents constipation

Smoothes skin

Reduces risk of stroke

# Oats

• • • • • • • • • •

English writer Samuel Johnson, in his 1755 *Dictionary of the English Language,* defined oats as "a grain, which in England is generally given to horses, but in Scotland appears to support the people."

Johnson's Scottish biographer James Boswell countered, "Yes, and that is why in England you have such fine horses and in Scotland we have such fine people."

Well, healthy people anyway. The Scots knew a good thing when they saw it. Oats and oat products have many health benefits, largely because of their soluble fiber beta-glucan. They also provide protein and key minerals like potassium, magnesium, phosphorus, manganese, copper, and zinc. Eating a healthy portion each day can help you lower your cholesterol, manage diabetes, prevent cancer, and cure constipation. Oats can even relieve itchy skin, which is why you'll see oat extract listed on many bath products.

Of course, you don't have to be Scottish to enjoy this healthy grain. (Or a horse either.) Whether you eat oatmeal for breakfast or sprinkle oat bran on your cereal or baked goods, you'll benefit from getting more oats into your diet.

Just think of it as having good old-fashioned horse sense.

## 4 ways oats keep you healthy

**Battles cholesterol.** You've probably heard all the fuss about oat bran and its ability to lower cholesterol. Normally, you shouldn't believe everything you hear — but in this case, it's true. Oat bran does lower cholesterol.

That's because oat bran, the outer husk of the oat grain, contains tons of beta-glucan. This sticky soluble fiber works by slowing down your food as it passes through your stomach and small intestine, explains Dr. Barbara Schneeman, a researcher at the USDA Agricultural Research Service and a professor at the University of California-Davis. This gives high-density lipoprotein (HDL) more time to pick up cholesterol and whisk it to the liver and out of the body. It also gives low-density lipoprotein (LDL) less chance to move cholesterol to your artery walls, where it can build up and cause problems.

Some studies have reported that oats slashed total cholesterol by as much as 26 percent and LDL, or "bad," cholesterol by 24 percent, but most experts are more cautious.

Researchers who studied several trials involving oat products concluded that 3 grams of beta-glucan could slightly lower cholesterol. Since even a modest reduction in cholesterol leads to a lower risk of heart disease, this is big news. Even the Food and Drug Administration (FDA) has endorsed oat products for their cholesterol-lowering ability. The U.S. Department of Agriculture and the American Heart Association also recommend this heart-healthy grain.

However, not everyone gets the same benefit from oats. If you have high cholesterol, you'll see a more dramatic dip than if your cholesterol levels are normal or low. Adding just one serving of oats to your diet should help if you have high cholesterol. Otherwise, the amount you need depends on the form of oats you choose. For example, you have to eat three packets of instant oatmeal to get 3 grams of beta-glucan, but you only need one large bowl of oat bran cereal. Check food labels for "soluble fiber," and choose oat products with the most.

**Manages diabetes.** If you're struggling with diabetes, you know you should watch your carbohydrates. One good way to do that is to eat more soluble fiber.

The viscosity, or stickiness, of the beta-glucan in oats bogs down your food as it travels through your stomach and small intestine. This not only helps lower cholesterol, it also slows absorption of carbohydrates. Your blood doesn't get flooded with glucose all at once, so you don't have an immediate and urgent demand for insulin.

Many experts have recommended a high-fiber diet, with an emphasis on soluble and cereal fibers, as an effective way to deal with diabetes. A study in *The New England Journal of Medicine* found that a diet with 50 grams of daily fiber (25 grams each of soluble and insoluble) helped keep blood sugar, insulin, and cholesterol under control in people with type 2 diabetes. It also showed you could achieve this type of diet without taking fiber supplements or eating special fiber-fortified foods.

**Prevents cancer.** Wheat bran gets most of the attention when it comes to colon cancer, but oats may have some anti-cancer powers, too.

Again, the soluble fiber beta-glucan does the dirty work. Like the insoluble fiber of wheat bran, beta-glucan speeds food through the large intestine. It may also react with tiny organisms to form compounds that protect the colon wall and tame carcinogens. Wheat bran and other insoluble fibers help by adding bulk to the stool to dilute the cancer-causing substances.

### A word of caution

Oats contain gluten, a sticky protein that can be dangerous if you have celiac disease or a gluten allergy. Gluten can cause cramps, diarrhea, or even severe intestinal damage. People with celiac disease should also avoid wheat, rye, and barley products.

New research also suggests these same cereal grains could increase the risk of rheumatoid arthritis (RA) in people whose genes make them susceptible to this disease. The theory is that lectins, a type of plant protein found in oats and other grains, spur your immune system to attack your body's own joints, leading to inflammation. If you already suffer from RA, try eliminating cereal grains like barley, oats, and wheat from your diet. Your symptoms may improve.

"Rather than saying one is better than the other, there are two different ways they are operating," Schneeman says of the two broad categories of fiber. "When all is said and done, it may not come down to one or the other. Both mechanisms might play a role."

In other words, try getting different types of fiber into your diet for maximum cancer protection.

**Cures constipation.** Fighting cancer and other diseases is only part of fiber's job. Oats and other sources of fiber also help you day to day by keeping your digestive system running smoothly and preventing constipation. When you eat enough fiber (and drink enough water), your colon forms stools that can pass easily out of your body.

"You need this stuff for a healthy gut," Schneeman says. "That's where eating a diet high in fiber is a positive."

## Pantry pointers

Most oats you can buy are some form of oat groats, which are formed by removing the outer layer, toasting, and cleaning the oat. They can be cooked as a side dish like rice or used in salads and stuffings. Rolled oats, also known as old-fashioned oats, are simply oat groats that have been steamed and flattened. They usually take about 15 minutes to cook. Instant oatmeal might be quicker, but it also contains added sugar and salt.

Other varieties include Scotch oats, steel-cut oats, or Irish oatmeal, which are all names for oats that have been cut but not rolled. You can also buy oat bran or oat flour. If you can't locate these products in your supermarket, try your local health food store.

## Benefits

Strengthens bones

Protects your heart

Eases arthritis

Controls blood pressure

Enhances blood flow

# Okra

• • • • • • • •

How okra made its way into dishes all over the world is quite a tale. People first grew the little green pod in Africa hundreds of years ago, but then it spread to the Middle East, India, Asia, and eventually with the slave trade, all the way to the New World. Some historians say North Americans should thank the French Creoles of Louisiana for making okra a popular ingredient in many delicious recipes. If you're an okra lover, you might want to try dried okra, okra oil, or ground okra seed as a coffee substitute.

Okra may not be a commonplace vegetable, but it's no secret how good it tastes stewed with tomatoes, or how thick and delicious gumbo is with the little green pod in it. Okra is so celebrated now that it even has its own holiday — the Okra Strut in Irmo, South Carolina.

You'll find many vitamins and nutrients in okra, including potassium, vitamin C, magnesium, folate, and manganese. These make this tasty vegetable a potent weapon against osteoporosis, arthritis, and heart disease.

## 3 ways okra keeps you healthy

**Socks it to heart disease.** For a triple-powered punch against heart disease, eat some okra. It strikes first with an antioxidant jab to atherosclerosis — that dangerous hardening and clogging of your blood vessels. The top antioxidant in okra's arsenal is vitamin C which the World Health Organization has linked to a reduced risk of fatal heart disease. One cup of sliced okra has more C than a whole tomato. Although you can't rely on okra as a single source of this important vitamin, it makes an interesting and nutritious addition to your diet.

With a healthy dose of folate — about 40 percent of your daily requirement in each cup — okra then gives heart disease a left hook. Without this B vitamin, your body leaves behind loose amino acids, called homocysteine, when it metabolizes protein. Too much homocysteine built up in your blood damages your arteries and can lead to heart disease and stroke.

Okra gives a final knockout blow with its wealth of minerals — mainly potassium and magnesium. For lowering blood pressure, experts say eating potassium-rich foods may be as important as losing weight and cutting back on salt. And just the right amount of magnesium is especially important to seniors, who may not absorb it as well as they used to and may excrete more of it as waste. Magnesium helps control cholesterol and blood pressure, regulates your heart rhythm, and may even improve your odds of surviving heart disease and heart attacks.

**Arms you against osteoporosis.** Don't forget okra when you're planning a bone-building menu. It's full of four osteoporosis-fighting nutrients — potassium, magnesium, vitamin C, and beta carotene. People who eat foods high in these nutrients, according to research from the United Kingdom, may slow down the bone loss that can lead to osteoporosis. To top it off, a cup of okra gives you over 10 percent of the recommended dietary allowance (RDA) of the most famous bone-building mineral of all — calcium.

**Eases osteoarthritis.** Doctors used to think osteoarthritis (OA), the most common type of joint disease, was unstoppable, but now natural alternatives give new hope.

Foods like okra contain both vitamin C and manganese, nutrients your body needs to build up joints and cartilage. Experts who looked at a variety of research suggest a diet high in vitamin C may slow down the development of OA. They also remind us that manganese is a necessary component of cartilage.

## Pantry pointers

Even though okra has a sticky reputation, don't judge this little veggie until you've enjoyed it cooked properly. The chemical compounds that make okra gummy stay safely trapped inside each pod, unless you slice them. Steam whole pods or add them to stews for extra flavor. If you're making a gumbo, cut up the pod and let the natural juices thicken your dish. For a different taste, slice okra raw into a salad or coat the little wagon wheels with cornmeal and fry them up crisp.

No matter how you eat your okra, remember two things. Rub off the outer fuzz with a towel if you don't like the roughness. And if you cook okra in a pot made of brass, iron, or copper, the pods will darken.

# Olive oil

• • • • • • • • • • • • • •

### Benefits

Protects your heart

Promotes weight loss

Eases arthritis

Combats cancer

Battles diabetes

Smoothes skin

Greeks know how to eat well. Their typical diet includes lots of fruits, vegetables, and grains — and fat. But not just any fat. Unlike the standard American diet, where most of the fat comes from animal products, the Mediterranean diet uses olive oil as its main source of fat.

Olive oil, made by pressing ripe olives, is 77 percent monounsaturated fat, the good kind that helps rather than hurts your body. It's also rich in Vitamin E and has several compounds scientists believe resist cancer. This flavorful oil fights heart disease, rheumatoid arthritis, and diabetes, and as a mild laxative, olive oil may also help with gallbladder problems. Now here's what you don't get with olive oil: cholesterol, salt, or gluten. And it has very little saturated or "bad" fat that can raise cholesterol and cause all sorts of health problems.

But olive oil is not some new miracle cure. It's been around — and prized for both cooking and healing — for thousands of years. The Cretes grew rich from exporting olive oil as far back as 2475 B.C., and both the Bible and Greek mythology refer to it. Now exported mainly from France, Spain, Italy, and Greece, you can find olive oil in any supermarket. Try substituting olive oil for butter, margarine or other vegetable oils when you cook. By pouring out some olive oil, you'll be pouring on the health benefits.

## 5 ways olive oil keeps you healthy

**Trumps heart disease.** In spite of their high-fat diet, the Greeks hardly ever develop heart disease or hardening of the arteries,

263

called arteriosclerosis. This is partly because their diet includes foods rich in fiber like grains, fruits, and vegetables; protein from fish and very rarely from red meat; and moderate amounts of red wine. But another important part is the monounsaturated fat from olive oil.

Unlike people, not all fats or cholesterols are created equal. Monounsaturated fat, the kind you find in olive oil, gives you the biggest benefit because it cuts down on the bad cholesterol without harming the good cholesterol. And experts think olive oil decreases your blood's stickiness — making it less likely to clot. This lowers your blood pressure and your risk for stroke. Remember high blood pressure contributes to heart disease because your heart has to work harder than it should.

Don't start eating high-fat meals thinking olive oil will save the day. Just continue to eat sensibly and add olive oil to your diet whenever possible. Your taste buds and your heart will approve.

**Halts those hunger pangs.** The type of fat you eat at lunch could affect how hungry you are at dinner. Anyone battling extra pounds knows the growl in your belly is hard to ignore. But if you are 20 to 30 percent over the average weight for your age, sex, and height, it is vitally important you take back control of your weight. Not only are you a prime candidate for high blood pressure and diabetes, but some cancers, as well.

> ## Olive oil: a skin-deep beauty
>
> Even if you don't eat it, olive oil is an amazing health remedy. According to Japanese researchers, putting extra virgin olive oil on your skin after sunbathing could protect you from ultraviolet radiation. It is not a sunscreen, but vitamin E and other antioxidants nab free radicals caused by the sun before they do too much harm. Just make sure you use extra virgin — regular olive oil isn't as effective.
>
> And its healing powers don't stop there. It's great for relaxing massages and for centuries olive oil has treated wounds, minor burns, eczema, and psoriasis. It also softens earwax and relieves ringing or pain in your ears. Just see your doctor before treating any kind of serious condition.

No one considers oil a diet food, since most, including olive oil, contain about 120 calories a tablespoon. But there are two reasons why substituting olive oil for others could help you lose weight.

Researchers at Penn State University found oils rich in monounsaturated fat, like olive oil, fill you up more than others. In their study, people who ate mashed potatoes prepared with monounsaturated oils were less hungry later in the day than people who ate the same food cooked with polyunsaturated oils. If you're less hungry, you're less likely to snack, overeat, and put on unwanted extra pounds. And because olive oil has such a rich flavor, you don't need to use as much of it.

**Takes aim against arthritis.** The next time you bring home a bag of produce, stir-fry it in olive oil and you may ward off rheumatoid arthritis. Perhaps it's the monounsaturated fat that stops inflammation in your joints, or it might be the antioxidants that lock up dangerous free radicals. Whatever the reason, those who ate the least olive oil in a clinical study were more than twice as likely to develop this painful condition. The combination of fresh vegetables and olive oil seemed to be especially beneficial.

**Keeps cancer at bay.** Free radicals roam throughout your body causing potential damage, including cancer. Fortunately, olive oil contains antioxidants, which keep free radicals in check. Studies show that adding olive oil to your diet may reduce your risk of breast, colorectal, prostate, and esophageal cancers.

### So good it's in the Good Book

You'll find olive oil in practically every cookbook and healthy living guide. But did you know there are plenty of references to olives and olive oil in the Bible?

In the Book of Exodus, God tells Moses how to make an anointing oil out of spices and olive oil. The Hebrews used olive oil in some of their offerings, for burning in lamps, and for anointing the dead. The olive branch became a lasting symbol of peace when the dove Noah sent from the ark returned with one. And Gethsemane, the site of the Last Supper, means "oil press" in Aramaic.

**Defends against diabetes.** Because olive oil can slash the amount of LDL and total cholesterol as well as triglycerides, or fats, in your blood, it helps reduce your risk for developing Type 2 (non-insulin-dependent) diabetes. It also seems to lower your blood sugar, or glucose, levels. High blood sugar is a key symptom of diabetes. Once again, the benefit comes from monounsaturated fat. However, if you are diabetic, avoid too much of a good thing. A high-fat diet can lead to obesity and other health risks.

## Pantry pointers

To get the most from your olive oil, look for the "Extra Virgin" variety. In addition to the strongest flavor, this less-refined product has the most of what makes olive oil good for you. If you want a milder taste, buy olive oil labeled "Virgin" or "Light." This refers to color and flavor and not calories or fat.

Olive oil kept in a tightly capped container, away from heat and light, can last about two years. You can refrigerate it, but it will become cloudy. As soon as it reaches room temperature again, the cloudiness will vanish.

---

### Benefits

Reduces risk of heart attack

Combats cancer

Kills bacteria

Lowers cholesterol

Fights fungus

Helps stop strokes

---

# Onions

• • • • • • • • • • • •

Onions might make you cry, but they certainly don't give you any reason to be sad. On the contrary, onions offer a bounty of health benefits along with the tears.

A member of the *allium* family — like garlic, leeks, and chives — the onion has been appreciated for thousands of years. Egyptian slaves building the pyramids were fed a diet that included onions, and onions were a prized food of the well-to-do in ancient China.

During the Civil War, Union general Ulysses S. Grant showed how essential onions were by sending a message to Washington that read, "I will not move my armies without onions." He got the onions — and his side won the war.

Coincidence? Maybe not. Thanks to the powerful flavonoid quercetin and a host of sulfur compounds, onions can make anyone a winner. Onions, which also have some potassium, vitamin C, and B vitamins, kill germs, help your heart, and fight cancer. Plus, they add great flavor and a pleasant aroma to almost any dish.

Peel an onion and start chopping. When you think of the onion's delicious taste and mighty health powers, the only tears you'll cry will be tears of joy.

## 3 ways onions keep you healthy

**Zaps heart disease.** Japanese women rarely get heart disease. That could be because they get plenty of flavonoids, including quercetin, in their diet. About 83 percent of their quercetin comes from onions. A recent study determined that quercetin intake led to lower levels of total cholesterol and "bad" low-density lipoprotein, also called LDL, cholesterol.

The Dutch Zutphen Elderly Study also demonstrated the beneficial effects of flavonoids. Men who ate the most flavonoids, mainly quercetin, were much less likely to die of heart disease. More specifically, men who ate onions cut their risk by 15 percent compared with those who didn't.

Quercetin in onions helps by stopping LDL cholesterol from becoming oxidized and, hence, more dangerous. Oxidized LDL carries cholesterol to your artery walls more quickly. Once there, it can build up and block your arteries, increasing your risk for a heart attack or stroke.

Getting your quercetin from onions seems especially helpful because your body absorbs it more quickly and retains it longer than quercetin from other food sources.

The sulfur compounds in onions may also lower your blood pressure and prevent blood clots by keeping the platelets in your blood from clumping together.

**Wipes out cancer.** Half an onion a day keeps stomach cancer away. That's what Dutch researchers discovered in a study of more than 120,000 men and women. People who ate at least half an onion a day were half as likely to get stomach cancer as those who never ate onions.

University of Hawaii researchers found similar results in their study of lung cancer. Those who ate the most onions were half as likely to get lung cancer as those who ate the least. A French study even indicated that onions and garlic might protect you from breast cancer.

> ### Stop crying over onions
>
> Ever wonder why you cry when you chop an onion? When you crush the cells of an onion, you release a sulfur compound. When this compound reacts with the moisture in your eyes, it turns into sulfuric acid, which irritates your eyes. Your eyes then produce tears to flush the sulfuric acid out.
>
> You can try many tricks to avoid crying. Refrigerating an onion for an hour before you chop it or chopping the onion under running water are some options. Or try chopping the onion while chewing on a piece of onion or a stick of gum. Your best bet, though, might be to wear goggles or glasses to protect your eyes.

The reason onions are so effective is probably because of their high levels of quercetin, which acts like an antioxidant. Antioxidants capture dangerous free radicals that can damage your cells and cause cancer. The sulfur compounds in onions may also inhibit tumors.

**Kills bacteria.** Planning a cookout? Plan to bring some onions. A Japanese study found that adding onions to ground beef helped neutralize *Salmonella* and prevent the formation of potential cancer-causing compounds called heterocyclic amines. Although quercetin might help, most of the credit goes to the sugars in onions. For tastier — and safer — burgers, just add a half-cup to one cup of chopped onion to each pound of ground beef you're grilling.

Even when applied to the skin, onions have healing powers. People have used onions to kill funguses, yeasts, and parasites; soothe the sting of insect bites; and even to ward off infection from stingray wounds.

## Pantry pointers

Onions come in many varieties. Some are seasonal, like the sweet Vidalia onion from Georgia, while others are available year round. You can find red, yellow, or white onions in a wide range of sizes. Try different ones to discover what you like best. You can also buy canned or frozen onions, which are usually smaller pearl onions.

Look for firm onions with papery skin that's free of spots. You can store onions in a cool, dry place for about two months. If you don't use all of an onion, wrap the leftover portion and refrigerate it for up to four days.

# Oranges

· · · · · · · · · · · · · ·

| Benefits |
| --- |
| Supports immune system |
| Combats cancer |
| Protects your heart |
| Strengthens respiratory system |

Oddly enough, the orange didn't get its name from its color but rather from an ancient Sanskrit word meaning "fragrant." In fact, people have prized this golden fruit for its beauty and scent for thousands of years.

Originally from Southeast Asia, oranges made their way to warm-weather areas of Europe, North Africa, and the United States. In 1513, Ponce de Leon planted the first orange tree in Florida, an area that now produces most of the world's oranges.

In the 1700s, oranges became even more popular when a Scottish naval surgeon discovered oranges and other citrus fruits cured scurvy, the plague of seamen everywhere.

Of course, oranges do much more than ward off that nutritional deficiency. Because they're loaded with vitamin C and contain carotenoids, folate, fiber, and potassium, they also strengthen your immune system, help your heart, and protect you from cancer. And don't forget how sweet, juicy, and delicious they are.

Peel an orange and sink your teeth into this tasty, healthy fruit ... now "orange" you glad you did?

## 4 ways oranges keep you healthy

**Boosts your immune system.** You may never get cancer or have a heart attack, but you will catch a cold. This pesky inconvenience strikes everyone at one time or another.

But thanks to oranges and their high levels of vitamin C, your cold won't stick around long. Vitamin C spurs your body's immune system into action so you can fight off germs. Although experts say vitamin C doesn't reduce the number of colds you get, it does cut down on how long and how seriously you're sick.

If you're extremely active, you may benefit even more from vitamin C. Some studies show people under heavy physical stress cut their risk of catching a cold in half if they take vitamin C. You'll see even more dramatic effects if your diet is low in vitamin C.

Even though many fruits and vegetables contain this nutrient, oranges are a great source, averaging more than 69 milligrams (mg) — close to a full day's recommended amount. So start eating oranges, and stop sniffling, sneezing, and coughing.

**Banishes pneumonia and bronchitis.** Even if you have a respiratory problem more serious than the common cold, vitamin C can help.

Several studies show extra vitamin C can cut your risk of developing pneumonia — by up to 80 percent. And with just 200 mg of vitamin C each day, elderly pneumonia or chronic bronchitis patients had fewer symptoms and recovered more easily. That's three oranges or less than two glasses of orange juice a day.

This eye-popping protection may come from vitamin C's ability to strengthen your immune system or from its antioxidant powers.

**Guards your heart.** Just as a single orange has several juicy sections, all oranges have many powerful weapons to fight heart disease.

◆ Fiber, especially the soluble kind in fruit, helps lower cholesterol. Too much cholesterol can clog or block your arteries, leading to atherosclerosis, heart attack, or stroke. You get 3 grams of fiber per orange, or about 12 percent of the RDA.

◆ Folate neutralizes homocysteine, a dangerous substance that increases clotting and can damage the lining of your blood vessels. One orange provides around 20 percent of the RDA for folate.

◆ Potassium helps keep your blood pressure under control — especially when you limit your sodium intake — and lowers your risk for stroke. An orange has 237 mg of potassium (nearly 12 percent of the RDA) and no sodium.

◆ Vitamin C may lower your blood pressure, improve blood flow, and shrink your risk of stroke. Because it's an antioxidant, it may fight cholesterol by preventing the low-density lipoprotein (LDL or "bad") cholesterol from becoming oxidized and, consequently, more dangerous to your artery walls.

**Thwarts cancer.** Cancer might be called "the Big C," but that title rightfully belongs to vitamin C, which looms large in the battle against the disease.

Although some tests have shown large doses (10 grams) of vitamin C can treat people with cancer and help them live longer, the antioxidant vitamin mainly shields you from free radicals that can cause cancer. Studies indicate vitamin C may protect you from stomach, throat, lung, bladder, and pancreas cancers.

Oranges also provide fiber, folate, flavonoids, and the carotenoid beta-cryptoxanthin — all dedicated cancer enemies. With all that protection, it's easy to see why eating more of this fruit is a sensible anti-cancer strategy.

## Pantry pointers

When shopping for oranges, choose firm, heavy fruits without any signs of mold. Don't be fooled by a bright color — often food coloring makes oranges look more appealing. Keep oranges at room temperature for a day or two or store them in the refrigerator for two weeks.

You can find fresh oranges year-round at the supermarket. Some varieties, like the navel or Valencia, taste sweeter, while the Mandarin is easier to peel. Bitter oranges, like the Seville, are used for marmalade but are too sour to eat raw.

### A word of caution

Vitamin C is good, but it's possible to get too much of a good thing. Taking more than 2,000 mg of C could lead to diarrhea or other stomach problems. Because vitamin C helps your body absorb iron, high doses could lead to too much iron. Excess vitamin C may also cause kidney stones or erode the enamel on your teeth.

Fortunately, if you stick to eating whole fruits you won't have to worry. It would take about 29 oranges to get 2,000 mg of vitamin C. So put away the pills and reach for some healthy fruits and vegetables. It's safer — and much tastier.

# Osteoarthritis

· · · · · · · · · · · · · · · · · · · · ·

| Eat | |
|---|---|
| Skim milk | Oranges |
| Broccoli | Grapefruit |
| Strawberries | Apples |
| Pears | Raisins |
| Ginger | Turmeric |
| Water | Parsley |

**Avoid**

Any food that seems to inflame your arthritis

High-fat foods

Osteoarthritis (OA) is the most common form of arthritis. Four out of five adults age 50 or older suffer from one form of OA or another.

The "wear and tear" of a long life plays a big part in developing this disease. Years of moving your joints can rub away your cartilage. This soft tissue normally buffers the end of your bones and prevents them from rubbing together. Without it, your bones scrape together, causing terrible pain. But some scientists also believe an enzyme imbalance in your joints might contribute to the problem. If you have too much of certain enzymes, your cartilage will break down faster than it's rebuilt.

Although people used to believe it was just a normal part of aging, some experts now think you can prevent this type of arthritis by living a healthy lifestyle. Everyday nutrients appear to be a winning weapon in the battle against osteoarthritis. It's possible the foods you eat could slow and even stop the damage to your joints. Although not all experts agree, boosting these nutrients in your diet can only help your overall health.

Shedding some pounds if you are overweight might also be a way to halt OA. Those extra pounds add up to more wear and tear on your knees, ankles, hips, back, and other joints that support you. So it's a good idea to eat foods like fruits, vegetables, and whole grains, which will help you manage your weight. And limit your intake of fatty and sugary foods, while getting your protein from legumes and fish instead of red meats.

Eating a healthy diet can't replace your doctor's advice and treatment, but it can give new hope for a future without painkillers and canes.

## Nutritional blockbusters that fight osteoarthritis

**Vitamin C.** You might think of a bowl of oranges as a toolbox for your joints. Experts say the vitamin C in those juicy treats seems to slow the damage of OA. It might even repair damaged cartilage. The reason behind it is simple: your body needs vitamin C to make collagen, a protein that builds new cartilage and bone.

Besides oranges, eat fresh uncooked foods like broccoli, grapefruit, and strawberries. Also, make it a practice to sprinkle lemon juice or parsley on cooked foods to replace the vitamin C lost in the oven.

**Boron.** You're probably not getting your fill of this trace element. Most people only get 1 to 2 milligrams (mg) a day. But according to British scientist Dr. Rex E. Newnham, 3 to 10 mg a day could help prevent arthritis. That same amount could also relieve morning stiffness and other arthritis symptoms.

Newnham's research suggests boron is an essential ingredient to bone and joint health. It could also help your body stop calcium loss. Either way, its effects are plain to see. In comparing people who got a lot of boron in their diets to those who didn't, Newnham found that people in boron-rich countries were less likely to develop osteoarthritis.

Snack on non-citrus fruits like apples and pears, a few tablespoons of peanut butter, and a handful of raisins or prunes to make your joint-saving quota of boron. You might not see results for a month or two, but be patient, and you may reap the benefits of boron's positive effects.

**Vitamin D.** Research has shown that without enough of this fat-soluble nutrient, you may be more at risk for osteoarthritis of the hip. If you already have OA, vitamin D might slow the condition's progression. Ample amounts of vitamin D can help your body reg-ulate its calcium levels and help regrow new cartilage.

Getting your daily dose of "the sunshine vitamin" could be as easy as fishing or golfing on a sunny day. Your body can make this vitamin when enough sunlight hits your skin. But you can still get this essential vitamin if you live in a cloudy part of the world like New England or Vancouver. Just eat plenty of low-fat dairy, eggs, and seafood to get your full supply of vitamin D.

**Ginger and turmeric.** Try these spices and you might be able to cut back on your painkillers. Both contain curcumin, a phyto-chemical with proven anti-inflammatory powers. It may even work as well as nonsteroidal anti-inflammatory drugs (NSAIDs) like aspirin and ibuprofen, according to the latest research. Brewing ginger tea is a painless way to add curcumin to your diet. Or toss some fresh ginger or ground turmeric into your next stir-fry.

It's a good idea to talk with your doctor first if you have gall-bladder trouble or take NSAIDs or blood thinning medication like warfarin.

**Water.** Making new cartilage for your joints could be as easy as drinking eight 6-ounce glasses of water each day. This pure bev-erage is a key ingredient in that bone-protecting tissue, besides hydrating you.

To make your daily eight, stick with simple water. Sugary drinks can lead to weight gain, and remember — you want to stress your joints as little as possible.

---

### A word of caution

Keep away from certain foods, and you may do your joints a favor. Some experts believe food allergies can inflame your arthritis. Top suspects include tomatoes, peppers, red meat, citrus fruits, and aspartame. This link is still controversial so talk with your doctor before making major changes in your diet. But you could stop eating one specific food at a time to see if it helps.

**Eat**

| | |
|---|---|
| Kale | Almonds |
| Bananas | Potatoes |
| Oranges | Tea |
| Yogurt | Apricots |
| Strawberries | Collard |
| Bok choy | greens |
| Milk | |

**Avoid**

Salt and high-protein foods in large amounts

# Osteoporosis

• • • • • • • • • • • • • • • • • • • • •

You might have heard your grandmother say an elderly lady had "dowager's hump," referring to her stooped posture and rounded back. What she really had was osteoporosis, or brittle bone disease. In the advanced stages, the spine can weaken enough to collapse, making the person appear shorter and hunched over. Unfortunately, the effects of osteoporosis are not always that visible. You can have this disease for years without any symptoms or pain.

If you are a woman, your bones are strongest when you're about 25 years old. Until that time, your body uses calcium and other minerals to strengthen your bones. But then the process tapers off. By the time you reach your 30s, you're losing a small amount of bone each year. And after menopause, hormonal changes can make you lose bone at an alarming rate, causing brittle bones that break easily.

Having osteoporosis means you can fracture a rib just by coughing or break a hip simply by stepping off a curb. By age 90, one out of three white men and women will break a hip. (The risk is a little less for blacks and Hispanics.) Frighteningly, one out of four will die from complications within six months of the break. But you don't have to be a statistic. You can declare war against osteoporosis and win.

Connie Weaver, Ph.D., head of Purdue University's Department of Food and Nutrition and an expert in calcium absorption, believes you can easily prevent this terrible disease. "The most important thing a woman can do to prevent osteoporosis," she says, "is good nutrition and good exercise habits, ideally before puberty." But you need to follow the same advice after menopause, she adds, and talk to your doctor about hormone replacement.

Men also can have brittle bones, but women — especially thin women who are past menopause — are at greater risk. If you're thin, you have less weight bearing down on your bones during normal activity, and that means your bones will weaken faster. It's particularly important for you to start a regular program of weight-bearing exercises such as walking, jogging, or strength training. Studies have found gardening is also good at pumping up your bones so if you enjoy that activity, keep it up. The fresh air and sunshine are an added bonus.

## Nutritional blockbusters that fight osteoporosis

**Calcium.** You know you need calcium for strong bones and teeth. The problem is packing the recommended 1,200 milligrams (mg) into each day's menu while trying to watch your weight. But it can be done. You can get more than your day's requirement of calcium by drinking two cups of skim milk (300 mg each) and one cup of a calcium-fortified juice (300 mg), and eating three quarters of a cup of low-fat yogurt (450 mg).

If you don't like milk, you can eat a half cup of Chinese cabbage or Chinese mustard greens instead. Kale and bok choy are also good sources of this important mineral. Try mixing these leafy greens into a soup for an easy way to add taste as well as calcium. And if you like nuts, an ounce of almonds (about 24 nuts) gives you 70 mg of calcium and 206 mg of potassium, which is also important for your bones.

**Potassium and magnesium.** Scientists have found a link between eating fruits and vegetables and having strong bones. Amazingly, fruits and vegetables are just as important to a child's future bone health as milk. That's because fruits and vegetables are full of potassium and magnesium. Without these minerals, your bones can't make use of calcium even if you faithfully drain your milk glass. Good sources of potassium are bananas, potatoes, oranges, and dried apricots. You'll find magnesium in bananas, oranges, grains, nuts, seeds, legumes, and unprocessed cereals.

**Vitamin C.** Your body needs vitamin C to build collagen — a fiber that holds bones, teeth, and cartilage together. Vitamin C also helps keep calcium in your skeleton instead of being reabsorbed into your blood. Citrus fruits, strawberries, red and green peppers, broccoli, and collard greens are all good sources of vitamin C. For a one-two knockout punch against osteoporosis, buy orange juice with calcium added. Try drinking it in place of soft drinks, which supply no nutrition and can make bones even weaker.

**Vitamin D.** Sometimes called the "sunshine vitamin," this vitamin is essential for building strong bones. Your body can make vitamin D on its own if you get out in the sun regularly. But if you live in a climate where it's often overcast or too cold to go outdoors, you'll need to get your vitamin D from food. The best sources for vitamin D are fortified milk and breakfast cereals.

**Tea.** Researchers have found that women tea drinkers have thicker bones than women who don't drink tea. It's possible the antioxidants in both black and green tea can protect your bones. Try drinking tea in place of colas or coffee, which can make your bones weaker. The high amounts of caffeine in those beverages keep your body from absorbing calcium.

---

### A word of caution

You can sabotage your efforts to get more calcium by eating too much protein and salt. High-protein foods like meat make your blood more acidic, and your bones will send some of their stored calcium to buffer the acid. If you eat too much salt, the extra sodium links up with calcium in your kidneys, and the calcium gets washed away in your urine. Eat just one serving of meat daily and cut down on salt, and your body will do a better job of hanging on to this critical mineral.

# Parkinson's disease

· · · · · · · · · · · · · · ·

| Eat | |
|---|---|
| Apricots | Mangoes |
| Sweet | Rice |
| potatoes | Almonds |
| Wheat germ | High-fiber |
| Apples | cereal |
| Coffee | Olive oil |

**Avoid**

Foods high in protein, such as red meat, cheese, and eggs

Scientific breakthroughs, along with celebrities like actor Michael J. Fox, boxer Muhammad Ali, and evangelist Billy Graham, have made Parkinson's disease (PD) frequent front-page news. Yet the experts still aren't sure why people get this muscle-weakening condition.

It's possible you may inherit it, or environmental chemicals might cause it. But somehow the brain cells that control your muscles break down, and you begin to lose control of your movements.

PD comes on slowly. In the beginning, you might feel anxious and have trouble sleeping. Trembling hands, stiff muscles, and slow movement are likely to follow. You may shuffle your feet when you walk and have trouble keeping your balance.

Nonetheless, most people with Parkinson's disease continue to lead a productive life. More than 90 percent of those who have it live at home with their families. That says a lot when you consider it mostly occurs in older folks. But PD can strike younger people as well. Fox's condition was diagnosed at age 30, and it sometimes even affects people in their 20s. But it is most likely to occur after age 50.

There's no cure yet, but there are effective medications to help control the symptoms. And your diet can influence how well the medicine works. More importantly, the foods you eat may help you avoid getting PD in the first place.

## Nutritional blockbusters that fight PD

**Vitamin E.** Eat a lot of foods containing vitamin E, and you are less likely to get PD. That's what researchers found in a study of more than 5,000 older people in a suburb of Rotterdam in the Netherlands.

How this vitamin protects you from PD is not yet clear. The experts think it may be that, as an antioxidant, it helps prevent the breakdown of nerve cells that affect movement.

You can get this vitamin E protection by eating lots of fresh fruits and vegetables like apricots, avocados, mangoes, kale, and sweet potatoes. Include bran, rice, wheat germ, almonds, peanut butter, and sunflower seeds in your diet as well.

Getting most of your vitamin E from these plant foods rather than from animal sources is a doubly good idea. That's because eating a lot of animal fat can increase your chances of getting PD. Substitute plant protein like beans and nuts for some of the meat in your diet. And when you do eat meat, stick to lean cuts.

Vegetable oil is another good source of vitamin E. Use olive and canola — two of the healthiest oils — on salads and in other uncooked dishes. Unfortunately, heat destroys vitamin E. But you can still lower the animal fat in your diet by cooking with these oils rather than butter or lard.

**Caffeine.** Jump-start your morning with a cup of Java, and you may help protect yourself from Parkinson's disease. A recent study published in the *Journal of the American Medical Association* found that Japanese-American men who drank no coffee were about five times more likely to get PD than those who drank four to five 6-ounce cups of coffee each day.

The researchers who did this study believe it's most likely the caffeine, not some other ingredient, that gives coffee drinkers this edge. But you may want to wait for further research before you start drinking coffee or increase the amount you presently drink.

> ## A word of caution
>
> If you have Parkinson's disease, chances are you take a medication called levodopa. Unfortunately, the protein in the foods you eat can interfere with its ability to control your symptoms.
>
> It may help to cut back on the meat, eggs, cheese, and other protein foods in your diet. But to maintain your weight, replace the lost calories by eating more carbohydrates. And you might need extra calcium if you cut out dairy products.

Other studies have found similar protection for those who smoke cigarettes and drink alcohol. This leads some experts to question whether any of these are really protective. They think it's possible the brain chemistry of people who get PD makes them less likely to be heavy users of these substances.

**Fiber.** Constipation is a common problem for people with Parkinson's disease. But by eating lots of fresh leafy greens, beans, apples, and other fibrous fruits and vegetables, you can help your bowels work smoothly. For additional fiber, munch on seeds and whole grain breads and cereals, or stir some unprocessed bran into casseroles or salads. Just be sure to drink plenty of water to aid digestion.

# Parsley

· · · · · · · · · · · · ·

**Benefits**

Protects your heart

Combats cancer

Strengthens bones

Fights urinary tract infections

Freshens breath

Parsley may look pretty on your plate, but if you simply leave it there, you've missed out on one of the best ways to punch up the vitamin C in any meal.

Ancient Romans ate parsley for its sharp flavor and to freshen their breath. Then in the Middle Ages people began to use parsley as a medicine. They nibbled on it to ease their stomach problems, rubbed it on insect bites and bruises to relieve the swelling and itch, and even brewed it into a tea to ward off gallstones and dysentery. Believe it or not, men even scrubbed parsley onto their scalps to cure baldness.

Though parsley doesn't really help baldness or dysentery, it can improve your health. Like its cousin the carrot, parsley's packed with vitamins and minerals — beta carotene, folate, and iron, to name a few. Plus, like other tasty greens, it's brimming with flavonoids, powerful plant chemicals that may prevent cancer and fight heart disease.

## 4 ways parsley keeps you healthy

**Holds off heart disease.** Experts say you might be at a greater risk of dying from heart disease if you don't eat enough flavonoids, those natural antioxidants found in fruits and vegetables. Flavonoids work, scientists believe, by guarding your arteries against cholesterol build-up and by lowering blood pressure. That makes parsley pretty important, since it's full of key flavonoids like apigenin. A good start to a healthier heart would be a bowl of tabbouleh salad, a Middle Eastern delicacy that's heaping with parsley.

**Outsmarts breast and prostate cancer.** Here's some good news for both women and men. Eating parsley may reduce your risk of hormone-related cancers, like breast and prostate tumors. According to a groundbreaking study from Canada, the flavonoid apigenin in parsley appears to work like estrogen and progesterone. Your body uses the weaker apigenin instead of these stronger, built-in hormones, which are known to trigger cancerous growth. Although the experts haven't said how much of this flavonoid will do the trick, munching on some extra apigenin-rich parsley is a smart decision.

In addition, half a cup of parsley has the same vitamin C boost as half a cup of broccoli. While there's no question vitamin C combats cancer, it's also proven that cooking destroys the C in food before it can even start protecting you. That's where parsley comes in. Sprinkle some on your hot dishes right before you eat them and you'll replace any C that's been lost in the oven.

**Irons out your iron deficiency.** Millions of women are iron deficient and don't even know it. If you're low on iron, it's harder to exercise, work, and even do chores around the house. More importantly, chronic iron deficiency can lead to anemia. Just to be on the safe side, add parsley to your diet on a regular basis. A half-cup fresh or one tablespoon dried has about 10 percent of your iron daily requirements. Plus, parsley has the C your body needs to absorb that iron.

**Cuts down on bone breaks.** A few sprigs of parsley may keep you walking strong. A new study from three top American universities and the National Heart, Lung, and Blood Institute found that getting at least 100 micrograms of vitamin K a day can cut your risk of hip fracture. Vitamin K is necessary for bones to get the minerals they need to form properly. And since parsley is tops when it comes to K — with over 180 micrograms in just a half cup — it's a hip idea to have parsley around all the time. Top off your sandwiches with it, dress up your salads with it, or better yet, toss it into simmering stews and sauces. Cooking parsley nearly doubles its vitamin K.

## Pantry pointers

What could be better than one kind of parsley? Two. Your first choice has frilly, curly leaves, almost like the fronds of a fern, and it's best used as a garnish. Its flat-leafed or "Italian" brother may be plainer looking, but it has the flavor genes of the family. Because of this type's stronger taste, it's better suited to cooking.

---

### A word of caution

Although most people can enjoy parsley without any side effects, check with your doctor before making it a regular addition to your diet if you take blood-thinning medication like warfarin. The vitamin K in parsley may counteract the medicine's effects.

---

Like any other herb, parsley should be crisp and dark green when you buy it. Avoid taking home any limp, yellow parsley with dried, brown spots or slimy patches.

If you plan to eat your parsley soon, keep just the stems in a water-filled container in your fridge. For longer-term storage, chop and rinse the herb, and then freeze it in a plastic bag.

Or try dried parsley as a condiment. It doesn't have nearly as much vitamin C as the fresh stuff, but it makes up for it with a more concentrated dose of iron.

### Benefits

Prevents constipation

Combats cancer

Helps stop strokes

Aids digestion

Helps hemorrhoids

Boosts your immune system

# Peaches

· · · · · · · · · · · · · · ·

The fuzzy peach and its clean-shaven brother, the nectarine, are members of the rose family. Perhaps that's why they smell so good. You can find peaches and nectarines growing in warm climates all over the world these days, but experts believe these fruits got their start in China.

Peaches and nectarines are divided into two categories — clingstone, in which the fruit hangs onto the pit, and freestone, in which the flesh of the fruit pulls away from the pit. They also come in three flesh colors — red, white, and yellow — and in thousands of varieties. The yellow ones are highest in vitamin A, although all are good sources of vitamins A and C.

Most people prefer smooth peaches so the fuzz is brushed off by machines before they're sent to the store. Don't confuse these with nectarines — naturally fuzzless fruits with the same nutritional value. Whether you prefer peaches or nectarines, though, you can't go wrong with this sweet, delicious, 40-calorie treat.

You can add peaches to hot or cold cereal, or stick one in your lunch bag for a late-afternoon snack. Peaches are also good in cobblers, pies, and jams.

When you can't get fresh peaches, don't be afraid to buy canned or frozen. They are still a good choice, says Melanie Polk, M.M.Sc., R.D., Director of Nutrition Education at the American Institute for Cancer Research.

"Flash freezing and other new technologies trap nutrients and phytochemicals immediately after harvest while the produce is at its peak," she says.

If you do your grocery shopping weekly, Polk suggests buying canned fruits and vegetables for the latter part of the week, after you've used up your fresh produce. A rule of thumb, she says, is to buy as many fresh fruits and vegetables as you expect to use in three days.

"After about three days of sitting in your pantry or refrigerator, many fresh produce items lose enough nutritive value that you're better served by frozen and canned alternatives," she explains.

## 3 ways peaches keep you healthy

**Keeps your colon peachy clean.** Peaches are more than 80 percent water and are a good source of dietary fiber. This combination makes them a perfect remedy for constipation. One medium size peach has 7 percent of the dietary fiber you need each day. Adding fruits like peaches to your diet can keep you regular and prevent straining during bowel movements. Straining has been linked to hemorrhoids, diverticular disease, hiatal hernia, and even varicose veins. So skip the potato chips, and grab a juicy peach the next time you wander into the kitchen looking for a snack.

**Strikes out cancer.** Eating a variety of fruits and vegetables, avoiding fat, and not smoking can help prevent many types of cancer.

Cancer of the mouth has been increasing in the past several years, and experts think diet could play an important role in this disease. Luckily, you can protect yourself. A study in China showed that men and women who ate peaches more than twice a week had less risk of developing cancers of the mouth than those who didn't eat peaches. This study focused on oral cancer, but peaches, like other fruits and vegetables with vitamins, minerals and antioxidants, are a good way to steer clear of all kinds of cancers.

**Staves off stroke in smokers.** Are you or a loved one trying to quit smoking? Kicking the habit will make a huge difference in your health. In the meantime, though, you probably should know that foods like peaches might help smokers avoid strokes. Strokes happen when the flow of blood to your brain is interrupted, or when a blood vessel breaks or leaks in your brain. Researchers aren't sure why, but they're guessing a combination of beta carotene — which forms vitamin A — plus vitamin C and other antioxidants may be at work.

## Pantry pointers

Peaches should be soft to the touch, but not mushy. And don't squeeze them — they bruise easily. Don't choose rock hard or greenish peaches since they were probably picked too early. Although they might look fine, they'll never be very sweet. Also, avoid peaches with tan spots on them, a sign of decay.

---

### A word of caution

The U.S. Department of Agriculture has said U.S. peach growers are among the worst offenders in pesticide overuse, sometimes using thousands of times more than what it considers safe.

Protect yourself from pesticides that can cause health problems and even cancer. Try to buy organically grown peaches whenever possible. If you can't buy organic — grown without pesticides — remove the skin before eating.

Canned peaches have only one thousandth of the pesticides found on fresh peaches, possibly because they're peeled before processing. So buy organic, peel them, or stock up on the canned fruit for the healthiest benefits.

---

Because peaches keep ripening after being picked, they may need a couple of days on the counter to soften up. If you refrigerate ripe peaches in a paper bag, they'll keep for about a week.

To peel peaches easily, drop them into boiling water for one minute, then immediately put them into very cold water. The skins should come right off.

When buying canned peaches, be sure to buy ones packed in their own juice to avoid lots of added sugar and extra calories.

# Peanuts

• • • • • • • • • • • • • •

### Benefits

Protects against heart disease

Promotes weight loss

Combats prostate cancer

Lowers cholesterol

Increases your energy

Comedian Bill Cosby once said, "Man cannot live by bread alone. He must have peanut butter." Cosby may be known as a funny man, but he's also a very smart man.

Although they are sometimes called "ground nuts" because they grow underground, technically, peanuts are not even nuts. They're legumes, like beans, and have many of the same nutritional qualities. They're high in protein and fiber, and are a good source of many important vitamins and minerals, including vitamin E, niacin, manganese, folate, magnesium, and potassium.

Former President Jimmy Carter, a peanut farmer with a keen interest in their health benefits, is always eager to defend the lowly peanut. "They contain zero cholesterol and are highly nutritious. Even for people that are losing weight, eating peanuts can help them to control their diet. In addition, eating peanuts can prevent heart disease."

## 3 ways peanuts keep you healthy

**Keeps your heart hardy.** Too much fat and cholesterol can really do a number on your heart. And although one cup of peanuts contains almost a full day's quota of fat, it's the good kind — monounsaturated fatty acids (MUFAs).

MUFAs are actually healthy for your heart since they help control cholesterol. In fact, a diet high in MUFAs can reduce cholesterol levels more than the American Heart Association Step II diet — an eating plan designed specifically to lower cholesterol.

Based on clinical studies, the American Heart Association now recommends you replace some of the fat in your diet with monounsaturated fats. "These studies are telling us that the type of fat may be as important as how much of it is eaten," says Penny M. Kris-Etherton, PhD., R.D., member of the American Heart Association Nutrition Committee.

The heart-healthy properties of peanuts don't end with MUFAs, either. Eat just 3 ounces a day and you've gotten half the amount of folate you need to fight artery-damaging homocysteine. And if you're looking for resveratrol, the plant estrogen that works like an antioxidant to combat heart disease, the Peanut Institute says to look no further than a handful of peanuts. One ounce, they say, contains about as much resveratrol as 2 pounds of grapes.

**Helps shed unwanted pounds.** But what about your waistline? Peanuts are still high in fat, even if it is heart-healthy fat. Experts say, however, you don't have to give up these crunchy tidbits. They are full of protein and fiber and give a lot of energy bang for the buck. In short, peanuts can be an important part of your total weight loss plan.

As any veteran dieter will testify, if you don't feel hungry, it's easier to eat less. A recent study published in the International Journal of Obesity says after you eat less than a cup of peanuts, you're not as likely to want other foods high in fat, protein, or carbohydrates.

And who wouldn't want a little more energy? Female soccer players who ate a higher-fat diet including peanuts, were able to work out harder and longer. This means munching on a few peanuts every day may enable you to step up your own exercise program and burn more calories.

Of course, you can't just add a few peanuts to your regular diet and watch the pounds magically melt off. You still have to exercise and watch your calories.

**Puts a lid on cancer.** Legumes, including peanuts, are a rich source of beta-sitosterol, one of the estrogen-like plant compounds called phytosterols. Experts believe these may help protect you from colon, breast, ovarian, or prostate cancer.

Part of the evidence is gathered from people eating an Asian or vegetarian diet, normally teeming with legumes. They're not only getting five times as many phytosterols as people eating a typical Western diet, but they're also less likely to suffer from these types of cancer.

Boost your odds by snacking on peanuts and peanut butter and start cooking with peanut oil and flour.

### A word of caution

Peanuts are one of the most common sources of food allergy, affecting over three million people and often causing severe, even fatal, reactions.

If you discover you're allergic to peanuts or any other food, protect yourself by becoming a conscientious label reader. Nicole Cheeks of the Food Allergy Network, says, "We stress that EVERY label on EVERY food product purchased must be read." Even a small amount of peanut or peanut oil can cause a serious reaction in sensitive people.

Ask your doctor for a prescription for epinephrine (an emergency anti-allergy injection) and make sure you carry it with you at all times, in case you're accidentally exposed to peanuts.

## Pantry pointers

If you're a peanut-lover, you can get satisfaction year-round. When buying them unshelled, look for clean, unbroken shells that don't rattle. They'll store in your refrigerator for up to six months.

Shelled peanuts are often sold vacuum-packed in cans or jars. Store them unopened at room temperature for up to a year. Once opened, keep them in the refrigerator, tightly sealed, and eat them within three months.

The most popular way to buy peanuts may not be shelled or unshelled, but mashed — as peanut butter. Although America leads the world in peanut butter consumption, it's also a favorite in Canada, Holland, England, Germany, Saudi Arabia, and is gaining popularity throughout Eastern Europe.

You can store most commercial peanut butter at room temperature for up to six months. Natural peanut butter, however, contains only peanuts and oil — no preservatives — so you must refrigerate it after opening. For a fun and healthy treat, make your own natural peanut butter at home with a blender or food processor.

Despite the huge quantity of peanut butter consumed, not everyone is a PB lover. It may be one of the few foods that has a specific phobia attached to it. "Arachibutyrophobia" (pronounced I-RA-KI-BU-TI-RO-PHO-BEE-A) is the fear of getting peanut butter stuck to the roof of your mouth.

# Pineapple

· · · · · · · · · · · · · · · · · ·

**Benefits**

Strengthens bones

Relieves cold
  symptoms

Aids digestion

Dissolves warts

Blocks diarrhea

Think "pineapple," and you probably think of Hawaii. This island state is one of the world's leading producers of pineapple, but interestingly, it wasn't even grown there until the late 1700s. Pineapple probably originated in South America in the area that is now Brazil and Paraguay. From there, it was transplanted to the Caribbean islands where it was discovered by Columbus in 1493.

Columbus took pineapples back to Europe, where its sweet flavor made it an instant royal favorite. The English called it pineapple because of its resemblance to a pinecone, but most other Europeans used the original Indian name "anana," which meant "excellent fruit." It was almost two centuries before Europeans devised a way to grow pineapples in hothouses, so the fruit remained a rare and coveted treat. Because it was such an honor to be served pineapple, the fruit eventually became a universal symbol of hospitality.

You may eat pineapple for its taste, but you can feel equally good about its health benefits. Pineapple has been used as a folk remedy for centuries for a variety of ailments, particularly digestive problems. Modern research indicates that bromelain, an enzyme found in both the stem and fruit, may be responsible for many of pineapple's reputed health benefits. In addition, pineapple contains substantial amounts of vitamin C and manganese.

## 2 ways pineapple keeps you healthy

**Helps build healthy bones.** Eat a cup of fresh pineapple chunks, and you've given your body 73 percent of the manganese it needs for the day. That's important for your bones, because manganese, a trace mineral, is needed for your body to build bone and connective tissues. And a recent study found that a combination of glucosamine, chondroitin sulfate, and manganese resulted in significant improvement for people with mild to moderate osteoarthritis of the knee.

**Soothes coughs and colds.** When you get the sniffles, you probably reach for a glass of orange juice. That's good, but maybe you should consider pineapple juice instead. It has vitamin C like its orange cousin, but it also has bromelain, which helps suppress coughs and loosens the mucus that often accompanies colds. Studies have found bromelain is effective in treating upper respiratory conditions and acute sinusitis.

> ### Warding off warts
>
> Pineapple's enzyme power seems good for a variety of ills, but its oddest use may be to dissolve warts. While most warts eventually go away on their own, if you want to speed up the process, try soaking a cotton ball with fresh pineapple juice and applying it to the wart.
>
> Pineapple isn't the only food you can try either. Some people say rubbing a raw potato on a wart several times a day will make it go away. Others tape a piece of banana peel on it, with the inside of the peel against the wart. Though not scientifically proven, these solutions are said to work as well as medical treatments.

The next time you get a cold, try making your own natural cough syrup, and take advantage of the tasty and soothing powers of pineapple. Combine 8 ounces of warm pineapple juice and 2 teaspoons of honey, and sip for soothing relief.

## Pantry pointers

Choosing a good pineapple can be a prickly process. Unlike some fruits, the color of the shell does not tell you how ripe it is.

A pineapple with a green shell is as likely to be ripe as one with a shell that is golden yellow.

You can try sniffing the pineapple at the stem end or choosing one with fresh-looking green leaves, but it wouldn't hurt to check the tag as well. If it says it has been jet-shipped, it's more likely to be ripe. That's because pineapples don't get any riper or sweeter once they're picked — they just get older. So the faster it gets to you, the better it will taste.

Once you bring your pineapple home, refrigerate it to keep it fresh.

Pineapple is ideal for many dishes, from pineapple upside-down cake to sweet and sour pork, but don't use fresh pineapple in gelatin dishes. The enzyme bromelain prevents gelatin from setting properly. In fact, the amount of bromelain in foods is sometimes measured in GDUs — gelatin dissolving units.

Cooked or canned pineapple will work fine in gelatin dishes. But if you're eating it for the health benefits, fresh is better.

# Prostate problems
. . . . . . . . . . . . . . . .

| Eat | |
|---|---|
| Tomatoes | Pumpkin |
| Oysters | seeds |
| Wheat germ | Watermelon |
| Pink | Soybeans |
| grapefruit | Green tea |
| Garlic | Broccoli |

**Avoid**

Foods high in saturated fat, such as red meat and whole-milk dairy products

It only weighs about an ounce, but your walnut-sized prostate can cause super-sized problems. This gland makes semen, the fluid that carries sperm. It's located just below your bladder, and it wraps around your urethra, the tube that carries urine out of your body.

This location contributes to some of the problems your prostate can cause. Prostate problems fall into three general categories.

**Prostatitis.** You can have two forms of prostate infection — acute and chronic. Acute prostatitis causes fever, chills, and pain between your legs and in your lower back. You may also find it difficult or painful to urinate. Antibiotic treatment usually clears it up.

Chronic prostatitis is an infection that returns repeatedly. The symptoms are similar to acute prostatitis, except that you probably won't have a fever, and the symptoms tend to be milder. Unfortunately, chronic prostatitis is also more difficult to treat because bacteria may not be the cause.

**Enlarged prostate.** This common condition, called benign prostatic hyperplasia (BPH), affects almost half of all men over age 40 along with 75 percent of men over age 60. Because it surrounds your urethra, an enlarged prostate can cause urinary problems like frequent urination, difficulty urinating, or dribbling. Medical treatments for BPH include drugs, surgery, heat or freezing therapy, and laser therapy.

**Prostate cancer.** Prostate cancer is the most common form of cancer among men and is second only to lung cancer as the leading cause of cancer deaths for men. It tends to be a slow-growing cancer, but it can sometimes be aggressive and spread quickly. Early stages of prostate cancer may not cause any symptoms so it's important to get regular prostate screenings. The American Urological Society recommends a yearly prostate examination for all men over age 40.

Prostate problems can be just an annoyance, or they can be deadly — prostate cancer kills about 40,000 men a year. And treatments for prostate problems can cause serious side effects. Recent information suggests about 60 percent of men who have prostate cancer surgery are impotent a year and a half later. Preventing prostate problems is obviously your best option, and the right foods can provide some natural help.

## Nutritional blockbusters that fight prostate problems

**Lycopene.** Harvard researchers created a stir several years ago when they discovered that eating 10 servings of tomato products weekly could dramatically cut your risk of prostate cancer. Lycopene, a carotenoid that gives tomatoes their brilliant red color, is probably responsible for this protective effect.

Processed tomato products such as tomato sauce and ketchup may be more beneficial than fresh tomatoes. This is probably because chopping and cooking the tomatoes helps break down cell walls, making the lycopene easier for your body to absorb. Other sources of lycopene include watermelon, pink grapefruit, and guava.

**Vitamin E.** A recent study found that men with the highest blood levels of gamma-tocopherol, a form of vitamin E, were five times less likely to develop prostate cancer.

Gamma-tocopherol appears to work with alpha-tocopherol (another form of vitamin E) and selenium to fight cancer. To get a good balance of both forms of vitamin E, eat a variety of vitamin E-rich foods — seed and vegetable oils, nuts, green leafy vegetables, and whole grains.

**Zinc.** Pumpkin seeds, which are high in zinc, have been used for centuries as a folk remedy for problematic prostates. The mineral may help shrink an enlarged prostate or reduce the inflammation of chronic prostatitis. Good food sources of zinc include oysters and other shellfish, chicken, beans, and whole grains.

**Vitamin D.** This "sunshine vitamin" may be useful in preventing or treating prostate cancer. However, vitamin D can also be toxic in large doses, so don't use supplements without a doctor's guidance. Instead, eat foods rich in vitamin D, such as dairy foods or fortified cereals, and get out and soak up some sun. Your body can make its own vitamin D from the sunlight on your skin.

**Soy and green tea.** China has the lowest rate of prostate cancer in the world, and Japanese men are also less likely to develop the disease. It could be that something in the Asian diet helps prevent prostate cancer, and research points to two possibilities — soy and green tea.

Researchers at Loma Linda University found that Seventh-day Adventist men who drank soy milk at least once a day were 70 percent less likely to develop prostate cancer. And an earlier study on Japanese men living in Hawaii found those who ate tofu (another soy product) were less likely to develop the disease.

Asians also drink lots of green tea, which may protect against several types of cancer. Green tea contains antioxidants called polyphenols that may be responsible for its cancer-protective effect.

A recent study suggests a combination of these two Asian staples could be the secret. Scientists found that the polyphenol in green tea did not fight prostate cancer cells in the laboratory by itself. But when combined with genistein, a substance found in soy, the solution halted the growth of prostate cancer cells.

One possible drawback to soy is that it may make your brain age faster, new research claims. For more information, see the *Memory loss* chapter.

**Garlic.** This favorite of Italian cooks contains more than just a strong flavor and odor. It may contain strong cancer protection as well. Garlic is loaded with antioxidants and other substances that act to boost your immune system and protect against cancer.

**Cruciferous vegetables.** Broccoli, cauliflower, and brussels sprouts can help you put the squeeze on prostate cancer. Eat just

---

### A word of caution

Couch potatoes, beware! You could be encouraging cancer to invade your prostate as you munch chips and watch television. A high-fat diet and sedentary lifestyle increase your risk of prostate cancer.

Fight back by eating less fat and making wise fat choices. Research finds that monounsaturated fats, which include olive, canola, and peanut oils, may help lower your risk of prostate cancer.

three servings of these cruciferous veggies every week, and you could cut your risk of prostate cancer in half.

# Prunes

• • • • • • • • • • • • •

| Benefits |
| :---: |
| Slows aging process |
| Prevents constipation |
| Lowers cholesterol |
| Boosts memory |
| Promotes weight loss |
| Protects against heart disease |

Movie stars frequently change their ordinary, given names to something more glamorous once they're in the spotlight. That's happened with your old friend the prune.

Ever since researchers discovered that prunes are packed with antioxidants, this dried fruit has gotten lots of attention. Who knew so much goodness was hiding inside that black, wrinkly package?

Like the star it hopes to become, the prune has changed its name and is now known as a "dried plum." The Food and Drug Administration approved the change, which was recommended by the California Prune Board. It hopes to shed the prune's image of a food for the elderly and target it to the young and health conscious. Market surveys show the name change is a winner, and this new celebrity should appear soon at a grocery near you.

But a prune by any name would taste as sweet. It would also give you lots of fiber, protect you from free radical damage, and maybe even lower your cholesterol. Prunes are also a good source of potassium — important for a healthy heart and strong bones. And you can eat 10 sweet, chewy dried plums filled with nutrition for only 200 calories. Not bad for a food that was rescued from hospital and nursing home cafeterias.

# 3 ways prunes keep you healthy

**Chases away aging.** For years, scientists have wondered what people can do to hold on to the health and vitality of their youth. The latest thinking is that antioxidants — free radical fighters found mainly in fruits and vegetables — are the key to keeping young and avoiding cell damage.

Researchers have measured and studied antioxidants in food at the Jean Mayer USDA Human Nutrition Research Center on Aging at Tufts University in Boston. Of all the foods tested, the prune had the highest Oxygen Radical Absorbance Capacity (ORAC) score. At 5,770 ORACs per 3 1/2-ounce serving, it registered more than twice as many antioxidants as the next highest food — its wrinkled cousin, the raisin.

When animals were given foods high in antioxidants, they showed less sign of aging on memory tests. Scientists think antioxidants may be an important key to protecting yourself from diseases of aging and even cancer. In fact, the loss of brain function in certain diseases like Parkinson's and Alzheimer's seems to be from free radical damage. If these high antioxidant foods can protect you from free radicals, imagine all the sickness you might avoid.

The USDA's Agricultural Research Service Administrator Floyd P. Horn has seen the future of treating age-related diseases, and it looks a lot like your grandma's vegetable garden.

"If these findings are borne out in further research," he says, "young and middle-aged people may be able to reduce risk of diseases of aging — including senility — simply by adding high-ORAC foods to their diets."

By studying blood samples from different groups of people, the researchers concluded that you can raise the levels of antioxidants in your blood by eating more fruits and vegetables. For now, they're recommending you eat enough fruits and vegetables to total between 3,000 and 5,000 ORAC units of antioxidants daily. Since most of the foods tested scored in the hundreds, you'd have to eat many servings to reach 3,000.

But chew on this: eating just seven prunes a day can put you well over the 3,000 mark. All the other fruits and vegetables you eat would be gravy. Make sure you eat a variety, though, because each fruit and vegetable has different protective nutrients.

**Revs up sluggish bowels.** Prunes can help keep you regular. That's why nursing homes and hospitals always have them on the menu. In addition to being a good source of fiber, they also contain a natural laxative ingredient. The combination is perfect if you don't get a lot of exercise or tend to have constipation. If you don't like chewing your fiber, prune juice works well, too.

In rural parts of Africa, people eat diets high in fruits, vegetables, and grains. Not surprisingly, constipation is rare. What might surprise you, though, is that hemorrhoids, hiatal hernias, varicose veins, and diverticular disease are also very rare in those places. And that's no coincidence. It looks like staying regular is a big part of staying healthy.

**Knocks down high cholesterol.** Eating a diet high in fiber can help lower your cholesterol, and a study of prunes helped prove it.

Researchers in the Department of Nutrition at the University of California, Davis, gave a group of 41 men with mildly high cholesterol 12 prunes each day for four weeks. They then gave the same men a couple of glasses of grape juice daily for four more

---

**Prunes can replace fat**

You can use prunes to make a puree substitution for oil or butter in recipes.

Just puree about 1 1/3 cups of pitted prunes with 6 tablespoons of hot water. This should make about a cup of prune puree that will keep in the refrigerator for up to one month. Use half the recommended fat in a recipe, then add half that amount of pureed prunes.

For example, if a recipe calls for a cup of oil or butter, use 1/2 cup of oil, then add 1/4 cup of prune puree. You can use this puree in cakes, muffins, cookies — even brownies.

weeks. The men were told not to change their eating or exercise habits during the study.

Tests showed that LDL cholesterol — the kind you want to keep low — was significantly lower during the prune period than during the grape juice period. This is great news if your cholesterol is starting to creep upwards and you don't want to take medicine. Lower cholesterol means you're less likely to develop heart disease.

## Pantry pointers

Like orange juice, prunes aren't just for breakfast anymore. You can add diced prunes to salads for added fiber and nutrition, or pack some in your lunchbox to satisfy your sweet tooth. Or try topping a hot cereal with prune bits for some variety.

Chopped prunes are great in baked goods, too. Add them to muffins, cookies, and breads the way you would use raisins. They'll keep in your pantry for a few months, or longer if you refrigerate them.

| Benefits |
| --- |
| Protects prostate |
| Preserves sexual function |
| Eases arthritis |
| Protects your heart |
| Lowers cholesterol |

# Pumpkin

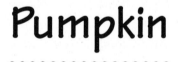

Thanksgiving was once postponed in Connecticut during Colonial times because the molasses needed to make pumpkin pies wasn't available. Pumpkin pie is still an important part of the holiday celebration, but if you only eat pumpkin at Thanksgiving, you're missing out on the many health benefits of this colorful fruit.

Pumpkin contains loads of beta carotene and alpha carotene, which are converted to vitamin A in your body. It's high in fiber, low in calories, and a good source of several important minerals, including iron, potassium, and magnesium.

The word "pumpkin" comes from the Greek word "pepon," which means "large melon," even though pumpkins are actually a member of the gourd family. The biggest pumpkin ever weighed over 1,000 pounds! That would make one really frightening jack-o-lantern. Speaking of jack-o-lanterns, the first ones were made from turnips, not pumpkins and were based on an Irish folktale about Jack of the Lantern. People used them to frighten away spirits on Halloween. When the Irish immigrated to America in the 1800s, they found that pumpkins were more plentiful and easier to carve.

The first pumpkin pie was a bit different than the one you may slice up on Thanksgiving. American colonists filled a pumpkin with milk, spices, and honey then baked it in hot ashes.

## 4 ways pumpkin keeps you healthy

**Protects prostate.** Munch a handful of pumpkin seeds every day, as men in the Ukraine do, and you may be able to sidestep prostate problems.

Scientists say the seeds may work because they contain zinc and chemicals called cucurbitacins, which interfere with the production of dihydrotestosterone (DHT), a hormone responsible for prostate growth.

Benign prostatic hyperplasia (BPH), a nonmalignant enlargement of the prostate gland, is so common that 90 percent of men who reach age 85 will have at least a mild case of BPH.

In one recent study, researchers found that a combination of pumpkin seed extracts and saw palmetto, another herbal remedy for prostate problems, improved BPH symptoms significantly.

**Boosts sexual drive.** Pumpkin seeds can improve your sex life by helping to prevent BPH, and its high zinc content helps ensure that levels of testosterone remain at peak performance levels.

**Eases arthritis.** If your joints ache, try adding a little pumpkin seed oil to your diet. The essential fatty acids in pumpkin seed oil, linoleic acid (omega-6) and linolenic acid (omega-3), may help fight arthritis. One study on arthritic rats found that supplements of pumpkin seed oil reduced signs of arthritis. The rats given pumpkin seed oil also had 44 percent less swelling in their paws. While no recent studies have been done on the effect of pumpkin seed oil on arthritis in humans, it may be a natural, easy way to get a little relief. You can buy pumpkin seed oil for cooking or in supplement form. (See *An unusual cooking discovery* in the box at left.)

**Helps your heart.** Pumpkin may help protect your heart because of its high beta carotene content. One study of almost 5,000 elderly people in the Netherlands found that the people who ate the most foods rich in beta carotene were 45 percent less likely to have a heart attack than those who ate the least amount. If you are thinking of taking beta carotene supplements, better think again. Researchers say supplements may not have the same effects.

---

### An unusual cooking discovery

The same area of Austria that gave the world Arnold Schwarzenegger is famous for another strong product — pumpkin seed oil.

The Styria region of south central Austria grows a type of pumpkin that is cultivated just for its seeds. The oil that is produced from those seeds is sometimes called "green gold," although its color is black, like motor oil.

Chefs call this pumpkin seed oil a "culinary discovery" because of its strong nutty flavor. It is most often used as an ingredient in salad dressings. You may not be able to find this unusual, nutritious oil in your grocery store, but you can get it through the mail. Contact Green Gold in Austria by e-mail (info@green gold.net) or visit their Web site at <http://www.greengold.net>.

You can also write to Peter Pumpkin Enterprises, P.O. Box 491, Picton, Ont., K0K 2T0 Canada or call Austria's Finest Naturally at 800-348-5766.

Two separate animal studies recently showed that pumpkin seed oil may improve the effectiveness of medications used to treat high blood pressure and high cholesterol levels.

## Pantry pointers

Fresh pumpkins are plentiful in fall and early winter — just in time for Halloween and Thanksgiving. While you may want to choose a jumbo-sized pumpkin to carve for Halloween, smaller ones will be more tender and tasty if you in-tend to eat them.

Whole pumpkins can be stored at room temperature for up to a month, or up to three months if you keep them in the refrigerator. For convenience, you can also buy canned pumpkin.

Whether you choose fresh or canned, don't limit your use of this versatile food to pies. Marsha Weaver, a County Extension Agent for Kansas State University, says, "Pies are just one way to use pump-kin. It's also delicious in chilled or hot soups, or in place of mashed potatoes in a shepherd's pie. Or try sautéing or stir-frying strips of fresh pumpkin." Weaver also recommends combining pumpkin with other foods for maximum nutritional value. Here are a few clever ideas:

> ### How to roast pumpkin seeds
>
> Pumpkin seeds have been a popular snack in many countries for centuries. You can buy roasted pumpkin seeds, but if you'd like to do it yourself, it's a snap. Remove the seeds from the pumpkin and rinse in a colander. Blot them dry with paper towels and then coat them lightly with olive oil or sesame oil. Spread on a cookie sheet and sprinkle with salt. Roast for about 45 minutes at 375 degrees. After the seeds cool, store them in an airtight container.

◆ Try adding one-fourth to one-half cup pumpkin pulp to two cups of mashed potatoes.

◆ Add two tablespoons pumpkin per serving to hot oatmeal or cream of wheat. Then serve with brown sugar or sprinkle with cinnamon-sugar.

◆ Thicken soups, sauces, beans, and chili with mashed pumpkin. Add one-fourth to one-half cup pumpkin to about 16 ounces of spaghetti sauce, baked beans, or chili.

◆ Add one-fourth cup pumpkin to the liquid ingredients of your favorite gingerbread mix (14-ounce size).

◆ Combine contents of one 3-ounce package of butterscotch or vanilla pudding and pie filling mix, two cups of milk, and one-half cup mashed pumpkin. Cook as directed on package.

◆ Stir together one cup vanilla low-fat yogurt, one-half cup pumpkin, and one-fourth teaspoon cinnamon.

| Benefits |
| --- |
| Combats cancer |
| Protects your heart |
| Ends anemia |
| Increases energy |
| Strengthens bones |
| Saves your eyesight |

# Quinoa

• • • • • • • • • • • •

Never heard of quinoa? This "super-grain" may be one of the healthiest foods you'll find. Pronounced "keen-wah," it was a staple of the Inca diet.

Quinoa can grow in high altitudes under terrible conditions. It flourishes even in poor soil with little rainfall and cold temperatures. If this grain sounds more like a weed, that's because it's technically not a grain at all but a member of the same family as spinach, beets, and Swiss chard.

It's no surprise quinoa differs from other grains. It has more protein, iron, and unsaturated fats but fewer carbohydrates. In fact, it is considered a complete protein because it provides all eight essential amino acids. And it's packed with minerals, B vitamins, and fiber.

When you also consider its versatility and interesting texture, which is both creamy and crunchy, it's no wonder this healthy grain is gaining in popularity. Quinoa is also cropping up in new places. Once limited to South and Central American countries like Peru, Bolivia, and Ecuador, quinoa is now being grown in Colorado, New Mexico, California, and Canada.

Go on a quest for quinoa, and you'll find this tough grain is tough on disease.

## 5 ways quinoa keeps you healthy

**Prevents cancer.** Fiber may be one of your best defenses against cancer. Luckily, quinoa comes with 4 grams of this valuable stuff per serving.

Quinoa is a good source of insoluble and soluble fiber. Both may fight colon cancer in different ways. Insoluble fiber, the kind found in wheat bran, adds bulk to your stool and dilutes the cancer-causing substances it contains.

Soluble fiber, the main kind in oat bran and barley, may work by reacting with the tiny organisms, called microflora, in your large intestine to form compounds that protect your colon. Both also speed stool through your body, which helps with cancer protection and constipation.

**Helps your heart.** As mighty as the Incas were, they couldn't compete with the superior firepower of the Spanish conquistadors. Quinoa, like the European conquerors, has quite an arsenal at its disposal — especially when it comes to heart disease.

With 4 grams of fiber per serving, quinoa can battle high cholesterol, heart disease, and stroke. In fact, one study determined that for every extra 10 grams of fiber consumed a day, women lowered their risk of heart disease by 19 percent.

Quinoa has about 2 grams of fat per serving, too. But before you decide to pass on the quinoa, consider that most of the fat is unsaturated, the kind that helps lower cholesterol. Too much cholesterol can lead to clogged arteries, high blood pressure, stroke, and heart attack.

What's more, quinoa is a good source of folate, the B-vitamin that keeps the dangerous substance homocysteine under wraps. And add potassium and magnesium, which help keep your blood pressure under control and reduce your risk of stroke, and quinoa seems well-armed.

There's even evidence that suggests protein — often linked to an increased risk of heart problems — may actually slightly lessen your chance for heart disease. But that doesn't mean you should eat more meat and eggs to get more protein. You don't want all that saturated fat and cholesterol. Quinoa, on the other hand, gives you the protein without the drawbacks.

**Irons out anemia.** If somebody told you to guess the most common chronic disease, chances are you wouldn't come up with iron-deficiency anemia. But this form of anemia just might take top honors. At least 18 million people in the United States alone are iron deficient.

Anemia makes you pale, weak, and drowsy and could cause headaches, stomach disorders, and a loss of sex drive. It happens when you don't have enough red blood cells or enough hemoglobin in those red blood cells to carry oxygen from your lungs to your body's tissues. You can get anemia for a number of reasons, including loss of blood or an inability to absorb iron properly, but not getting enough iron in your diet can increase your risk.

That's where quinoa can help. Loaded with 4 milligrams of iron per serving, quinoa provides plenty of iron to keep anemia at bay.

Even if you don't have anemia, you can be affected by an iron deficiency. For instance, if you're not getting enough iron, you might have less stamina and use up more energy to do simple tasks. Iron deficiency might also trigger restless legs syndrome. People with this condition get strange sensations in their legs and feel as if they must move them to stop the uncomfortable feelings.

**Boosts your energy.** You don't have to be anemic to feel sluggish. Fatigue strikes many people, and elderly people are especially vulnerable because they often take medication that can cause fatigue.

Once again, quinoa comes to the rescue. It's a good source of protein, which can give you a burst of energy to help you make it through the day. Besides energy, your body also needs protein for building new tissue and repairing injured or worn-out tissue.

Foods rich in B vitamins help your body use the fuel you get from carbohydrates, fats, and proteins. The result is more energy. So if you're not getting enough B vitamins, you may feel tired and drained. Quinoa is an excellent source of B1 (thiamin), B2 (riboflavin), B3 (niacin), B6, and folate. While no one food can provide all the nutrients you need, for a little more get-up-and-go, add enriched cereals, liver, and beans to your weekly menu.

**Strengthens bones, teeth, and muscles.** Miners can spend years searching for precious minerals. All you have to do is search for some quinoa, which is chock-full of minerals your body needs.

For strong bones, teeth, and muscles, there's calcium, magnesium, manganese, and phosphorus. Quinoa also gives you plenty

---

### Crush cataracts with quinoa

Don't look now, but quinoa might even protect your eyes. According to the Australian Blue Mountains Eye Study, protein and polyunsaturated fats — both found in quinoa — may help you avoid cataracts.

In the study, the people who ate the most protein, about 99 grams a day, were only half as likely as those who ate the least to develop a nuclear cataract. With a nuclear cataract, light has trouble passing through the center of your eye's lens.

Meanwhile, those who ate the most polyunsaturated fat, about 17 grams a day, were 30 percent less likely to get a cortical cataract, which affects the outer lens.

of zinc, to sharpen your senses, and copper, which helps form oxygen-carrying hemoglobin. All these minerals help keep your body working properly. When it comes to precious minerals, eating quinoa is like hitting the mother lode.

## Pantry pointers

Quinoa can be cooked like rice and used in place of it and other grains. It's great if you're in a hurry because it takes half as long to cook as rice. One drawback is that quinoa is harder to find (look in health food stores or in the health food section of your supermarket) and more expensive than other grains. However, since it expands to four times its size when it cooks, you get more bang for your buck.

You can use quinoa in soups, salads, side dishes, main courses, desserts, or even as a hot breakfast cereal, like oatmeal.

Just make sure you rinse it thoroughly before you cook it because it's coated with saponin, a bitter substance that keeps away birds and insects. Most of the saponin is removed before you buy it, but there may be some residue left. Your quinoa will taste soapy if you don't rinse it carefully.

| Eat | |
| --- | --- |
| Olive oil | Salmon |
| Mackerel | Ginger |
| Pumpkin seed oil | Turmeric |
| | Water |
| Flaxseed | Peanuts |
| Grapes | Mushrooms |
| Tuna | |

**Avoid**

Any food that seems to inflame your arthritis

# Rheumatoid arthritis

• • • • • • • • • • • • • • •

Your body literally turns on itself when you have rheumatoid arthritis (RA). That's why this devastating condition is called an autoimmune illness. White blood cells, which normally hunt harmful bacteria and viruses in your blood, seem to invade and attack the soft tissues of your joints. Experts aren't sure why the white blood cells go haywire, but they know the symptoms — swollen and throbbing joints.

Like osteoarthritis, RA can lead to permanent damage to your bones, cartilage, and other joint parts. In time, it can even hurt internal organs, like your heart and lungs.

RA tends to attack matching joints at the same time — both knees or both elbows, for example, or your hand's small joints. The best way to prevent the disease from going that far is by getting treatment early. The sooner you begin therapy, the less the condition will disfigure your joints. Rheumatologists — doctors specializing in arthritis — usually prescribe nonsteroidal anti-inflammatory drugs (NSAIDs) or other strong medications. These can quiet your RA, but they can cause side effects.

Relief, however, could be as painless as eating a healthy, balanced diet. "Certainly," says Dr. David S. Pisetsky, author of *The Duke University Medical Center Book of Arthritis,* "a patient with rheumatoid arthritis who may not be eating well would benefit from a nutritious and well-balanced diet."

Eating high-fiber, low-fat foods will also help you manage your weight, and keeping the pounds off leads to better bone health. Remember — extra ounces equals added stress to your joints. As Pisetsky states, "Rheumatologists believe that body weight does influence arthritis."

The right foods, together with regular exercise, could make it easier for your body to fight RA. That makes them the perfect complement to your doctor's treatment plan.

## Nutritional blockbusters that fight RA

**Omega-3.** According to the Arthritis Foundation, eating fish at least two or three times a week can soothe your stiff, achy joints.

You can thank the omega-3, or linolenic, fatty acids. Omega-3 appears to relieve the symptoms of RA so well that some people can cut back on NSAIDs. Stick with cold-water, fatty fish, like salmon, mackerel, albacore tuna, and herring, for the biggest boost. Between seafood suppers, try cooking with canola oil and making salad dressings with flaxseed oil.

Cut back on omega-6, or linoleic, fatty acids, too. While omega-3 reduces the number of enzymes in your body that promote inflammation, omega-6 encourages your body to make more. This is a tug-of-war you want omega-3 to win. To help it win, limit your intake of foods rich in omega-6, like meats, processed and fast foods, and vegetable oils, like safflower, corn, and soybean.

**Olive oil.** This fragrant oil turned up the big winner in a recent study from Greece. The researchers surveyed the eating habits of over 300 people in search of foods that can benefit people suffering with RA. Of over 100 different types of food, olive oil came out the winner.

The monounsaturated fatty acids in olive oil appeared to work like omega-3 fatty acids by helping to reduce joint swelling at the source. The oil's antioxidants could play some role, too.

Try to work olive oil into your diet almost every day. The more you use, the better. In the study, the people who consumed the least olive oil had a two and a half times greater risk of getting RA than the top olive oil eaters, who averaged three tablespoons more per day.

**Antioxidants.** Speaking of free radical fighters, exciting new research suggests all antioxidants might relieve, or even prevent, RA. Rheumatoid sufferers tend to be overloaded with free radicals and low on antioxidants. This imbalance leads experts to believe free radicals have a hand in causing joint damage. Eating antioxidant-rich foods could give the edge back to the good guys — the antioxidants.

There are a few leaders in the antioxidant army — selenium, vitamin E, and resveratrol. In a recent study from Sweden, low selenium levels appeared to increase a person's risk for getting a certain kind of RA. Some experts think raising your selenium intake might even help to reduce your swelling and pain. Low vitamin E levels, on the other hand, raised the risk for all types of RA.

Boost your selenium levels with seafood, mushrooms, dairy, and whole wheat. Rich sources of vitamin E include fortified cereals, vegetable oils, peanuts, and fish.

Resveratrol mainly comes from grapes. Many researchers think it inhibits inflammation, making it a weapon against RA, heart disease, and cancer.

**Pumpkin seed oil.** You can profit simultaneously from the powers of antioxidants and fatty acids when you cook with pumpkin seed oil. Sometimes called "green gold," this unusual oil contains omega-3 fatty acids, as well as selenium, vitamin E, beta carotene, and other antioxidants called polyphenols. When you put all of these ingredients together, you get a potent anti-inflammatory remedy. You can cook with it or use it to make your favorite salad dressing. Chefs prize "green gold" because of its unique nutty taste. If you have trouble finding this oil in your grocery store, you can order it through the mail. (See the *Pumpkin* chapter for more information.)

> ### To be a vegetarian or not to be
>
> Eating vegetarian could be the key to a life free from RA. According to a European study, cutting meats from your diet appears to promote a balance of bacteria in your digestive system. That means less bad bacteria get absorbed into your blood through your intestinal wall. Without these bad bacteria, some experts believe, your white blood cells might not begin the RA process.
>
> Then again, strict vegetarian diets can also lead to nutritional deficiencies. Make sure you talk with your doctor before going vegetarian.

**Ginger and turmeric.** Ease the inflammation and ache of your next flare-up with a pot of ginger tea or a heaping plate of curry. Turmeric, the leading spice in curry, and ginger both contain curcumin, an antioxidant with pain-fighting powers. In laboratory studies, curcumin appeared to be as potent as NSAIDs, like ibuprofen.

---

### A word of caution

Many RA sufferers blame food allergies for their arthritis. The biggest culprits seem to be tomatoes, red meats, citrus fruits, legumes, and coffee. And yet, scientific evidence hasn't been able to show a connection. Cutting one suspicious food from your diet won't hurt, but it's a good idea to check with your doctor before making any drastic food changes.

---

The Arthritis Foundation even lists turmeric and ginger as alternative therapies for RA.

**Water.** Soothing your fiery joints could be as easy as drinking six 8-ounce glasses of water each day. Water lubricates and cushions your joints. But stay away from sugary drinks. They can lead to weight gain, which could make your arthritis worse.

### Benefits

Protects your heart

Battles diabetes

Helps stop strokes

Conquers kidney stones

Combats cancer

# Rice

· · · · · · · ·

For you it's just a side dish. But for half the people on earth, rice is the main course.

Originating somewhere in Asia, historians know farmers grew rice in China over 6,000 years ago. When western explorers finally visited the Far East, they brought this interesting little grain back with them. Now you can find rice paddies on every continent except Antarctica.

Rice actually comes in three basic varieties — short, long, and basamati. Short grain rice is sticky when cooked and grows mainly in Asia. The longer grain is native to India but is the kind most people in the world eat. Basamati, from the northern plains of

India, is extra long and more difficult to grow. Don't be fooled by wild rice, though — it's not really a rice at all, but related to oats.

All rice starts off brown. But milling, or polishing, removes the outer hull and bran along with nearly all the fiber and nutrients, including an important B vitamin, thiamine. If you don't get enough thiamine, you can develop a serious illness called beriberi. This disease can lead to loss of muscle tone, nerve and heart damage — even death. Most modern countries now enrich polished rice with thiamine making beriberi almost unheard of.

But why not eat rice the way nature intended — brown, natural, and full of fiber. Alice H. Lichtenstein, D.Sc., a professor of nutrition at Tufts University in Boston, suggests passing up refined foods for healthier, whole grains like brown rice. "Increasing dietary fiber," she says, "is just one more component of a healthy dietary regimen that can help reduce your risk for heart disease, as well as other diseases such as cancer and diabetes."

## 4 ways rice keeps you healthy

**Blocks heart disease.** Refined foods are like books with every other page ripped out — you can't get much out of them. But we still insist on processing and refining most of the nutrition out of foods. If you're looking for extra protection against serious health problems like heart disease, add whole, unrefined grains to your diet.

A study of more than 75,000 nurses over 10 years showed whole grains including cereal bran might protect you from heart disease. The nurses who ate foods like whole-wheat bread and brown rice were less likely to develop heart disease than those who ate mostly refined foods like white bread and white rice.

**Defends against diabetes.** Whole grains rich in fiber and magnesium mean added protection against adult-onset (type 2) diabetes, especially for older women. With diabetes, your body becomes less and less sensitive to insulin and your blood sugar keeps going up. But even the American Heart Association is recommending more fiber — 25 grams a day — based on research proving high fiber foods can improve your blood sugar control.

Make brown rice part of a three-servings-a-day-plan to cut your risk of developing diabetes. However six helpings of whole-grain foods every day is better.

**Sidesteps stroke.** More women die from strokes than men. And many stroke survivors end up with permanent disability. Don't let this happen to you. Eat just a little more than one serving of whole grains every day and you could reduce your risk of having a stroke by 30 to 40 percent. (If you've never been a smoker, your risk is even lower.) That translates into about a cup of cooked brown rice — easy enough to fit into your lunch or dinner menu.

**Blocks kidney stones.** Kidney stones are hard, rock-like deposits formed from too much calcium in your blood. If you've ever had one, you know how incredibly painful they can be. But a painless solution is as simple as adding rice bran to your diet.

Less than two tablespoons of rice bran with breakfast and dinner protected 60 percent of the people in a Japanese study from new kidney stones. And the group, as a whole, formed fewer stones than before the study.

Doctors think rice bran reduces how much calcium your body absorbs through your intestines. You can buy it at most health food stores and even at some supermarkets.

## Pantry pointers

If you're used to instant rice, at only five minutes from stove to table, you'll have some adjusting to do with long grain brown rice. It takes about 25 minutes to cook and short grain takes more than half an hour. But it's worth the wait.

To prepare, start with two cups of boiling water. Add a cup of rice, cover, and simmer. Instead of a bland side dish you have to drown in butter, you'll serve up a nutty, chewy grain that adds interest and nutrition to your plate.

# Sea vegetables
· · · · · · · · · · · · · · · · · · · ·

**Benefits**

Combats cancer

Supports immune
system

Protects your heart

Ends anemia

Defends against
viruses

You may only think about seaweed or algae when you go to the beach, but around the world people have been eating sea vegetables for eons. Today they are more popular than ever as a health food.

In places like Iceland, Africa, Mexico, and Japan, sea vegetables share the plate with potatoes, salad, and other landlubber fare. And actually you can find a variety of sea vegetables right under your nose. Check the label on your toothpaste, chocolate milk, ice cream, or pudding. They all probably contain a seaweed fiber called carrageenan or perhaps agar. These make certain products thicker and help ingredients in mixtures — like the chocolate and the milk — stay together.

But the sea vegetables you might add to your menu come in a variety of shapes, colors, and sizes. And not only are they a flavorful ingredient in sushi, soups, or snacks, but they are chock-full of minerals like selenium, iodine, magnesium, calcium, and iron. Plus, don't forget beta carotene, antioxidants, fiber, and protein. All together, these nutrients make sea vegetables a weapon against cancer, heart disease, and certain nutritional deficiencies.

# 4 ways sea vegetables keep you healthy

**Beats breast cancer.** Stephen Cann, associate researcher at the University of British Columbia, gives advice to women who want to fight breast cancer with diet, "Eat different types of seaweed." These include wakame, kombu, and the more common nori — sea vegetables that might fight cancer because of their iodine and selenium.

"We think it's very important for the breast," Cann says about iodine. This mineral, he believes, may prevent and even shrink breast tumors by combining with certain fatty acids and stopping cancerous cells from multiplying. And without the selenium, iodine doesn't do its job properly.

You can see the power of this dynamic duo in Japan, where people eat about 5 grams of sea vegetables virtually every day. Cann points out the Japanese have one of the highest life expectancies and a very low rate of breast cancer.

To get in on seaweed's protection, look for dried sheets of wakame or kombu at your local health food store. The nori used to wrap sushi is a slightly less potent source of these benefits.

---

**To supplement or not to supplement**

In the past few years, sea vegetable supplements have become all the rage. Spirulina, chlorella, wild blue-green algae, and kelp are all available in pills and powders. You'll read claims these products can help you lose weight, clean out toxins, boost your energy, and treat diseases from diabetes to hepatitis.

Many herbal experts disagree, however, since most of these claims are unproven. Some algae supplements can actually do more harm than good. For instance, those made with wild blue-green algae may contain stray unhealthy algae. Your best bet — discuss these supplements with your doctor.

---

**Neutralizes bugs.** If you are ready to launch an attack on colds, flu, and other pesky viruses, see about sea vegetables. Eating wakame and kombu may punch up your body's B cells, white blood cells that rush to the scene of infection. There they give off antibodies that kill what ails you. Though most research comes from test-tube or animal studies, adding a tablespoon or two of dried sea vegetables to your favorite recipe couldn't hurt.

**Heals heart disease.** Experts say postmenopausal women may be able to protect themselves from cardiovascular disease — one of the greatest risks to their health — by eating sea vegetables and other foods rich in phytoestrogens. These plant chemicals resemble the actual hormone estrogen, since they lower cholesterol, thin blood, and in general, prevent heart disease. But unlike hormone replacement therapy (HRT), phytoestrogens may not have dangerous side effects. If you are interested in making phytoestrogens part of your menopause treatment, talk with your doctor.

Sea vegetables also have a load of other nutrients to boost anyone's heart health — magnesium, potassium, fiber, and beta carotene. Eating them can lower your blood pressure, keep free radicals in check, and deal with your cholesterol.

**Defends against B12 deficiency.** Many vegetarians don't get enough vitamin B12. Without meat, the main source of this nutrient, you're at risk of pernicious anemia, nerve damage, and even memory loss. Add nori to your diet and you may never miss that hamburger. This special sushi ingredient is loaded with B12. Just two or three (8-inch square) sheets have a whole day's supply.

## Pantry pointers

Like their landlocked relatives, sea vegetables are natural and versatile. Some are so small you can't see them, while others blanket vast parts of the ocean. Of course, before you start munching, you'll want to know exactly what you're eating. Here are the four main varieties of sea veggies.

- ◆ **Brown algae.** These like to live in the deep, cold waters of the ocean. Some edible kinds include wakame, kombu, and a stringy kind called sea spaghetti. You can also find another type — kelp — as a supplement in your local health food store.

- ◆ **Red algae.** People use this variety the most for foods. One type, nori, is used to make sushi, the Japanese delicacy. You'll also find dulse in many foods, including snack chips, in certain parts of the United States and Canada. Try this cooking tip from Iceland — fold dulse into mashed potatoes.

◆ **Green algae.** You might find this type next time you take a walk on the beach. On your plate, though, keep an eye out for sea lettuce, the kind most commonly eaten.

◆ **Blue-green algae.** Unlike the other three varieties, these algae are microscopic — too small to see with the naked eye. Some kinds, though, grow together in huge clumps. You can find spirulina and chlorella in health food stores as pills or powders.

To add some undersea plant life to your diet, visit you local health food store or Asian market. There you'll most likely find dried sheets of nori, dulse, or any other popular sea vegetable. These can make your next soup or salad a totally different experience.

---

### A word of caution

Though sea vegetables can be a unique treat, they have some drawbacks. Most are high in both iodine and sodium. If you're on a low-salt diet, stay away from them. And according to the American Thyroid Association, rich sources of iodine, like sea vegetables, put adults at risk for thyroid dysfunction. Moderation is the key. If you are already taking thyroid medication, don't eat sea vegetables since the iodine can interfere with the effects of your prescription.

"The other complication," says Cann, "is where the seaweed is harvested." Certain parts of the world — like Europe — have more polluted oceans than others. In these waters sea vegetables can pick up toxic chemicals such as cadmium, lead, and mercury.

# Sinusitis

. . . . . . . . . . . . . .

<table>
<tr><td colspan="2">Eat</td></tr>
<tr><td>Apricots</td><td>Cantaloupe</td></tr>
<tr><td>Strawberries</td><td>Kale</td></tr>
<tr><td>Parsley</td><td>Sweet</td></tr>
<tr><td>Mangoes</td><td>  potatoes</td></tr>
<tr><td>Liver</td><td>Water</td></tr>
<tr><td>Whole-wheat</td><td>Broccoli</td></tr>
<tr><td>  bread</td><td>Black beans</td></tr>
<tr><td colspan="2">Avoid</td></tr>
<tr><td colspan="2">Dairy products, sugar, and alcohol in large amounts</td></tr>
</table>

Have you ever had a cold that just wouldn't quit? Chances are, your "cold" was actually infected sinuses.

The confusion is common. In one study of college students, 87 percent thought they had colds when they really had sinusitis. A sinus infection often follows a cold, however, so it's sometimes hard to tell when one ends and the other begins.

Your sinuses are hollow spaces located above, behind, and below your eyes. Very narrow passageways connect them to the inside of your nose. They act like air filters, protecting your lungs by producing mucus that traps bacteria and pollutants. When you have a cold, the lining of these cavities becomes inflamed and swollen.

"As a result," says Dr. Robert S. Ivker, author of the book *Sinus Survival,* "the mucus being produced in the sinuses cannot drain properly, and the sinuses become a breeding ground for bacteria." This can easily lead to a sinus infection.

You'll know you have a sinus infection if you feel stuffed-up and tired, if your face is tender and swollen, and if headache pain and pressure increase when you bend over. Thick, yellow-green mucus is another sign. With a simple cold, the mucus is generally clear.

Dr. Ivker has been treating people with sinus problems for over thirty years. In that time, he's seen sinusitis increase to epidemic proportions, and he places the blame on air pollution.

Breathing smoke or fumes can trigger a bout with sinusitis even if your sinuses are healthy. But if your membranes are already weakened by pollution, you are even more likely to get infections.

This chronic irritation to nasal passages, Ivker believes, might lead to nasal allergies, a major cause of sinusitis.

Fungi are another prime cause of sinus problems. Researchers at the Mayo Clinic recently found 96 percent of those with chronic sinusitis in their study had one or more types of mold or fungus in their mucus.

Ivker however, hesitates to place all the blame on fungal organisms. He says it's normal to have them — candida, or yeast, as well as good bacteria — in your nose, sinuses, and throat. "They usually coexist in a harmonious balance," he says.

The problem, Ivker thinks, is more likely caused by taking a lot of antibiotics that can destroy the good bacteria, making the way clear for an overgrowth of fungi.

"The body reacts to this imbalance," says Ivker, "by sending white blood cells to the nose and sinuses to combat the problem and this results in inflammation, increased swelling of the mucous membranes, and sinusitis."

Ivker believes, however, the right diet can help heal your sinuses by protecting and healing mucous membranes, strengthening your immune system, and reducing the growth of yeast. He discusses additional ways to fight sinusitis on his Web site at <www.sinussurvival.com>.

## Nutritional blockbusters that fight sinusitis

**Vitamins and minerals.** Colorful fruits and vegetables — like apricots, cantaloupe, strawberries, red and green peppers, kale, parsley, and broccoli — get high praise from Ivker. They contain lots of vitamin C, which, he says, fends off colds, allergies, and sinus infections.

You also need vitamin A to keep your mucous membranes healthy. If you eat carrots, sweet potatoes, mangoes, and winter squash, you'll get lots of beta carotene, which your body converts to vitamin A.

Zinc, found in beef liver, dark turkey meat, and black beans, helps change beta carotene to vitamin A. It also helps build up your immunity and reduces the risk of respiratory infections that can lead to colds.

Ivker recommends vitamin E, too, for preventing allergies and sinusitis. And its power, he says, is doubled when you get selenium with it. Whole grains grown in the rich soil of the United States and Canada provide both these nutrients.

**Water.** Keeping your mucous membranes moist will increase your resistance to infection and allow your sinuses to drain more easily. So drink lots of water — even more than the recommended six 8-ounce glasses a day. For adults who aren't very active, Ivker suggests half an ounce of water per pound of body weight. If you get a lot of exercise, increase the amount to two-thirds an ounce per pound.

For example, if you weigh 130 pounds, you need between eight and 13 8-ounce glasses a day. You can drink less if you eat a lot of fresh fruits and vegetables.

For variety, Ivker suggests herbal teas, natural fruit juices diluted 50 percent with water, or thin soups. Choose products low in salt and without added sugar.

Avoid coffee, regular tea, and cola. "Caffeine is a diuretic that can contribute to dehydration and increased mucus production," says Ivker.

---

### A word of caution

You may think of milk, sweets, and alcoholic beverages as comfort foods, but if you are battling sinusitis, they may be adding to your discomfort.

"The change I recommend most," says sinus expert, Dr. Robert Ivker, "is to avoid milk and dairy products. The protein in milk tends to increase and thicken mucus secretions."

**Benefits**

Saves your eyesight

Strengthens bones

Protects your heart

Combats cancer

Helps stop strokes

Boosts your immune
system

# Spinach

• • • • • • • • • • • • • • •

Spinach may be the best kept secret in the produce department. It's loaded with nutrients, including many antioxidant powerhouses. It's rich in carotenoids, and is a good source of iron, magnesium, manganese, folate, and vitamins A, C, and K. It's also a dieter's dream.

Just don't think like Popeye and reach for the spinach when you've run out of other options. Make this nutritional knockout part of your everyday menu and you could reap major health benefits.

## 4 ways spinach keeps you healthy

**Maintains your vision.** The two most common causes of losing eyesight in your senior years are macular degeneration which affects your retina and cataracts which affect your lens. Spinach may help ward off both these sight stealers.

Your eye's retina is extremely rich in the carotenoids lutein and zeaxanthin. Experts believe these antioxidants protect your eye from light damage and also support the blood vessels to your retina. Boosting the amount of lutein and zeaxanthin in your body can keep your retina strong and efficient — able to fight off the damage that may cause macular degeneration. In fact, research found that people who took in more carotenoids decreased their risk of developing age-related macular degeneration by 43 percent. Spinach and collard greens, both containing high amounts of lutein and zeaxanthin, were the foods most closely linked to this protection.

Damage from free radicals may also cause cataracts, a clouding of your lens. But once again, lutein and zeaxanthin come to the rescue. A 10-year study of 36,000 men discovered those who ate the most spinach were protected.

For the best vision defense, eat these leafy greens at least twice a week — more if possible. And if you want to get the most lutein from your spinach, do what Southern cooks have been doing for years — add a little fat. Although too much is bad for you, a small amount of fat will really increase how much lutein your body can absorb.

**Beefs up your bones.** Just one-half cup of raw spinach a day could help you cross the finish line. If you want to keep your bones strong and cut your risk of suffering a hip fracture, get more vitamin K in your diet. And spinach is a great way to do it.

Just be careful if you suddenly begin eating lots of leafy vegetables while on the blood-thinning drug warfarin. Your doctor may have prescribed this drug to prevent blood clotting if you're at risk for stroke or certain heart problems. Too much vitamin K could seriously affect the way warfarin works. Eat spinach and other leafy greens in moderation and talk to your doctor about any major changes in your diet.

> ### Spinach tastes better with age
>
> Fine wines may taste better as they age, but spinach may taste better as you age.
>
> If you decided as a child that spinach wasn't for you, give it another try. Nutritionists have found the older you get, the more likely you are to enjoy the slightly bitter taste of vegetables like spinach and broccoli. And if that's not enough good news, you're less likely to crave sweets, too.

**Halts heart damage.** High levels of a substance called homocysteine in your blood means you're more likely to develop heart disease. Fortunately, folate, a B vitamin, can help lower levels of heart-damaging homocysteine. Studies have found that supplements and folate-fortified cereals will do the job, but if you prefer more natural sources, spinach and other leafy greens are a good choice. Fresh is best when it comes to folate since cooking and processing tend to drain this important nutrient from foods.

### A word of caution

Spinach may be a wonder food, but it isn't perfect. It contains oxalic acid, which gives it that slightly bitter taste some people love and some people hate. Besides that, oxalic acid blocks calcium absorption — your body can only use 5 percent of the calcium in spinach. You'd have to eat 8 cups of spinach a day to equal the calcium in one cup of milk. So eat your spinach for its other outstanding nutritional qualities, but when it comes to calcium, the dairy case is still where it's at.

**Cramps cancer's style.** It's common knowledge. Eat your fruits and vegetables and you'll lower your risk of cancer. Generally, spinach is a smart side dish to fight all types of cancer, but experts believe it's particularly powerful against these:

◆ **Colon cancer.** Spinach may provide a one-two punch against colon cancer through lutein, an antioxidant, and folate, a B vitamin. People who get plenty of these nutrients are less likely to develop colon cancer.

◆ **Stomach cancer.** Korea has a high rate of stomach cancer, so researchers examined whether certain foods or cooking methods common in that country might be responsible. They found broiled meats and salty foods increased the risk of stomach cancer, while eating lots of spinach, tofu, and cabbage decreased risk.

◆ **Breast cancer.** Toss a spinach salad three times a week and you could cut your risk of breast cancer in half. All fruits and vegetables are beneficial, but carrots and spinach are dynamite.

## Pantry pointers

Fresh spinach is at your grocer's year-round. Look for leaves that are crisp and dark green, and avoid wilted leaves or yellow spots.

Spinach will keep just fine in a sealed container for up to three days in your refrigerator. Before eating, however, wash it to get rid of any dirt. Even bagged spinach can still have grit clinging to the leaves.

Raw veggies are usually more nutritious, but in this case, your body can absorb beta carotene and iron better from cooked spinach. To make the most of this leafy green, include both fresh and cooked spinach in your diet.

# Strawberries

. . . . . . . . . . . . . . . . . . . . . . . .

| **Benefits** |
| --- |
| Combats cancer |
| Protects your heart |
| Boosts memory |
| Calms stress |
| Shields against Alzheimer's |

A strawberry just might be the perfect berry. At least that's what people have believed for hundreds of years. Medieval stonemasons carved their shape into the altars and pillars of churches as a symbol of perfection and virtue. People ate them at festivals in hopes of a peaceful and happy future. Newlyweds celebrated with them and queens bathed in them.

If strawberries aren't the perfect food, they're close. Just one cup of medium berries has a full day's requirement of vitamin C. This delicious snack also fills you up with over 3 grams of fiber — almost as much as in an apple. In addition, strawberries come with hearty supplies of folate and potassium.

Just these nutrients alone could put you on your way to better heart health and cancer prevention. But strawberries also boost your well-being with antioxidants. They have more of these chemical superheroes than most other foods, according to the USDA-ARS Human Nutrition Research Center on Aging — which places them among the top five antioxidant-rich fruits.

With all their wholesome ingredients, strawberries are undeniably "berry" good for you.

## 4 ways strawberries keep you healthy

**Corrals cancer.** According to Dr. Gary Stoner, Chair of the Division of Environmental Health Sciences at Ohio State University, research proves that strawberries act as antioxidants and cut down on free radical mischief.

"They reduce the levels of genetic (DNA) damage caused by carcinogens and inhibit tumor progression," Stoner explains. In other words — strawberries are a topnotch cancer fighter.

They owe much of this power to ellagic acid, a natural chemical that's in only a handful of fruits. But that's not all. Stoner adds, "Berries contain many potential protective substances including vitamins C and E, folic acid, other phenols (besides ellagic acid), various carotenoids, and anthocyanins." All of these substances work together, he believes, to nip cancer in the bud.

**Heals your heart.** Those same antioxidants that fight cancer, Stoner's findings suggest, also make strawberries tough against heart disease. "The berries reduce levels of blood cholesterol by about 10 percent," Stoner says, "so they could have some protective effect on cardiovascular disease."

Although this connection comes only from animal studies, tossing a handful of strawberries onto your breakfast cereal will probably do more than just perk up your morning — you'll perk up your heart, too.

**Enhances your memory.** A bowl of strawberries could be the best-kept secret for a sharper mind. According to research at Tufts University, the antioxidants in strawberries could prevent or even reverse problems like memory loss, Alzheimer's, and Parkinson's disease — all conditions blamed on free radical damage.

**Soothes away stress.** Feeling anxious? Pop a strawberry and your brain might pump out more dopamine. This brain chemical is an ingredient in norepinephrine, which controls how well you deal with stress. These findings came from animal studies, but it can't hurt to add strawberries to your menu before a big meeting at work or other stressful situation.

## Pantry pointers

Whether you buy locally grown strawberries or ones from a supermarket, there are a few simple secrets for picking the best of the bunch. Remember that size doesn't matter. Just look for plump berries with bright red skins and green caps. Discard any that are soft or discolored. If you're buying by the carton, check the bottom of the container. If it's stained or wet, the strawberries on bottom may be moldy or mashed.

When you bring your berries home, dump them out of their container and look for any overripe ones. Eat these right away — not a hard task at all. Keep the rest in the refrigerator, either in a covered container or wrapped in paper towels. Don't store them too long though, since strawberries keep only about a week.

### A word of caution

The headline was frightening — "Frozen strawberries give schoolchildren hepatitis." This is not just newspaper hype. It's reality. Imported produce can carry harmful bacteria, mostly because food safety laws vary from country to country. But there are simple ways you can defend yourself.

If possible, buy from a strawberry farm near you and ask about fertilizing and processing methods. Always wash your hands in hot, soapy water before handling any food. Then wash your berries under running water, and use a vegetable brush to scrub away dirt and bugs.

### Eat

High-fiber        Oats
  cereal          Cantaloupe
Bananas           Black-eyed
Sunflower           peas
  seeds           Tea

### Avoid

Foods high in saturated
fat, such as red meat

Salt and alcohol in large
amounts

# Stroke

• • • • • • • • • • • •

Every minute, someone has a stroke.

That means a blood vessel becomes blocked (an ischemic stroke) or one bursts (a hemorrhagic stroke), cutting off blood flow to part of your brain. Without the oxygen in the blood, your brain cells die — and never come back. Depending on which part of your brain is affected, you could be paralyzed on one side of your body, lose feeling, balance, bladder control, or sight, or have trouble swallowing, talking, or remembering things. That's if you survive. Stroke is the third leading cause of death in developed countries, ranked behind only heart disease and cancer.

Because of the serious damage it can do, stroke sometimes goes by a more serious name — brain attack. If you feel a sudden numbness or weakness on one side of your body, have unexpected difficulty speaking, understanding, seeing, walking, and keeping your balance, or a sudden severe headache, you should call for emergency help right away.

Dr. Vladimir C. Hachinski, a Canadian neurologist who coined the term "brain attack," believes only if you respond to strokes as urgently as you do heart attacks, will you have a chance to limit their damage.

Older people should be extra cautious. Two-thirds of all stroke victims are over 65 years old. In fact, your risk of stroke doubles every decade after you turn 55. Other risk factors include high blood pressure, high cholesterol, smoking, diabetes, obesity, and transient ischemic attacks (TIAs). Often called "mini-strokes," TIAs happen when the blood supply to an area of the brain is cut off temporarily. Although you have no permanent damage from a TIA, you are 10 times more likely to have a real stroke later.

Fighting stroke means more than dialing quickly for help. You should also watch what you eat. Cut down on salt and fat and load up on fruits, vegetables, and fiber to lower your risk. Add foods full of these nutrients to your diet and strike out against stroke.

## Nutritional blockbusters that fight stroke

**Fiber.** Cholesterol build-up can block blood vessels, causing an ischemic stroke. About 80 percent of all strokes fall under this category. High blood pressure increases your risk of a hemorrhagic stroke — when a blood vessel in or near your brain bursts. Because fiber can lower blood pressure and cholesterol, it can also reduce your risk of both types of stroke.

One study showed men who ate 29 grams of fiber a day — roughly the amount in three cups of Grape Nuts cereal — were 43 percent less likely to have a stroke as those who ate only about half that much. Cereal fiber, the kind in oats, wheat, rye, and barley, gave the most protection. Rich sources of fiber include whole-grain foods, bran flakes, beans, fruits, leafy vegetables, nuts, and prunes.

> ### Herbs and spice are twice as nice
>
> Garlic and ginger, two tasty ways to perk up a meal, may also perk up your defense against stroke.
>
> A substance in garlic called ajoene stops your platelets from clumping together, reducing the risk of clots. Garlic also lowers cholesterol and blood pressure, two big risk factors in stroke.
>
> Ginger, thanks to natural phytochemicals called gingerol and shogaol, may also prevent blood clots. Add both fresh and dried ginger to your everyday dishes and do your health a favor.

**Potassium.** If you have high blood pressure, you're probably already on the lookout for ways to get more potassium into your diet. Don't give up, because potassium also guards against brain attacks.

Say the only potassium you got each day was from a medium-sized cantaloupe and a banana (totaling about 2 grams). If you doubled that amount, you might lower your chances of having a stroke by 41 percent. Eating a large cantaloupe, a cup of prunes, and a banana each day gives you more than the 4 grams you need.

Cereals, peas, beans, dried apricots, dried figs, oranges, and peaches also give you potassium.

**Magnesium.** As another mineral that helps keep your blood pressure under control, magnesium can be a valuable addition to an anti-stroke diet. In fact, make sure you get more than 450 milligrams (mg) of this mineral every day and you might reduce your risk of stroke by one-third. A baked potato with skin, two cups of a ready-to-eat cereal with wheat germ, and an avocado are all you need.

> ## Alcohol + moderation = lower stroke risk
>
> A drink a day might keep stroke away. Too many, though, might prove deadly.
>
> One study conducted by Columbia University College of Physicians and Surgeons found that people who drank up to two alcoholic drinks a day cut their risk of stroke in half. However, drink more and you could double — even triple — your risk. Similar results came from a recent study of women in the Baltimore-Washington D.C. area. Two glasses of wine a day lowered their risk of stroke by 60 percent.
>
> Don't take up drinking just to protect yourself from stroke, but if you already drink, remember to say "when."

You'll also find magnesium in black-eyed peas, almonds, spinach, broccoli, squash, oatmeal, steamed oysters, sunflower seeds, and pinto beans.

**Antioxidants.** A diet rich in fruits and vegetables gives you plenty of antioxidants. These natural compounds stop free radicals from oxidizing low-density lipoprotein (LDL), or "bad," cholesterol. That means the LDL cholesterol has less chance to stick to your artery walls and form plaque. Without plaque, which can block arteries or break off into clots and travel toward your brain, you have less risk of a stroke. The following nutrients act as antioxidants in your body.

◆ Flavonoids, found in a variety of fruits and vegetables, keep LDL particles from oxidizing and the platelets in your blood from sticking together to form clots. A 15-year Dutch study found men whose diets included lots of flavonoids — especially from black tea — had a 73 percent less chance of stroke than those who ate very few flavonoids.

◆ Beta carotene also has anti-stroke power. It's plentiful in brightly colored fruits and vegetables. Munch on a carrot a day, especially if you smoke, and you could slash your stroke risk.

◆ Vitamin C gets support from long-term clinical research. For example, a British study found people who got at least 45 mg of vitamin C every day had a 60 percent less chance of dying from a stroke than those who got half that amount. One cup of tomato juice, half a cup of brussels sprouts, or half a grapefruit each give you enough to make this difference.

◆ Vitamin E, because of its potential to stop LDL oxidation, also may reduce stroke risk. Avocados, nuts, seeds, and wheat germ are great sources of E.

**Unsaturated fats.** Although slashing fat from your diet can help prevent stroke, certain fats are protective. Omega-3 fatty acids, those found in cold-water fish like tuna, mackerel, and salmon, and monounsaturated fat, the kind in olive oil, give stroke a fat chance.

Researchers in The Netherlands discovered men who ate just 20 grams (less than an ounce) of fish a day were half as likely to have a stroke as those who ate less. You would get that much fish by eating a serving of salmon every week.

Olive oil, which lowers cholesterol and blood pressure, also works against clots. Make olive oil your primary oil for cooking, and you'll make your heart and brain safer.

**Folate.** This member of the B vitamin family takes on a dangerous substance called homocysteine, known to encourage blood clots and hardening of your arteries. If your diet doesn't have enough folate, you might have too much homocysteine, and therefore a higher risk of heart disease and stroke.

Put the brakes on this villain, dubbed "the cholesterol of the '90s," with folate-rich foods such as green leafy vegetables and legumes.

| Benefits |
| --- |
| Saves your eyesight |
| Combats cancer |
| Protects your heart |
| Strengthens bones |
| Lifts mood |
| Boosts your immune system |

# Sweet potatoes

• • • • • • • • • • • • • • • • •

Sweet potatoes are naturally delicious because of their high sugar content. An average-sized sweet potato has a little more than 100 calories, virtually no fat, and absolutely no cholesterol. Instead, it's loaded with vitamins, minerals, and fiber.

With all its nutrients, the colorful tuber is more than just a tasty side dish. A sweet potato has what it takes to brighten your mood, prevent cancer, heal heart disease, and clear up eye ailments.

## 5 ways sweet potatoes keep you healthy

**Packs a triple punch against cancer.** Three of the toughest cancer fighters in the nutrient world — folate, vitamin C, and beta carotene (which turns into vitamin A) — are packed into a sweet potato. One sweet potato gives you almost three times the recommended daily amount of vitamin A and almost half the suggested amount of vitamin C. That's a lot of cancer prevention packed into one potato.

And don't forget folate. You need at least 400 micrograms (mcg) of this B vitamin each day, and a sweet potato will contribute more than 25 mcg. Your body needs folate to build and repair its DNA, and if you don't get enough, experts believe you may increase your risk of certain types of cancer.

**Heads off heart disease.** If you want a healthy heart, enjoy a steaming, baked sweet potato. Inside that hearty treat are potassium, beta carotene, folate, and vitamins C and B6 — five keys to lowering your blood pressure and keeping your arteries flowing smoothly. On top of all these nutrients, a sweet potato has more than 3 grams of fiber. You can help protect yourself from chronic heart disease by including fiber-rich fruits and vegetables in your daily diet.

**Controls cataracts.** A sweet potato's bright orange color means it has lots of beta carotene, which your body turns into vitamin A. And this particular vitamin may be critical to the health of your eyes.

"Vitamin A is an antioxidant," explains Dr. Richard G. Cumming, head researcher of the Blue Mountains Eye Study in Sydney, Australia. "Our study supports the view that antioxidant vitamins might help prevent cataracts. However, it suggests that other nutrients are also important." A good way to keep your eyes healthy, says Cumming, is to eat a well-balanced diet. The sweet potato is an excellent food to include because it is rich in beta carotene and other important nutrients.

**Bats 5 for 5 against osteoporosis.** It's never too late to go to bat against osteoporosis. To prevent or slow down the disease, just eat a diet packed with five ingredients — potassium, magnesium, fiber, vitamin C, and beta carotene. Unlike many other foods, sweet potatoes contain all five, and all but magnesium in abundance.

To add even more bone-building power, top a baked sweet potato with a slice of your favorite low-fat cheese and a handful of chopped parsley. The cheese will add calcium, the original osteoporosis fighter. The parsley will replace the vitamin C lost in baking.

**Sweetens your mood.** Snack on a sweet potato, and you may lift yourself out of the doldrums. Experts say eating foods high in vitamin B6 may be a key to beating the blues. Your body needs the nutrient to balance chemicals in your brain that may control whether you're happy or sad. If you are a vegetarian, sweet potatoes and other plant sources high in B6 — like navy beans, spinach, and bananas — are especially important. Most people get their B6 from chicken, liver, and other meats.

## Pantry pointers

Some people call sweet potatoes "yams," but they're actually two separate vegetables. The yam belongs to the lily plant family and is found mainly in Latin America and the Caribbean. The sweet potato you're familiar with comes from the root of the morning glory vine.

What's more important than the name is their color — pale yellow or deep orange. Those with darker skins, according to sweet potato connoisseurs, have a bright orange inside that's moister and sweeter than its lighter cousin.

Take both types home and try for yourself. Just make sure to buy potatoes that are hard to the touch with blemish-free skins. Once you've brought them home, you can leave them out in the open where they'll last up to 10 days. If you want them to keep them longer, store them in a cool, dark place.

# Thyroid disease

· · · · · · · · · · · · · ·

### Eat

| | |
|---|---|
| Spinach | Sea |
| Iodized salt | vegetables |
| Skim milk | Whole-wheat |
| Carrots | bread |
| Apricots | Liver |
| Oysters | Olive oil |

### Avoid

Foods high in goitrogens, such as peaches and cabbage

If you're feeling tired and depressed and perhaps finding it hard to sleep or enjoy your food, don't chalk it up to simple aging — you could have a problem with your thyroid. It's hard to believe thyroid disease affects millions when most people don't even know where their thyroid is or what it does. Although some thyroid disorders are beyond your control, a proper diet can help keep you and your thyroid safe and healthy.

Located in the base of your neck and shaped like a butterfly, the thyroid gland keeps your body's metabolism running smoothly. It sends out hormones to all your major organs — an important job for your complete health. That also means when things go wrong with your thyroid, many parts of your body feel the effects.

If your thyroid produces more hormones than it should, your metabolism increases. You might suffer from nervousness, bulging eyes, tremors, weight loss, and a rapid heart rate. This condition is called hyperthyroidism.

On the other hand, if your gland is not pumping out enough hormones, you could experience depression, memory loss, fatigue, high cholesterol, muscle aches, hair loss, weight gain, and constipation. This is called hypothyroidism. A high-fiber, low-calorie diet can help combat some of these symptoms.

The most obvious warning sign of a thyroid problem is a swollen thyroid gland or goiter, which appears as a bulge in your throat. The American Association of Clinical Endocrinologists (AACE) suggests a simple at-home goiter test. Tip your head back and drink a glass of water while watching your throat in a mirror. Be alert for swelling just above your collarbone but below your Adam's apple. Notify your doctor if you see something. A blood test can tell for sure if you have thyroid disease.

> ### High cholesterol could mean thyroid disease
>
> According to the National Cholesterol Education Program (NCEP), hypothyroidism is a major cause of high cholesterol.
>
> You may not be treating your cholesterol problems correctly unless you get your thyroid checked.

Although seniors and adult women are especially at risk — about 20 percent of women over 60 suffer from thyroid disease — it can strike anyone. That's why the American Thyroid Association recommends all adults over 35 have a thyroid blood test every five years.

## Nutritional blockbusters that fight thyroid disease

**Iodine.** Without this trace mineral, your thyroid can't make its hormones. Disturbing new data suggest iodine deficiency is on the rise — and not just in countries like Africa and Asia. It's becoming more common in developed nations, too.

The public's love-hate relationship with salt is a major reason for this. Most Western countries add iodine to their salt to prevent just such a deficiency. But more and more people are cutting back on salt for health reasons. Reducing salt intake is still a great idea. Just make sure you use iodized salt when you do sprinkle it on.

If you're on a no-salt diet, try getting your iodine from whole foods. High-powered iodine sources include seafood, sea vegetables, low-fat dairy foods, and spinach.

Still, remember to practice moderation with these foods, especially if you're also using salt. Too much iodine can be dangerous, especially to iodine-sensitive people. Excess iodine can cause hypo-thyroidism, hyperthyroidism, goiter, or even shut your thyroid down completely.

**Selenium.** Even with the right amount of iodine, if your body isn't getting enough selenium, your thyroid can have trouble making hormones. Experts suggest the right amount of selenium might also guard your thyroid against free radicals.

It's fortunate many high-iodine foods, such as seafood and milk, are also good sources of selenium. Also, eat whole-wheat products and meat to help keep your thyroid safe.

**Vitamin A.** Vitamin A is essential for thyroid health since it helps you absorb iodine properly. Without it, you can develop a goiter even if you have safe iodine levels. Crunch on some carrots or serve up sweet potatoes, liver, apricots, spinach, or some other super source of beta carotene which your body turns into vitamin A.

**Iron.** Low iron levels mean your thyroid can't function as it should. Meat is one of your best resources for iron, but if you're a vegetarian or watching your fat intake, you can get your iron from other foods. Green leafy vegetables, legumes, and certain grains like quinoa are good choices. Top these foods with lemon juice or drink a glass of orange juice with your meal. The vitamin C helps your body digest iron from plants. Plus, you need C anyway to make thyroxine, a thyroid hormone.

**Zinc.** Levels of this mineral affect your thyroid function and oysters are a number one way to get it. If you're squeamish when it comes to shellfish, stick with lean meats, lima beans, and whole grains.

**Vitamin E.** Drizzle on the sunflower or olive oil for better thyroid health. These vegetable oils — as well as seeds, wheat germ, some nuts, and avocados — are great sources of vitamin E.

**Vitamin D.** A chronic deficiency of "the sunshine vitamin" can bring on hyperthyroidism. For those rainy days, plan ahead by eating fortified dairy products and seafood.

---

### A word of caution

All soy products contain goitrogens, natural chemicals that interfere with your thyroid hormones. Seniors and women — prime targets for hypothyroidism — should be especially careful about eating soy on a daily basis.

Peaches, almonds, peanuts, and cruciferous vegetables like turnips, rutabagas, and cabbage also contain small amounts of goitrogens. As long as these foods are part of a well-rounded diet, you shouldn't experience problems. Remember, moderation is the key. Cooking also helps by breaking down these potentially harmful compounds.

---

**Copper.** Your thyroid needs this trace mineral, though experts aren't sure why. Don't worry though, you'll probably get all the copper you need from a normal diet — especially if you're a fan of oysters, baked potatoes, lima beans, and mushrooms.

**Benefits**

Protects prostate

Combats cancer

Lowers cholesterol

Supports immune system

Protects your heart

# Tomatoes

• • • • • • • • • • • • • • • • • • •

Most people don't care if tomatoes are a fruit or a vegetable — as long as they're juicy and delicious. They're the most popular home-grown crop in the United States since not only are they great fresh, but they really punch up a homemade sauce, soup, or casserole.

Tomatoes weren't always so fashionable, however. When European explorers brought "love apples" from the New World back to their homelands, people were suspicious. Many thought tomatoes were poisonous because they are related to belladonna and nightshade, two deadly plants. In fact, the roots and leaves of the tomato plant are poisonous.

It wasn't until the 1900s that people in North America learned tasty tomatoes are a terrific health food. They contain lycopene, a unique nutrient that may ward off cancer, plus they're high in vitamin C, folate, and potassium. This means tomatoes are great protection against heart disease and can even boost your immune system.

And by the way, they're a fruit.

## 3 ways tomatoes keep you healthy

**Conquers cancer.** If you had to pick just one food as a cancer-fighting superstar, would it be tomatoes? If not you'd be missing out on the amazing carotenoid lycopene. Found only in a handful of plants, lycopene not only gives tomatoes their brilliant color, but may also lower your risk of developing cancer, according to a Harvard Medical School review of 72 different studies.

You've already heard how deadly tomatoes can be to prostate cancer — if you eat 10 or more servings a week, the lycopene could cut your risk of prostate cancer in half. But also the more tomatoes and tomato products you eat, the less likely you are to develop stomach, lung, breast, colon, mouth, or throat cancer, as well.

If the thought of 10 servings of tomatoes is daunting, just remember ketchup and pizza and spaghetti sauce count — maybe even more than eating a fresh tomato. The heat from cooking frees up tomato's lycopene and adding oil provides fat. Both steps make it easier for your body to absorb the lycopene.

**Heals your heart.** Tomatoes don't stop at cancer, either. An army of nutrients works at closing down one heart-stopping condition after another. Lycopene breaks down cholesterol in such a way that it keeps your arteries free-flowing. Folate cleans up homocysteine, an amino acid that links with cholesterol to give your heart double trouble. And in a study from Europe, drinking 11 ounces of tomato juice every day — about as much as in one soda can — really put the crunch on LDL or "bad" cholesterol. If that's not enough, tomatoes are chock-full of potassium, a mineral crucial for lowering blood pressure. So slice up a tomato and you're slicing your risk of heart disease and heart attack.

**Beats back bacteria.** Experts say, drink just one 11-ounce can of tomato juice and you've boosted your immune system more than by eating foods like spinach or carrots. Nutrients in the tomatoes first encourage your body to produce more T cells, white blood cells that direct attacks against foreign substances like bacteria and viruses. Then the antioxidants in the tomatoes protect these white blood cells from free radicals. The bottom line — tomatoes offer a double whammy against anything that tries to slow you down.

---

### A gardener's guide

Nothing says summer like a vine-ripened tomato. And if you grow your own, you're sure to have all you can eat — and more.

- Pick the right seeds. "Determinates" are good for small gardens. "Indeterminates" will grow as big as you let them.

- Plant in a nice sunny spot with good drainage — you'll get more tomatoes.

- Grow cabbage, carrots, celery, onions, and borage near your tomatoes to keep pests away, add flavor to the tomatoes, and return nutrients to the soil.

- Support your plants with 6-foot stakes. Tie each one up every 12 inches.

- Enrich your soil with manure and compost. Also mix in some lime — the calcium helps prevent deformities in the fruit.

---

## Pantry pointers

Tomatoes from your grocery store's produce section may look nice and red, but they're usually unripe — which means they're hard and tasteless. You may have to take them home like this, but you certainly don't have to eat them this way.

---

> ## A word of caution
>
> Heartburn after every meal, a chronic cough, sore throat, hoarseness —
> these are all the symptoms of acid-reflux disorder, an uncomfortable con-
> dition where stomach acid is forced up into your throat.
>
> If you have these problems, see your doctor. But in the meantime, the
> National Naval Medical Center says stop eating tomatoes and tomato
> products. Along with cigarettes, alcohol, caffeine, and large meals, toma-
> toes probably make your discomfort worse.

If you store your tomatoes in the refrigerator, they'll never get ripe and flavorful. But stick them in a paper bag and they'll release a natural gas that speeds up the ripening process. Before you can say "salsa," you'll have soft, juicy tomatoes.

# Turmeric

· · · · · · · · · · · · · · ·

| Benefits |
| --- |
| Reduces inflammation |
| Combats cancer |
| Aids digestion |
| Guards against liver disease |
| Eases arthritis |

Since the days of Marco Polo, people in Europe only reached for turmeric when they couldn't get their hands on saffron, a much tastier and more expensive spice. Sometimes people didn't even consider turmeric worthy of their food. Instead, they used it to dye fabric.

In Asia, on the other hand, people have always appreciated turmeric for its own sake. Curry, the spicy seasoning in Indian and Thai cooking, would not be the same without it. People also used turmeric in medicines — for colds, infections, and indigestion. Some even frightened off crocodiles with it, fed it to their sick ele-phants, or used it as makeup and perfume.

Turmeric may not really keep crocodiles away, but it might scare disease away — mainly because of curcumin, a powerful antioxidant. According to recent research, curcumin and other phytochemicals in turmeric may defeat cancerous tumors, reduce inflammation, fight heart disease, improve liver ailments, and ease indigestion. So who needs saffron anyway?

## 4 ways turmeric keeps you healthy

**Deflates inflammation.** Experts say, if you want relief from pain and swelling, try turmeric. It might work as well as ibuprofen and other nonsteroidal anti-inflammatory drugs (NSAIDs), but without their side effects. Turmeric might even be powerful enough to fight the stiffness and swelling of rheumatoid arthritis and osteoarthritis, according to the Arthritis Foundation.

**Wages war against cancer.** It's scary to think about, but cancer can grow inside of you for months or even years — without you even knowing it. Rest assured, there's something you can do to fight hidden tumors.

> ### A team player
>
> If you want to spice up turmeric's power to battle disease, don't leave it by itself on your dinner plate. Experts suggest teaming it with a shake of black pepper. Piperine, the main phytonutrient in pepper, can increase your body's intake of curcumin by an amazing 2,000 percent.
>
> And there's more — after you eat a dish spiced with pepper and turmeric, enjoy a cup of green tea. Green tea and curcumin, researchers at the Memorial Sloan-Kettering Cancer Center in New York discovered, team up as a cancer-fighting dynamic duo.

In an exciting new study of almost 30,000 Canadian women, anti-inflammatory substances, like turmeric, seemed to slow the growth of undetected breast tumors. When these cancers were eventually found, they were smaller and easier to treat.

You may also prevent cancer by spicing up your food with turmeric — thanks again to curcumin. This antioxidant, researchers suggest, may halt cancers of the skin, stomach, colon, mouth, and liver in their tracks. So far, evidence only comes from animal studies, but experts are now testing curcumin in people, too. Stay tuned.

**Safeguards your liver.** This incredible organ spends a lifetime keeping your blood clean. During all that time, what keeps your liver clean? One answer to that question could be turmeric and its team of antioxidants. They put the kabosh on free radicals and other toxic chemicals before they can harm your liver.

**Beefs up bile flow.** If you get stomach pain after eating fatty foods, turmeric might offer some relief. This type of indigestion results from a poor flow of bile from your liver to your gallbladder. Besides the stomach pain, symptoms include heartburn, bloating, nausea, and even light-colored stools. Turmeric gets your bile flowing, which could relieve your pain. It works so well that the German Commission E, experts in the field of herbal medicines, recommends taking up to a half tablespoon (about 3 grams) every day for this kind of indigestion.

However, if your symptoms are severe, they could indicate a more serious condition, like gallstones. Before you treat yourself with turmeric, check with your doctor.

## Pantry pointers

The easiest way to get turmeric in your diet is to order curry at your local Indian restaurant. For you chefs who want to cook with turmeric, finding it is easy. Most chain supermarkets carry powdered turmeric in their spice aisle. Or visit your local natural foods store or Indian grocer. Their spices might be fresher because they have a faster turnaround.

Enjoy experimenting with turmeric in your cooking, but remember — a little goes a long way. And there's one place you don't want to shake the spice — in your teacup. Curcumin and the

> ### A word of caution
>
> If you have a history of gallstones, think twice about ordering curry. Even a small amount of turmeric can aggravate a gallstone or other blockage of the bile duct. That's even truer for the pure turmeric spice.

other ingredients in turmeric won't dissolve in water, so forget about making a yellow-colored brew.

| Eat | |
|---|---|
| Honey | Yogurt |
| Garlic | Olive oil |
| Cranberries | Sunflower oil |
| Wine | Broccoli |
| Apples | Cantaloupe |
| Prunes | Barley |

**Avoid**

Spicy foods if they trigger ulcer pain

# Ulcers

• • • • • • • • • • •

What's eating you? If you frequently have a gnawing pain in your stomach, it's probably a peptic ulcer — a sore on the lining of your stomach or small intestine.

People once thought ulcers were caused by stress or spicy foods. But in the 1980s, research uncovered a more treatable cause — *Helicobacter pylori (H. pylori),* a corkscrew-shaped bacterium. The lining of your stomach normally protects it from pepsin and other digestive acids. But when *H. pylori* burrows into your stomach lining, it allows those digestive acids to eat into your stomach, creating a painful ulcer.

Not all ulcers are caused by bacteria, but ones that are can be treated with antibiotics — and it's a much more effective treatment than chewing over-the-counter antacids. Your doctor can perform a simple blood test or breath test to see if you have *H. pylori.*

This discovery is good news for people who thought they'd just have to live with their painful sores. And there could be even better news ahead. Research is beginning to show that certain foods may affect whether you develop ulcers.

## Nutritional blockbusters that fight ulcers

**Honey.** To get sweet relief from ulcer pain, try a spoonful of honey. This "liquid gold" acts as an antibacterial, and research shows it zooms right in on *H. pylori*. Early studies suggested only Manuka honey from New Zealand worked against *H. pylori*, but more recent studies found that American honeys also were effective. Try eating a tablespoon of honey an hour before meals and at bedtime to help soothe your discomfort.

**Garlic.** This "fragrant" bulb also acts as an antibacterial, and a Dutch study found that garlic slowed the growth of four different strains of *H. pylori* in the laboratory. Researchers used small amounts of garlic so this may mean the garlic you eat provides some protection against ulcers. More research needs to be done, but if you're a fan of garlic bread and spaghetti, you might be doing your stomach a favor.

**Polyunsaturated fats.** Use olive oil on your garlic bread instead of butter, and you could give *H. pylori* a double whammy. Polyunsaturated fats such as olive oil, fish oil, and sunflower oil prevented growth of *H. pylori* in the laboratory. While no studies have tested the effects of polyunsaturated fats on human ulcers, these fats are always a healthier choice than saturated fats like butter. And in this case, they may give your stomach an added boost of ulcer protection.

**Cranberries.** These tart berries are thought to protect against urinary tract infections by keeping bacteria from sticking to your cells. They also may prevent *H. pylori* from setting up housekeeping in your stomach the same way, says Dr. Ted Wilson, a professor at the University of Wisconsin-La Crosse and a leading researcher on the health benefits of cranberries. By drinking a glass of cranberry juice every day, you may help wash *H. pylori* out of your stomach and prevent an ulcer from occurring.

**Yogurt.** The "good bacteria" found in yogurt and other fermented dairy products may protect against *H. pylori*. *Lactobacillus casei,* one of these knights in shining armor, destroyed *H. pylori* in test tube studies. These helpful bacteria may also fight the side effects of antibiotics doctors prescribe to treat an *H. pylori* infection. Diarrhea is the most common side effect yogurt helps to control. If you have an ulcer, try eating several cups of this creamy treat each day to speed relief.

**Fiber.** Fill up on fiber-rich fruits and vegetables, and you could lower your risk of ulcers. People who eat a lot of fruits and vegetables are less likely to develop ulcers, and researchers think fiber could be the reason. Fiber seems to encourage the growth of the mucous layer that protects your stomach from digestive acids.

**Wine.** If you already have an ulcer, drinking alcohol is a definite no-no because it irritates your stomach. However, an occasional glass of wine may protect you against infection by *H. pylori*.

A study in Germany found that people who drank moderate amounts of alcohol were less likely to be infected with *H. pylori*. Wine was more protective than beer. People who drank three-and-a-half ounces or less of wine daily were 53 percent less likely to have an active *H. pylori* infection than people who didn't drink at all.

---

### A word of caution

Although stress and spicy foods are no longer considered causes of ulcers, they may trigger pain once you have an ulcer. Smoking and aspirin or other pain relievers may also aggravate an ulcer. Try to control stress and avoid triggers until your ulcer heals.

# Urinary tract infections

· · · · · · · · · · · · · · · · · ·

**Eat**

Cranberries   Blueberries
Water         Grapefruit
Parsley       Oranges
Lemons        Broccoli
Tomatoes      Sweet red
Strawberries   peppers

**Avoid**

Foods that may irritate
your bladder, such as
coffee and spicy foods

Visiting the bathroom is a routine part of every day. You probably don't give it a second thought — until it becomes painful. If you experience a burning, stinging feeling when you urinate, you may have a urinary tract infection (UTI).

Women are especially prone to urinary tract infections — one in five will have one sometime during her lifetime. Still, men over 50 can get UTIs from an enlarged prostate. Anything that interferes with urine flow causes urine to stay in the urinary tract longer. And bacteria have more time to get a grip and multiply.

Most urinary tract infections only cause temporary discomfort. If the infection spreads to your kidneys, however, it can cause permanent kidney damage or result in sometimes-fatal blood poisoning. Therefore, if you think you have a urinary tract infection, see your doctor right away — if you're right, he'll prescribe antibiotics.

Once you've had one urinary tract infection, you're likely to have more. Here are some natural nutritional strategies that may help prevent a painful infection in the future.

## Nutritional blockbusters that fight urinary tract infections

**Cranberries.** Modern medical research is beginning to confirm the healing powers of many home remedies, and that's certainly the case with cranberries. Studies show that cranberry juice really can prevent urinary tract infections. Some doctors think these tart little berries work by making your urine more acidic which slows the growth of bacteria. Other evidence suggests cranberries may work by keeping bacteria from clinging to your urinary tract.

To take advantage of cranberry's protective powers drink about 3 ounces of juice every day. One study found that the beneficial effects appeared only after four to eight weeks. So, for the most protection, drink cranberry juice regularly.

**Vitamin C.** Keep your refrigerator stocked with refreshing orange and grapefruit juice and you may keep UTIs at bay. Like the elements in cranberry juice, vitamin C and citric acid in citrus fruits may make your urine more acidic, thus making it more difficult for bacteria to grow.

**Water.** Ordinary water does an extraordinary job of washing bacteria out of your body before it has a chance to multiply. Drink at least six to eight glasses of water every day. Pale-colored urine is a good sign that you're getting enough. If your urine is dark, visit the water fountain a little more often.

**Parsley.** A green sprig of parsley on your plate doesn't just look good. It's a great source of vitamin C. What's more, it may act as a diuretic, which means it increases urine flow. And anything that increases urine flow may help reduce your chances of getting a urinary tract infection. So the next time a restaurant serves you a parsley garnish, don't just admire it — eat it for an extra bit of urinary protection.

---

### A word of caution

If you're prone to UTIs, avoid foods that may irritate your bladder. Common offenders include coffee, tea, alcohol, carbonated beverages, and spicy foods.

# Walnuts

· · · · · · · · · · · · · · ·

**Benefits**

Lowers cholesterol

Enhances blood flow

Combats cancer

Boosts your memory

Lifts your mood

Protects against heart disease

You don't have to be Sherlock Holmes to "crack" this case. Even Watson knows walnuts are good for you.

From the ancient Chinese to the American colonists, people have enjoyed these hard-shelled heroes for centuries. Roman grooms would toss walnuts at wedding guests to bring good health and fertility. During the Middle Ages, Europeans believed walnuts could ward off fever, epilepsy, lightning, and even protect them from witchcraft. When times were especially tough during the colonization of America, the settlers survived on walnuts.

That probably made for some pretty healthy colonists. Loaded with unsaturated fat, vitamin E, and ellagic acid, walnuts can lower cholesterol, fight cancer, and boost your brainpower. Use walnuts for baking or cooking, throw them in a salad for some crunch, or just munch on them for a tasty snack.

Crack open a walnut and crack the case of good health.

## 4 ways walnuts keep you healthy

**Conquers cholesterol.** If you don't care about your cholesterol, you must be nuts. If you want to lower your cholesterol, you should eat them.

In a six-week study in Spain, patients substituted walnuts for some of the olive oil and other fatty foods in their traditional Mediterranean diet. This simple change caused total and LDL or "bad" cholesterol to drop considerably. This research proved women, older people, and those with high cholesterol already at risk of heart disease can benefit from eating walnuts as much as young, healthy men.

"Walnuts lowered the risk of coronary heart disease by 11 percent," says Dr. Emilio Ros, a researcher at the Hospital Clinic of Barcelona and director of the study. "It's as simple as this: if you eat a handful of walnuts a day, you will lower your blood cholesterol, and therefore lower your cardiovascular risk."

> ### Walnut oil packs a punch without the crunch
>
> If you're tired of cooking with the same old oil, give your food a nutty change with walnut oil. It has a pleasant flavor that's great for salad dressings, cooking, baking, and sautéing. Although some supermarkets and gourmet food stores carry it, it's a bit pricier than ordinary oils — but worth it for that special dish. Just like the nut, walnut oil has lots of omega-3 fatty acid — a healthy alternative to soybean or corn oil.

Part of what makes walnuts so effective is their high fat content. An ounce of English walnuts (about a handful) contains more than 18 grams of fat. Most of it is polyunsaturated, including a form of omega-3 fatty acid called alpha-linolenic acid. Walnuts also contain some monounsaturated fat. Both lower cholesterol.

Walnuts also provide vitamin E, a powerful antioxidant that stops LDL particles from oxidizing and damaging your arteries.

**Smashes clots.** If someone told you a certain food could reduce your risk of heart disease, you might respond, "Nuts." And you'd be right. That same alpha-linolenic acid keeps the platelets in your blood from clumping together. Lumpy, sticky blood can lead to all sorts of problems, including atherosclerosis, high blood pressure, blood clots, heart attack, and stroke. In fact, four major studies found that eating nuts regularly can reduce your risk of heart disease by 30 to 50 percent.

**Puts the crunch on cancer.** Walnuts are one of the richest natural sources of ellagic acid, a flavonoid that fights cancerous tumors, especially of the lung, liver, skin, and esophagus.

In addition, men should know a few walnuts a day could safeguard their prostate. The University of Massachusetts Medical School gathered information on diet and prostate cancer from 59 countries. They found that nuts, along with grains and cereals, offered real protection. Plus, with the antioxidant vitamin E mopping up those dangerous free radicals, walnuts give you even more anti-cancer benefits.

**Brightens up your brain.** In the past, people thought walnuts look a bit like a brain and so believed they were a good food for your brain. Turns out they were right. The omega-3 fatty acid in these delicious nuts can improve brain function, boost your memory, and may even brighten your mood.

## Pantry pointers

You'll find English walnuts in most supermarkets. They come large, medium, or small, and with or without the shell. Walnuts in the shell shouldn't have any cracks or holes. Store them in a cool, dry place for three months. When shopping for shelled walnuts, look for plump, crisp nuts. Keep these in your refrigerator, covered, for six months or in your freezer for up to a year.

---

### A word of caution

As tasty and nutritious as walnuts are, they aren't the perfect food. Because of a certain protein, walnuts are among the most common source of food allergies. If you're allergic to walnuts, you could experience respiratory problems and stomach or skin irritation.

Another problem with walnuts, and all nuts for that matter, is that they limit the amount of iron your body absorbs. You can fix this easily, however, by getting an additional 50 milligrams of vitamin C — the amount in half a cup of orange juice.

Finally, if you're trying to lose weight, don't go overboard on walnuts. They still contain a lot of fat, even if it's the good kind.

**Benefits**

Promotes weight loss

Combats cancer

Smoothes skin

Eases arthritis

Conquers kidney
  stones

# Water

· · · · · · · · · ·

You could probably survive over a month without food, but 10 days without water and you're a goner.

Why is it so important? For one thing, about three-quarters of your body is made up of water. Your blood is 83 percent water, your 15 billion brain cells are mostly water, and 'dry as a bone' is a relative term — your skeleton is about 22 percent water.

Even if you're a couch potato, you lose up to 10 cups a day — through sweat, urine, even breathing. And if you're active, you lose even more. To stay healthy, you must constantly replenish your body's supply of water.

Drink about six full glasses a day, minimum — just don't count alcohol or caffeinated drinks, like coffee and soft drinks. These actually increase the rate your body loses water. And don't wait until you're thirsty to head for the water fountain since thirst is not always a reliable gauge of your body's needs. You can lose 2 percent of your body weight in fluids before you even begin to feel thirsty.

## 6 ways water keeps you healthy

**Flushes away cancer.** The solution to bladder and colorectal cancer may be as basic as water — drinking lots of water. Research proves it. One study found that drinking six 8-ounce glasses of water a day reduced the risk of bladder cancer by 50 percent. The bottom line is the more water that flows through your urinary tract, the healthier it will be. Carcinogens and other toxins are simply washed away or diluted.

**Helps keep you trim.** Drinking calorie-free water instead of sweetened cola, tea, or juice is one easy way to cut calories from your diet. And many waistline watchers believe that drinking a tall glass of ice water just before a meal dulls your appetite, fills your stomach, and helps you eat less.

While cutting calories is one part of a successful weight-control program, exercise is just as important. Drink water before and during exercise to avoid dehydration and to get more out of your workout.

**Shields your joints.** If you've ever slept on a water bed, you know water can be a comfortable cushion between your body and the hard floor. Water can also provide padding and lubrication for your joints — making them more comfortable, too. If you have arthritis, particularly gout, drink plenty of water. Not only does it cushion your joints, but it helps dilute and flush out the uric acid that causes gout.

**Prevents kidney stones.** If you need an incentive to drink more water, experience the pain of kidney stones and you'll be gulping away in no time. An Italian study divided people who had kidney stones into two groups. Researchers told one group to drink lots of water, while the other got no special instructions. During the five-year study, the high-water group developed half as many kidney stones. If you're at risk of kidney stones, water should be your first line of defense.

### When bottled is better

You may not need to keep bottled water in your refrigerator at home, but if you're planning a trip to Mexico, Africa, or South America, bottled water can be essential to your health.

The water supply in undeveloped countries is often contaminated with bacteria. Drinking it could make your vacation one you'll always remember — but wish you could forget.

To keep your vacation pleasant, use bottled water for drinking and brushing your teeth. Don't use ice unless you know it was made from boiled or filtered water, and don't eat raw fruits or vegetables.

**Cools your body.** One of water's most important jobs is to keep your body temperature within a safe range. If you're a senior, you're especially vulnerable to dangerous heat illness because of risky conditions like heart disease. You are also more likely to take medications that may keep your body from sweating properly — another risk factor.

Heat cramps and heat exhaustion are mild forms of heat illness, but heatstroke is a life threatening emergency. Symptoms include headache, slurred speech, dizziness, faintness, and hallucinations. If you suspect someone is suffering from heatstroke, act quickly to cool them off.

To prevent heat illness, try to stay cool, and make sure you drink extra water during hot weather or whenever you exercise.

**Moisturizes your skin.** Summertime isn't the only time you should drink lots of water. During cold months your skin can become dry and your lips chapped. Drinking lots of water helps keep your lips and your skin cells moist and comfortable.

> ## Water hikes blood pressure
>
> If you want to get an accurate reading on your blood pressure, before your next doctor's visit lay off the caffeine, cigarettes, alcohol — and water. A recent study found that seniors experienced a rise in blood pressure after drinking just 2 cups of ordinary tap water. The increase was similar to that caused by smoking two unfiltered cigarettes or taking 250 milligrams of caffeine. People with autonomic nervous system failure (a problem with the involuntary responses in certain muscles and glands) had an even greater increase. The largest effect was seen after 30 to 35 minutes. But the effect began to decrease after about an hour.

## Pantry pointers

Water, water everywhere ... but which kind should you drink? A hundred years ago, that would have been a silly question but today the choices in drinking water are almost overwhelming. The market is flooded with products — distilled water, spring water, flavored water, even fortified water with extra fiber or vitamins. Drinking plain old tap water may now seem a bit old-fashioned.

Fortunately for your pocketbook, there's no good reason to buy those fancy bottled waters, unless you just want to. Research finds they're not any cleaner than city water and you can get vitamins and other nutrients from the foods you eat.

# Watermelon

· · · · · · · · · · · · · · · · · · ·

| Benefits |
| :---: |
| Protects prostate |
| Promotes weight loss |
| Lowers cholesterol |
| Controls blood pressure |
| Helps stop strokes |

There's nothing quite like a refreshing slice of icy-cold watermelon on a hot summer day. Most agree it's the perfect picnic food — juicy, sweet, and tasting of sunshine. Grown in 96 countries, from China, the world's leading producer, to Africa, Egypt, and the United States, it's a warm weather favorite.

Watermelon is also a healthy food choice no matter where you live. It's low in calories — only about 51 per cup — and it will give you a nutritious dose of vitamins A and C, potassium, and the antioxidant lycopene.

## 3 ways watermelon keeps you healthy

**Provides prostate protection.** Watermelon is the fresh food champ when it comes to lycopene — even beating out fresh tomatoes. This naturally occurring chemical gives many fruits and vegetables their red color and is known to fight prostate cancer. But most people associate it with tomatoes. Although canned tomato products are highest in lycopene, watermelon beat out all other fresh fruits or vegetables. So enjoy a slice whenever you can for super prostate protection.

**Enhances heart health.** Watermelon has earned the American Heart Association's "heart check" seal of approval. This certification program was developed to help shoppers easily identify foods that are part of a heart-healthy diet. To qualify, a food must be low in total and saturated fat, cholesterol, and sodium. It also must contain at least 10 percent of the daily value of one or more key nutrients — protein, vitamin A, vitamin C, calcium, iron, or dietary fiber.

Watermelon not only meets, but exceeds these requirements. It also contains lycopene to help fight cholesterol, and potassium, a mineral that battles high blood pressure and stroke. All that adds up to first-rate heart protection.

**Watches your weight.** If you want to satisfy your sweet tooth, fill yourself up, and stay on your diet, slice up a watermelon. Experts know foods with a high water content help you lose weight, and watermelon is a staggering 92 percent water. What's more, one slice contains only a single gram of fat. So don't pass up dessert just because you're watching your weight — make for the melon.

## Pantry pointers

There are over 50 different types of watermelons, but two main varieties: picnic and ice box. Picnic watermelons are generally oblong and weigh from 12 to 50 pounds. Ice box varieties are smaller because they're designed to fit into a refrigerator.

Picking out the perfect melon is easy, according to the National Watermelon Promotion Board. First, choose one that is symmetrical and firm, without bruises, cuts, or dents. Next, pick it up. You're looking for one that's heavy for its size. Finally, turn it over. If you see a yellow area, the watermelon rested on the ground while it ripened in the sun, which means you'll get a sweeter, juicier melon. Contrary to popular belief, don't thump your melon — slap it. If it sounds hollow, it's ripe.

Once you take your watermelon home, keep it in the refrigerator for up to a week. After you cut it, wrap it tightly in plastic wrap and enjoy within a day or two.

# Weight control
• • • • • • • • • • • • •

| Eat | |
|---|---|
| Brown rice | Sweet |
| Beans | potatoes |
| Apples | Celery |
| Cucumbers | Tuna |
| Salmon | Grapefruit |

### Avoid

Foods high in saturated fat, such as red meat

Foods high in refined sugar, such as pastries

When you look in the mirror, you may long for a slimmer figure. But the best reason to lose weight is your health. Being overweight increases your risk of diabetes, high blood pressure, and heart disease. In fact, it puts you at risk for most everything from flat feet to some kinds of cancer.

If you're thinking of jumping into a fast weight loss diet, slow down. A "quick fix" won't work in the long run. Overeating is likely to follow, taking you right back to where you started.

Your best plan of action is to make moderate changes in your diet with the goal of losing one or two pounds a week. Decide how many calories you are presently eating, on average, each day. Then take steps to reduce that amount by 500 to 1,000 calories.

As a rule, weight loss experts don't recommend eating less than 1,200 calories. "However," says registered dietitian Kimberly Gaddy, "folks that need quick weight loss for health or motivation reasons — typically folks who need to lose 60 or more pounds —

may need to be on a calorie level of less than 1,200 for faster initial weight reduction."

Going lower than 800 calories can be dangerous — especially for people over 50. Have your doctor evaluate the risks and benefits of a very low calorie diet for you before taking this gamble. No matter what your age, you need medical supervision if you are on a diet this severe.

"It is important to focus on long-term behavior change," says Gaddy. If you want never to gain back the weight you lost, you have to form new habits. The key is to eat a healthy diet and exercise, taking in no more calories than you burn. One thing's for sure — a positive attitude also helps.

What if, after a few months of following a healthy eating plan, the weight still doesn't come off? Ask yourself if you are really getting enough exercise. The habits of a sedentary lifestyle — which may have been a cause of your weight gain in the first place — can be hard to change.

If, on the other hand, you are sure a lack of exercise isn't blocking your success, see your doctor. A thyroid condition could be causing your problem.

## Nutritional blockbusters that help weight control

**Carbohydrates.** Is it necessary to cut back on starchy foods, like rice and potatoes, if you want to lose weight? Actually, the opposite may be true. Carbohydrates, gram for gram, have less than half the calories of fat. What's more, your body can't burn the fat you eat without them. They also give you energy and help raise your metabolism, causing you to burn more calories.

Some diet experts say your metabolism speeds up enough to use most, if not all, of the calories you take in from carbohydrates. But any extras you don't burn, your body breaks down and stores as fat. Fortunately, about a fourth of these extra calories get used up in the process.

On the other hand, you burn up almost no calories storing the fat you eat. So you gain more weight from eating excess fat calories than you do from an equal number of extra carbohydrate calories.

Dieting or not, most nutritionists suggest getting at least 55 percent of your total calories from carbohydrates. That's not hard to do. Carbohydrates come mainly from plants — milk is the only animal source.

Unprocessed grains — like brown rice — are one of the best sources of carbohydrates. They haven't lost any of their nutrients and fiber to processing. And since they are whole and firm, it takes longer for your body to break them down. That means you may absorb less starch — and calories — during digestion.

Other "star" carbohydrates include vegetables like sweet potatoes, dry beans, corn, peas, and winter squash.

And, as long as you stay within your calorie limits, fruits are another good choice. Chopped apples, bananas, and strawberries, for example, make a healthy carbohydrate treat. But don't top it with shredded coconut. It's too high in saturated fat, which is bad for your heart and your figure.

"A little dab will undo you," say Dr. Ron and Nancy Goor, in their book, *Choose to Lose.* "Coconut is what scientists feed rats to give them heart disease."

The writers of some diet books suggest you may burn up more calories in digesting certain carbohydrates than you gain in eating them. They say foods like celery, cucumbers, and iceberg lettuce have "negative" calories. Others aren't quite sure this is possible. Nevertheless, filling up on these low-calorie, no-calorie, or negative-calorie foods — whatever you call them — can certainly help you toward your weight loss goal.

Sugar, also a carbohydrate, is not the friend of a trim waist-line. It adds calories but no nutrition. And desserts rich in sugar and fat are doubly dangerous to your dreams of good health and a slender figure.

**Fats.** The right kind of fat, believe it or not, can help you lose weight. That's what researchers in Australia found when they compared the results of two weight loss diets. Some people ate a serving of fish containing omega-3 fatty acids — like tuna or salmon — every day. They dropped almost four pounds more during the 16-week study than those whose diet didn't include any fish.

Weight loss isn't your only reward from eating fish. Other studies show this healthy fat helps protect you from diabetes, depression, heart disease, and cancer.

Fats from plant sources — like olive or canola oil, avocado, and nuts — are better for you than fats from meats and dairy foods. But remember, if you eat too much fat of any kind, you can ruin your chances of ditching those extra pounds. One gram of fat has the same number of calories, no matter what the source.

**Protein.** Your body needs the complete protein you get from meats, fish, and dairy products. Some plant foods, like beans and whole grains, provide incomplete proteins. Yet, if you eat them together, as in a dish of red beans and rice, you also get the complete protein.

High-protein diets have become popular recently, but these diets don't build muscle and burn fat as some claim. In fact, they may actually be dangerous.

These diets can put a strain on your liver and kidneys and contribute to artery disease and bone loss. They also lack some of the other nutrients you need. Most health organizations, including the American Heart Association and the American Dietetic Association, recommend avoiding high-protein diets.

---

**A word of caution**

Don't let worries about your weight lead you to drink alcohol — it's high in calories. As a matter of fact, an ounce of alcohol, the amount in an average drink, has about 130 calories, almost the same as half an ounce of fat.

Alcohol also slows down your ability to burn stored body fat. And it may even lead to the storage of fat in the "beer belly," where it is most dangerous.

---

**Fiber.** Eating fiber-rich fruits, vegetables, and whole grains can be a big help in taking off extra pounds. Just be sure to drink plenty of water. The liquid makes the fiber swell, causing you to feel full. And since it passes slowly through your upper digestive tract, you won't get hungry again right away. What's more, most fiber isn't digested, so it doesn't add many calories.

# Wheat germ and wheat bran

**Benefits**

Lowers cholesterol

Combats colon cancer

Prevents constipation

Helps stop strokes

Protects against heart disease

Improves digestion

The word "germ" probably makes you think of sickness and disease. But put the word "wheat" in front of it, and you have a whole new ball game.

Wheat germ, the heart of the wheat kernel, is packed with protein, fiber, polyunsaturated fat, vitamins, and minerals. It's the most nutritionally dense part of the wheat kernel, which also includes the endosperm and bran, or outer husk.

Second only to rice as a food staple, wheat was cultivated thousands of years ago by the ancient Chinese, Egyptians, and Greeks. Today, the world grows more wheat than any other cereal crop.

Chances are you get plenty of wheat in your diet since most breads are made with that grain. But you probably don't eat much wheat germ or bran, two of the healthiest parts of the kernel, which are often removed during milling. Wheat germ can lower cholesterol and help your heart, while the bran, which is loaded with fiber, can fight constipation and colon cancer.

## 3 ways wheat germ and wheat bran keep you healthy

**Dissolves cholesterol.** Cholesterol has the power to clog or block your arteries, trigger heart attacks, and cause stroke. But wheat germ has the raw power to stop it.

A French study found that eating 30 grams, or about a quarter of a cup, of raw wheat germ a day for 14 weeks lowered total cholesterol by 7.2 percent. It also lowered LDL or "bad" cholesterol by 15.4 percent and triglycerides, a type of fat in your blood, by 11.3 percent.

This is important because, according to another study, reducing cholesterol just 7 percent may lead to a 15 percent lower risk of heart disease.

Wheat germ's success against LDL cholesterol could stem from the antioxidant powers of vitamin E. Dr. Lori J. Mosca of the University of Michigan led a study that suggested vitamin E from foods, but not from supplements, prevented LDL particles from becoming oxidized. And oxidized LDL presents a much greater danger to your health.

"When a fat such as LDL undergoes oxidation, it is more prone to collect in blood vessels to form plaque," says Mosca, whose study involved postmenopausal women. "Over time, the plaque narrows the blood vessels or unleashes a clot, which can result in a heart attack or stroke. When LDL is not oxidized, it does not seem to cause problems."

Because vitamin E in supplements might not offer the same protection, your best bet is to get vitamin E through your diet.

"We can never be sure exactly which nutrient is providing the benefits, and it is likely that several different nutrients are involved," Mosca explains. "That's why we recommend getting vitamin E from foods."

**Fights heart disease.** The message that whole foods are better than supplements was sounded earlier by a *New England Journal of Medicine* study on the risk of heart disease in post-menopausal women.

In that study, women who got the most vitamin E from food sources were less than half as likely to develop heart disease as women who ate the least. However, the same relationship didn't exist for supplemental vitamin E. Another recent study suggested that, even after four to six years, vitamin E supplements had no effect on the risk of heart disease. Again, a better strategy is to get vitamin E through foods rather than pills.

When it comes to foods, whole-grain foods offer even more protection. A Harvard Medical School study of 75,521 nurses showed that eating about 2.5 servings of whole grains a day could lower your risk of heart disease by about 30 percent, an estimate the researchers said may be "conservative."

The whole-grain foods they studied included wheat germ and bran. Research data showed that eating about one serving of each per day dramatically reduced the risk of heart disease. People who ate a little less than one serving of wheat germ per day were 59 percent less likely to develop heart disease than people who rarely ate wheat germ. For bran, one serving per day reduced the risk of developing heart disease by 37 percent.

Of course, whole-grain foods have several heart-healthy things going for them, including fiber, folate, vitamin E, and potassium. But the beauty of eating whole foods is you don't have to figure out how each nutrient helps you — you get the combined benefits of them all.

**Defends against cancer.** When it comes to heavy hitters against colon cancer, wheat bran is Babe Ruth. Time and time again, wheat bran has knocked colon cancer out of the ballpark.

A cup of wheat bran gives you a whopping 25 grams of fiber. This kind of fiber, insoluble fiber, adds bulk to your stool and dilutes the carcinogens in it. It also speeds your stool through the gastrointestinal tract so it's not hanging around causing trouble. This makes wheat bran good for curing constipation and maintaining a healthy gut as well as protecting you against cancer.

But fiber might not be the only hero. Wheat bran also has a lot of phytic acid, a substance with antioxidant properties that may stop tumors. Those who doubt fiber's anticancer power point to phytic acid as a possible explanation for wheat bran's effectiveness against colon tumors.

Whether it's the fiber or the phytic acid, wheat bran works. Studies have shown wheat bran can inhibit both colon and intestinal tumors better than other brans such as oat or barley.

## A word of caution

Wheat contains gluten, a sticky protein that makes it ideal for baking bread. However, gluten also makes wheat dangerous for people with celiac disease or a gluten allergy.

If you have a gluten allergy, wheat products could give you cramps, diarrhea, and other problems. Celiac disease is even more serious, and eating wheat could severely damage the lining of your intestines. Usually, people with these conditions have to avoid all products containing wheat, rye, oats, or barley.

## Pantry pointers

You can find wheat germ in both toasted and natural forms. Use it soon after you buy it, though, because its oiliness makes it turn rancid quickly. You can also buy wheat germ oil, but it has a strong flavor and is fairly expensive.

Most wheat flours make use of the wheat endosperm, the main part of the wheat kernel, which contains starch, protein, and iron. Other forms of wheat you can buy include wheat berries (which are whole kernels), cracked wheat, and bulgur. These are usually found in health food stores.

# Yeast infections
. . . . . . . . . . . . . . . .

| Eat | |
| --- | --- |
| Yogurt | Asparagus |
| Cantaloupe | Spinach |
| Turnip greens | Liver |
| Apricots | Broccoli |

**Avoid**

Foods high in refined sugars, such as pastries

Foods containing yeast, such as breads and aged cheese

If you're a woman, you're likely to have at least one yeast infection in your lifetime. Yeast infections are just one type of vaginitis, an inflammation of your vagina. You always have a small amount of yeast in this area, but when it multiplies, it can cause itching, burning, and irritation. Pregnancy, diabetes, and the use of birth control pills or antibiotics increase your risk of getting this condition. Luckily, several key nutrients may help fight off the specific bacteria that cause these annoying infections.

## Nutritional blockbusters that fight yeast infections

**Folic acid.** This B vitamin protects you from vaginitis and may decrease your risk of cervical cancer as well. Researchers think low levels of folic acid may make it easier for cancer-causing substances to attack your tissues. So protect yourself by eating more cantaloupe, asparagus, beets, liver, and green, leafy vegetables like spinach and turnip greens. If possible, eat these fruits and vegetables raw since cooking destroys up to half of this important vitamin.

**Iron.** This mineral is especially important to a woman's health before menopause. Foods high in iron include shellfish, red meat, dried fruit, and spinach. Adding foods high in vitamin C will help your body absorb the iron better. For example, stir-fry some vitamin C-rich broccoli with your shrimp, or garnish your spinach salad with orange slices.

**Magnesium.** Research finds that women who have recurring yeast infections are likely to have low levels of magnesium. To make sure you get plenty of this mineral, eat nuts, whole grain foods, and dark green vegetables like spinach and broccoli.

**Zinc.** About half of all adult women in the United States get substantially less than the recommended daily amount of zinc. That's bad news for them because this mineral may help fight yeast infections. Foods rich in zinc include seafood, red meat, poultry, legumes, and whole grains.

**Selenium.** Scientists don't know how selenium fights vaginal infections, but they do know that women with chronic cases of vaginitis have low selenium levels. To get plenty of selenium, make sure you eat unprocessed foods like grains and fresh fruits and vegetables.

**Vitamin A.** The lining of your vagina acts as a protective barrier against bacteria. If cells die, bacteria can invade and cause infection. Vitamin A keeps these cells alive and well so it's your first line of defense against vaginal infections. Foods rich in vitamin A include liver, fortified dairy products, and eggs. You can also eat foods high in beta carotene, which your body turns into vitamin A, such as spinach, sweet potatoes, carrots, and papaya.

**Fatty acids.** Inflammation often goes hand-in-hand with yeast infections. To fight it, you need to eat more of the essential fatty acids omega-3 and omega-6. Have some fish two or three times a week, along with small amounts of vegetable oils like canola, safflower, sunflower, or olive oil. Seeds, nuts, poultry, and eggs contain good amounts of fatty acids as well.

**Yogurt.** Eating a cup of yogurt every day may be an easy and delicious way to sidestep yeast infections. *Lactobacillus acidophilus* is a good kind of bacteria found in the vagina. Scientists believe it may fight off the bad bacteria that result in yeast infections. Many yogurts also contain *L. acidophilus* cultures. In several studies, researchers had women eat 8 ounces of bacteria-rich yogurt every day for several months. Most of the women had fewer vaginal infections during that time.

### A word of caution

The bacteria that cause vaginal infections thrive in a high-sugar environment. That's why diabetics may be more likely to get yeast infections. You know you should cut out candy bars and desserts, but you may not know that many processed foods contain hidden sugar. Read the labels on your cereal boxes, canned fruits, spaghetti sauces, and diet products. You may be unpleasantly surprised.

And not all doctors agree, but some recommend eliminating yeast-containing foods if you tend to get yeast infections. Breads, aged cheese, vinegar, and beer are all high in yeast.

**Benefits**

Aids digestion

Guards against ulcers

Strengthens bones

Supports immune
 system

Lowers cholesterol

# Yogurt

• • • • • • • • • • • •

Legend has it yogurt was invented accidentally. Somewhere in Turkey, milk in a goatskin bag curdled — or fermented — during a desert journey. That brave nomad must have been pleasantly surprised when he tried the end result. Turkey is still famous for its yogurt, but it's different from the yogurt you buy at the supermarket.

You make commercial Western yogurt by adding bacteria, usually *Lactobacillus bulgaricus* and *Streptococcus thermophilus,* to pasteurized milk, then heating. These bacteria are responsible for many of yogurt's claims to health fame. Unfortunately, some processing steps destroy the bacteria. So, for the best nutritional benefit, make sure your yogurt label says "active yogurt cultures."

Yogurt is also a good source of calcium, riboflavin, protein, vitamin B12, and potassium.

## 6 ways yogurt keeps you healthy

**Aids digestive health.** Eat some creamy yogurt regularly, and you may be able to avoid unpleasant intestinal problems.

There are over 400 different kinds of bacteria in your digestive tract. Some of these are good ones, called probiotics, that help keep harmful bacteria in check. However, a round of antibiotics, a bout of food poisoning, or various illnesses often kill a lot of your good bacteria. The result can be intestinal upset, including diarrhea. You can help your body maintain the delicate balance between the good and bad bacteria by eating yogurt. With its wealth of probiotics, yogurt is a natural way to re-stock your inventory of good bacteria.

Research over the last 40 years confirms this. Yogurt can help treat and perhaps prevent intestinal infections or diarrhea caused by bacteria such as *Salmonella* and *E. coli.*

**Blocks ulcers.** Discovering that *Helicobacter pylori* bacteria cause ulcers was a major medical breakthrough. Dr. C. N. Wendakoon from the University of Alberta says, "*H. pylori* is a small bug, living in the stomach that causes chronic gastritis and peptic ulcer diseases in humans. It is sometimes involved in certain forms of gastric cancer." Since this discovery, antibiotics have been the standard treatment. However, antibiotics can cause side effects, and *H. pylori* is developing resistance to some of them. Wendakoon adds, "*H. pylori* has special adaptations to survive and is difficult to wipe out from the stomach." Now, many experts believe yogurt may be a natural solution.

Wendakoon's research determined that skim milk with *Lactobacillus casei,* a dairy starter bacterium, destroys *H. pylori* cells — at least in the laboratory. "Our results," she says, "would lead to the development of a new, safe, and effective therapeutic regimen (such as yogurt drink) against *Helicobacter* infection."

Because of differences in processing, your yogurt may or may not help fight *H. pylori,* but for now it's a natural and tasty way to try.

**Strengthens bones.** An 8-ounce serving of yogurt provides about a third of the calcium you need every day to strengthen your bones. And if you're lactose intolerant, you'll probably be able to digest yogurt much more easily than milk or other dairy foods.

**Boosts immune system.** A healthy immune system means you're better able to fight off a multitude of diseases, including cancer. And yogurt may be one food that helps. A University of California study found that eating two cups of yogurt daily increased an important immune system substance called gamma-interferon.

Researchers have tested other specific probiotics in yogurt and found many of them cause your body's defense system to kick in. To get this benefit, be sure your yogurt contains live and active cultures.

**May cut cholesterol.** It took a remote tribe in Africa to spark scientific interest in the cholesterol-lowering effect of yogurt. Despite the sort of diet that would typically raise cholesterol levels, including large amounts of meat, the Maasai people have low rates of heart disease. Further investigation uncovered a staple of their diet responsible for these unusual findings — fermented milk. Although there are several ways it could happen, experts believe more yogurt means less cholesterol circulating throughout your body.

Clinical studies have had mixed results, but most indicate that yogurt could have a modest cholesterol-lowering effect. The key seems to be eating yogurt with live cultures on a daily basis. And since yogurt is a good source of so many important nutrients, you've nothing to lose by making it part of your daily diet.

**Battles yeast infections.** Women seem to be more likely to eat yogurt than men, and perhaps for good reason. A cup or two a day may provide just the right amount of good bacteria to prevent or treat vaginal infections. So if you're prone to this type of complaint or if you're on a round of antibiotics, snack on this creamy treat.

---

### Drink to your good health

If yogurt is simply not your favorite food, you can still enjoy the benefits of probiotics, with acidophilus milk. The friendly bacteria *lactobacillus acidophilus* are added to milk where they produce lactic acid by fermenting the sugars in milk.

All this means you'll experience healthier digestion and a natural source of antibiotics to control harmful bacteria in your stomach, intestines, urinary tract, and vagina.

Especially if you've taken antibiotics to treat a bacterial infection, pour yourself a daily glass of acidophilus milk.

# Pantry pointers

If you want to get the most health benefits from commercial yogurt, you have to read the label. Look for kinds that contain live active cultures, and haven't been heat-treated, since heat kills the beneficial bacteria. Also check the expiration date — the probiotics in yogurt get weaker as the product ages.

Reading the label will also tell you how much sugar it contains. Some yogurts have up to seven teaspoons of added sugar — empty calories you don't need.

You can store yogurt in its original container for up to 10 days in the refrigerator. Most people enjoy eating it right out of the carton, but it's also good for cooking. Use it as a low-fat substitute for sour cream or mayonnaise. Remember, however, that heat kills the good bacteria, so use it in cooking for its other nutritional qualities.

# Index

●●●●●●●●●●